T0156068

Essentials of
Spinal Cord Medicine

Essentials of
Spinal Cord Medicine

Sunil Sabharwal, MD
Chief of Spinal Cord Injury
VA Boston Healthcare System
Assistant Professor of Physical Medicine
   and Rehabilitation
Harvard Medical School
Boston, Massachusetts

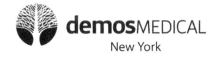

demosMEDICAL
New York

Visit our website at www.demosmedpub.com

ISBN: 978-1-936287-38-3
e-book ISBN: 978-1-61705-075-6

Acquisitions Editor: Beth Barry
Compositor: diacriTech

Medicine is an ever-changing science. Research and clinical experience are continually expanding our knowledge, in particular our understanding of proper treatment and drug therapy. The authors, editors, and publisher have made every effort to ensure that all information in this book is in accordance with the state of knowledge at the time of production of the book. Nevertheless, the authors, editors, and publisher are not responsible for errors or omissions or for any consequences from application of the information in this book and make no warranty, expressed or implied, with respect to the contents of the publication. Every reader should examine carefully the package inserts accompanying each drug and should carefully check whether the dosage schedules mentioned therein or the contraindications stated by the manufacturer differ from the statements made in this book. Such examination is particularly important with drugs that are either rarely used or have been newly released on the market.

Library of Congress Cataloging-in-Publication Data

Sabharwal, Sunil, author.
  Essentials of spinal cord medicine / Sunil Sabharwal.
    p. ; cm.
  ISBN 978-1-936287-38-3 — ISBN 978-1-61705-075-6 (e-book)
  I. Title.
  [DNLM: 1. Spinal Cord Injuries. 2. Spinal Cord—physiology. 3. Spinal Cord Diseases. WL 403]
  RD594.3
  617.4'82044—dc23
                          2013038404

Special discounts on bulk quantities of Demos Medical Publishing books are available to corporations, professional associations, pharmaceutical companies, health care organizations, and other qualifying groups. For details, please contact:

Special Sales Department
Demos Medical Publishing, LLC
11 West 42nd Street, 15th Floor
New York, NY 10036
Phone: 800-532-8663 or 212-683-0072
Fax: 212-941-7842
E-mail: specialsales@demosmedpub.com

Printed in the United States of America by Gasch Printing.

13 14 15 16 17 / 5 4 3 2 1

Contents

III. NONTRAUMATIC MYELOPATHIES

IV. PHYSICAL FUNCTION AND REHABILITATION

V. MEDICAL CONSEQUENCES AND COMPLICATIONS OF SCI

VI. PSYCHOSOCIAL ISSUES AND LIFE PARTICIPATION AFTER SCI

VII. SYSTEMS-BASED PRACTICE

Preface

There were two main goals for writing this book. The first goal, in keeping with the book title, was to distil the "essentials" of the rapidly growing knowledge in spinal cord medicine, and provide succinct yet comprehensive information that is relevant to clinicians who care for people with injuries and disorders of the spinal cord. This is an effort to bridge the gap between several good but encyclopedic texts on this topic and those that consist primarily of lists with restricted and limited coverage of material. The second goal was to make information user-friendly and easy to access and digest by using a consistent format, paragraphs with clarifying subtitles, appropriate cross-referencing, and a large number of tables that highlight and reinforce key material.

Given the broad scope of spinal cord medicine, this book should be of interest to a diverse group of clinicians and trainees. These include specialists in spinal cord medicine as well as those who encounter people with spinal cord injuries and disorders within a broader area of practice (physiatrists, neurologists, primary care physicians, internists, various medical and surgical subspecialists, and rehabilitation clinicians from multiple disciplines). It may also be of interest to researchers in the field who are looking for clinical context. The chapters are organized under the broad headings of general principles, clinical considerations, and knowledge gaps and emerging concepts, and include a select list of suggested readings that substantively informed the chapter or are good resources for additional information.

The book is organized into seven sections. Section I covers basic science fundamentals, but with a focus on clinical relevance. It includes information on applied anatomy and physiology, pathophysiology of spinal cord injury, and a concise summary of the rapidly growing research in neuroprotection, repair, and regeneration of the spinal cord. Section II covers various aspects of traumatic spinal cord injury ranging from prevention to assessment and management, and incorporates the most current guidelines on those topics. Section III covers nontraumatic myelopathies. In addition to a clinical overview and general approach, it includes separate chapters on various myelopathies. These vary in length and detail with more comprehensive coverage of commonly encountered conditions (such as multiple sclerosis, amyotrophic lateral sclerosis, and cervical spondylotic myelopathy) and briefer summaries with tables highlighting the pertinent facts about less frequently encountered conditions.

Section IV discusses physical function and rehabilitation. For this section an effort was made to include information that would be of broad interest to clinicians, rather than technical details that would primarily be relevant to physical or occupational therapists. Section V provides comprehensive coverage of the multiple medical consequences and complications of spinal cord injuries and disorders. The chapters in this section are organized by body system and incorporate clinical practice guidelines, practice pearls, and practical tips for assessment and management. Section VI summarizes psychosocial issues and life participation following spinal cord injury. Here again the focus is on practical information of broad clinical relevance, rather than details that may only be pertinent to psychologists or social workers. Section VII covers important aspects of systems-based practice that are often not covered elsewhere or are only covered generically. It includes chapters on systems of care, ethical issues, and patient safety, each with a specific focus on the practice of spinal cord medicine.

Many people made this book possible. Special thanks to the excellent team at Demos Medical Publishing for their professionalism and support throughout this process, to my family for their encouragement, humor, and understanding during the long hours spent on this book, and to the multiple mentors and patients who have taught me so much over the years.

Sunil Sabharwal, MD

I. Basic Science Fundamentals

CHAPTER 1

Applied Anatomy and Physiology of the Spinal Cord

GENERAL PRINCIPLES

External Anatomy of the Spinal Cord

The spinal cord is located within the vertebral canal and extends from the foramen magnum to the lower part of the first lumbar vertebra where it ends as the conus medullaris. There is a subtle enlargement in the cervical and lumbar regions of the spinal cord, where the neurons that innervate the upper and lower extremities, respectively, are located. Distal to the conus medullaris, the vertebral canal contains the collection of lumbar and sacral nerve roots that form the cauda equina.

Meningeal Coverings

The meningeal coverings of the spinal cord—the pia, arachnoid, and dura—are continuous with those of the brain. The dura ends caudally at the level of the second sacral vertebra and continues as the coccygeal ligament that serves to anchor the spinal cord to the vertebral canal. The epidural space is located between the dura mater and the vertebral canal. The arachnoid lines the dura and ends as a sac at the level of the second sacral vertebra. The subarachnoid space is filled with cerebrospinal fluid, and is largest inferiorly between the second lumbar and second sacral vertebral levels, where it surrounds the cauda equina and is known as the lumbar cistern. The pia tapers distal to the conus medullaris and continues inferiorly as a slender filament known as the filum terminale.

Relationship Between Spinal Cord and Vertebral Segments

The spinal cord has 31 segments:

- 8 cervical (C)
- 12 thoracic (T)
- 5 lumbar (L)
- 5 sacral (S)
- 1 coccygeal (Co)

Spinal segmentation is based on the sites where spinal nerves emerge from the spinal cord.

The vertebral column consists of 33 vertebrae:

- 7 cervical
- 12 thoracic
- 5 lumbar
- 5 sacral
- 4 coccygeal

The sacral and coccygeal vertebrae fuse in the adult to form the sacrum and coccyx.

The spinal cord is shorter than the vertebral column, ending between L1 and L2 so the spinal cord segment levels do not correspond to the vertebral levels below the upper cervical segments. This discrepancy between the spinal cord and vertebral levels becomes progressively more marked for the more caudal segments of the spinal cord (Table 1.1). The lumbar and sacral roots descending in the vertebral canal below the L1 vertebra form the cauda equina.

Spinal Nerves and Roots

There are 31 spinal nerves to which each spinal segment corresponds. Each spinal nerve consists of a sensory nerve root, which enters the spinal cord at that level, and a motor root, which emerges from the cord at each level. In the dorsal root of a typical spinal nerve lies a dorsal root ganglion, a swelling that contains nerve cell bodies. First order neurons of all ascending spinal cord tracts are located in the dorsal root ganglia. The sensory component of each spinal nerve is distributed to a dermatome, a well-defined segment of the skin (See Chapter 10 and Figure 10.1). The first cervical and coccygeal nerves typically have no dorsal root so do not have any dermatomal representation. The skeletal musculature innervated by motor axons in a given spinal root is called a myotome.

Table 1.1

Approximate Relationship Between Vertebral Bodies and Spinal Cord Levels	
Vertebral Body	**Corresponding Spinal Cord Level**
Upper cervical (C1–C4)	Same as vertebral level
Lower cervical (C5–C7)	Add 1 level
Upper thoracic (T1–T6)	Add 2 levels
Lower thoracic (T7–T10)	Add 3 levels
T11–T12	Lumbar
T12–L1	Sacral
L2 and below	Cauda equina (lumbosacral nerve roots)

The first seven pairs of cervical spinal nerves (C1–C7) exit above the same-numbered cervical vertebra. However, because there are 8 cervical spinal cord segments but only 7 cervical vertebrae, the C8 nerve emerges between the seventh cervical and first thoracic vertebrae and the remaining spinal nerves caudal to that level all emerge below their respective same-numbered vertebra.

The spinal dura forms dural root sleeves that follow the spinal nerve roots into each intervertebral foramen and blend with the epineurium covering of each spinal nerve. Within the subarachnoid space, nerve roots lack any dural covering.

Internal Structure of the Spinal Cord

On transverse section, the spinal cord includes outer white matter tracts containing ascending sensory and descending motor pathways, and inner butterfly-shaped gray matter with nerve cell bodies. It surrounds a central canal, which is anatomically an extension of the fourth ventricle, and is lined with ependymal cells and filled with cerebrospinal fluid.

Gray matter

The spinal cord plays a key role in integration of multiple peripheral and central inputs via the system of neurons in the gray matter. On cross-section, the gray matter in the spinal cord includes the dorsal, ventral, and an intermediolateral horns or columns. The gray matter is divided into 10 zones or laminae labeled from I to X.

- The dorsal, or posterior, horn is the entry point of sensory information into the central nervous system. Laminae I to VI are in the dorsal horn and receive different inputs. Laminae I, II (substantia gelatinosa), and V receive input from noxious stimuli; laminae III and IV (also referred to together as the nucleus proprius) receive light-touch and position-related inputs; and lamina VI responds to mechanical signals from the joints and skin.
- The intermediolateral horn, present in the thoracic and upper lumbar segments only (T1-L2), contains preganglionic cells for the sympathetic nervous system. In thoracic and upper lumbar segments, lamina VII of the gray matter contains the intermediolateral nucleus which has the cells from which preganglionic sympathetic fibers project. Lamina VII also contains the cells of the dorsal nucleus (Clarke's column) that give rise to the posterior spinocerebellar tract. A corresponding cell column is located at the S2-S4 levels with preganglionic parasympathetic neurons for pelvic visceral innervation.
- The ventral, or anterior, horn contains motor neurons (alpha and gamma) and interneurons. Lamina VIII and IX are located in the ventral horn. Neurons in these laminae are somatotopically arranged, with the more medial neurons innervating the axial and proximal limb musculature and the more laterally situated neurons primarily

innervating the distal limb muscles. Neurons innervating the extensor muscles are located ventral to the ones innervating the flexor muscles.

Lamina X represents the neurons surrounding the central canal.

White matter
The white matter includes ascending and descending tracts that are composed of axons. The white matter also has glial cells.

The amount of white matter increases at each successive higher spinal segment. Cervical spinal cord levels, therefore, contain more white matter because all neurons descending from the brain inferiorly or traveling up to the brain pass through the cervical spinal cord. The sacral spinal cord has the least amount of white matter because most ascending or descending fibers have entered or exited the spinal cord above that region of the spinal cord. The amount of gray matter is increased in the lumbar and cervical enlargements of the spinal cord.

The ascending tracts in the spinal cord white matter (also see Table 1.2) include:

- Fasciculus gracilis (FG) and fasciculus cuneatus (FC) (dorsal columns).
- Spinothalamic tracts (anterolateral system): The distinction between the lateral spinothalamic tracts that carry pain and temperature, and the anterior spinothalamic tract carrying nondiscriminative touch sensation is no longer universally accepted and the two tracts are often collectively referred to as the anterolateral system.
- Spinocerebellar tracts, including the dorsal and ventral spinocerebellar tracts, which transmit signals from muscle spindle and golgi tendon organs to the cerebellum.

The descending tracts in the white matter include:

- Corticospinal of which 90% are fibers that have crossed at the pyramidal decussation above the spinal cord and make up the lateral corticospinal tract that controls voluntary movements of the opposite side; the remaining uncrossed fibers make up the anterior corticospinal tract.
- Rubrospinal tract: arising from the red nucleus in the midbrain and play a role in motor function.
- Tectospinal tract: arising from the midbrain and involved in coordinating head and eye movements.
- Vestibulospinal tract: arising from the lateral and medial vestibular nuclei and involved in postural reflexes
- Reticulospinal tract: going from the brain stem reticular formation to both the dorsal and ventral horns; modulate sensory transmission (especially pain) and modulate spinal reflexes.

The most important tracts in humans whose function and effect of injury is best understood include the dorsal columns, spinothalamic tracts, and corticospinal tracts. Their function, location, and topography in the spinal cord is summarized in Table 1.2.

While neuron cell bodies are present in the gray matter, the white matter contains a variety of glial cells in addition to axonal tracts. Glial cells include: oligodendrocytes (form myelin in the CNS analogous to Schwann cells in peripheral nerves), astrocytes (regulate ionic environment, guidance of growing axons, and re-uptake of neurotransmitters), and microglia (have a role in immune surveillance; while some are always present, others enter from blood vessels in response to injury or inflammation).

Spinal Reflexes

In addition to being a conduit for motor and sensory information, the neural connections in the spinal cord mediate several reflexes. A spinal reflex involves discharge of an efferent motor neuron in response to afferent stimulation.

Autonomic Nervous System in Relation to the Spinal Cord

The autonomic nervous system (ANS) maintains the internal homeostasis or balance of the body and regulates various involuntary functions. It includes the sympathetic and parasympathetic divisions. Descending autonomic pathways from the brain travel in the spinal cord and terminate on the preganglionic sympathetic and parasympathetic neurons in the spinal cord that are located at T1 to L2 and S2 to S4, respectively.

The sympathetic preganglionic neurons are located in the intermediolateral horn at the T1 to L2 segments in the spinal cord. Axons of these preganglionic sympathetic neurons project, via the ventral roots and white rami communicans, to paravertebral sympathetic ganglia. These axons either synapse in the paravertebral ganglia (sympathetic chain ganglia) or pass through the sympathetic ganglia without synapsing to one of the prevertebral ganglia (celiac, superior mesenteric, or inferior mesenteric ganglia) where they then synapse. Postganglionic fibers travel with peripheral nerves to innervate target organs (also see Table 33.1).

The preganglionic neurons for the parasympathetic division of the ANS are located in the brainstem and the sacral region of the spinal cord (S2–S4). The parasympathetic control of much of the body, including the cardiovascular system and the proximal part of the gastrointestinal tract, is through the vagus nerve (cranial nerve X) so it bypasses the spinal cord. In the spinal cord, the preganglionic parasympathetic neurons are located in the S2 to S4 sacral segments along the lateral surface of the base of the anterior horn of the gray matter. These innervate the bladder, reproductive organs, and distal part of the gut. Axons of these cells exit through ventral roots and travel through the pelvic nerve to the postganglionic neurons that are located close to the organ being innervated.

Table 1.2

The Primary Motor and Sensory Spinal Cord Tracts*

Tract	Functions	Spinal Cord Location	Spinal Cord Topography	Effect of Lesion/ Injury
Fasciculus gracilis (FG) and fasciculus cuneatus (FC) (Dorsal column)	Carry fine touch, vibration, two-point discrimination, and proprioception (position sense); FG carries sensation from lower body and FC from the upper body (above T6 level)	Ascend in the dorsal column of the spinal cord without synapsing to terminate in the ipsilateral nucleus gracilis and cuneatus in the medulla; FG is medial to FC	Sacral (S) fibers are most medial, followed by lumbar (L), thoracic (T), and cervical (C) which are most lateral	Ipsilateral loss of sensation of fine touch, vibration, two-point discrimination, and proprioception
Spinothalamic tract (Antero-lateral system)	Pain, temperature, and tactile sensation	First order fibers synapse in the dorsal horn after ascending for 1-2 segments in the periphery of the dorsal horn (Lissauer's tract), second order fibers cross in the anterior commissure of the spinal cord, and then ascend in the opposite spinothalamic tract	Cervical fibers are most medial, sacral fibers are most lateral	Contralateral loss of pain, temperature, and touch sensation
Corticospinal tract	Voluntary control of motor function	90% of fibers decussate in the medulla and descend as the lateral corticospinal tract in the lateral column. The remaining uncrossed fibers descend in the anterior column. Descend to all levels of the spinal cord, terminate in spinal gray matter of both the dorsal and ventral horns	Cervical fibers are most medial, sacral fibers are most lateral	"Upper motor neuron" paralysis with loss of voluntary control of movement, Babinski sign, hyperreflexia, and spasticity

*See text for other spinal cord tracts that have a less well defined role in humans.

Blood Supply of the Spinal Cord

A single anterior spinal artery arises from the vertebral arteries and lies in the anterior median fissure of the spinal cord. Although it descends the entire length of the spinal cord it requires reinforcement through segmental connections from the radicular arteries. These connections can be quite variable and relatively sparse in the mid-thoracic region, where the anterior spinal artery is often less robust, making that region more vulnerable to ischemia. The artery of Adamkiewicz, is the major segmental artery supplying the lower spinal cord, and most commonly arises between T10 and T12 on the left, but may arise anywhere between T5 and L2.

The posterior spinal arteries are paired and arise from the vertebral artery. They receive contributions from the posterior radicular arteries, forming a vascular plexus on the posterior surface of the spinal cord. They supply the posterior third of the spinal cord.

Venous drainage is through six longitudinal veins that drain ultimately into the epidural venous plexus.

See Chapter 16 for further discussion on the blood supply of the spinal cord and its clinical implications.

CLINICAL CONSIDERATIONS

Anatomy and organization of the spinal cord has important clinical implications. Table 1.3 summarizes some important clinical correlations of the anatomy and organization of the spinal cord, spinal nerves, and blood supply.

Table 1.3

Applied Anatomy of the Spinal Cord and Important Clinical Correlations	
Anatomical Fact	**Clinical Significance**
Gross Anatomy of the Spinal Cord	
The spinal cord is shorter than the vertebral column, ending between L1 and L2 and occupying only the upper 2/3rd of the length of the vertebral canal.	There is a discrepancy between spinal cord segment levels and vertebral levels especially for the more caudal segments (Table 1.1). E.g., An injury or mass at the level of the L1 vertebra will affect the sacral S2–S5 spinal cord segments, not the L1 spinal cord segment.
10 spinal cord segments (L1–S5) are contained in relation to just 3 vertebrae (T11–L1).	Precise neurological level of injury from fractures or dislocations of T12–L1 vertebrae can vary considerably and is difficult to predict.

(continued)

Table 1.3

Applied Anatomy of the Spinal Cord and Important Clinical Correlations (*continued*)

Gross Anatomy of the Spinal Cord

The spinal cord typically ends between L1 and L2 in adults, and at the lower end of L3 in infants.	Lumbar puncture can be performed between L3–L4 in adults, but is performed between L4–L5 in young children.

Spinal Nerves/Roots

C1–C7 spinal nerves exit above the same-numbered vertebra, while the remaining spinal nerves emerge below the respective same-numbered vertebrae.	A herniated disk between C4–C5 impinges on the C5 spinal nerve, whereas a herniated disk between L4–L5 impinges on the L4 spinal nerve.
There is no dorsal root for the C1 spinal nerve.	There is no sensory testing or dermatomal representation for C1 spinal level
Spinal nerves have connective tissue covering in the form of epineurium, but nerve roots in the subarachnoid space lack protective dura mater covering.	Nerve roots within the subarachnoid space (e.g., the cauda equina) are more fragile and liable to injury than spinal nerves.

Spinal Cord Tracts

The second-order sensory fibers originating from the dorsal horn, that make up the spinothalamic tract, ascend for one or two levels before they cross to join the opposite side spinothalamic tract.	With a unilateral spinal cord lesion, the sensory level on the opposite side is often one to two segments lower than the site of the lesion. With a bilateral lesion, the loss is generally at the level of the lesion.
Second-order sensory fibers cross anterior to the central canal before joining opposite side spinothalamic tract.	A process such as syringomyelia, that results in expansion of the central canal along several spinal segments, can manifest with selective loss of pain and temperature sensation (dissociated sensory loss) due to involvement of these crossing fibers.
The spinothalamic tract has fibers that have crossed from the opposite side, but the fibers ascending in dorsal columns don't cross till they reach the brainstem, and descending corticospinal tract fibers also don't cross in the spinal cord for the most part.	A hemi-section, injury, or pathology involving one half of the spinal cord causes loss of pain and temperature sensation on the opposite side, but ipsilateral weakness and loss of position sense (*Brown-Sequard Syndrome*).
The main ascending and descending tracts are somatotopically organized with a laminated distribution. In the spinothalamic as well as the corticospinal tracts, the location of the cervical thoracic, lumbar, and sacral segments progresses from medial to lateral.	Pathology or injury involving predominantly the central part of the spinal cord often manifests with more pronounced upper limb than lower limb weakness, and sacral sensory sparing (*Central Cord Syndrome*).

(continued)

Spinal Cord Tracts	
The lateral corticospinal tract is in close proximity to the spinothalamic tract.	May partly explain why preserved pin-prick sensation is a particularly good predictor of functional motor recovery.

Autonomic Pathways (Also See Chapter 33)	
Sympathetic innervation to all viscera including the cardiovascular system is via preganglionic sympathetic neurons located in the T1–L2 spinal cord segments, whereas parasympathetic innervation of the cardiovascular system bypasses the spinal cord since it is via the vagus nerve whose neurons are in the brainstem.	Disproportionate loss of supra-spinal control of the sympathetic nervous system compared to the parasympathetic nervous system in cervical or high thoracic SCI contributes to cardiovascular problems such as low resting blood pressure, orthostatic hypotension, and limited cardiovascular responses to exercise.

Blood Supply of the Spinal Cord (Also See Chapter 16)	
A single anterior spinal artery with discontinuous reinforcement by segmental arteries supplies the anterior two-thirds of the cord, versus two posterior spinal arteries with relatively robust segmental reinforcement throughout the length of the spinal cord that supply the posterior third.	Spinal cord infarction often causes an anterior cord syndrome with paralysis and impaired pin-prick and temperature sensations, and relative sparing of the posterior columns with preserved touch, position, and vibration sensations.
There is a relatively avascular watershed area in the mid-thoracic region between the rostral region where the anterior spinal artery is more robust and the caudal region where blood supply is supplemented by the relatively large radicular artery of Adamkiewicz.	Mid-thoracic (T4–T8) level is the most common site of spinal cord infarction.

KNOWLEDGE GAPS AND EMERGING CONCEPTS

Emerging concepts about neuroplasticity of the spinal cord have important implications on the effect and potential therapeutic interventions for spinal cord injury (SCI), and this is an area of growing research. Newer techniques are enabling improved understanding of the structure, function, and organization of the spinal cord and its tracts.

SUGGESTED READING

Purves D, Augustine GJ, Fitzpatrick D, Hall WC, LaMantia AS, White LE, eds. *Neuroscience.* 5th ed. Sunderland, MA: Sinauer Associates; 2012.

Seigel A, Sapru HN. *Essential Neuroscience.* 2nd ed. Baltimore, MD: Lippincott William and Wilkins; 2011:381-406.

Waxman SG. Chapter 5. The spinal cord. In: Waxman SG, ed. *Clinical Neuroanatomy.* 26th ed. New York, NY: McGraw-Hill; 2010.

CHAPTER 2

Pathophysiology of Spinal Cord Injury

GENERAL PRINCIPLES

The majority of current understanding of the pathophysiological processes involved in spinal cord injury (SCI) comes from animal models, and very little is derived from human studies.

SCI involves both primary damage, occurring at the time of impact, and secondary damage that occurs due to pathophysiologic processes that follow.

Primary Injury

Primary injury is the initial tissue disruption and damage to the spinal cord that occurs at the time of impact. Forces related to flexion, extension, axial loading, rotation, and/or distraction produce a primary mechanical insult to the spine and spinal cord. The physical injury to the spinal cord results in laceration, contusion, compression, shear, and traction of the neural tissue. There may be traumatic severing of axons. Primary injury rarely transects the spinal cord, and often leaves an intact subpial rim of tissue on the outside.

The extent of both the primary injury and the subsequent secondary injury is likely related to the energy delivered to the spinal cord at the time of impact. The direction of the force also has a significant effect on the nature of the spinal injury (Table 2.1).

Secondary Injury

In addition to the immediate injury, SCI also causes delayed damage and death to cells that survive the original trauma. Studies of secondary damage after SCI performed in blunt injury animal models, for example, delivered via a precisely calibrated weight drop, have largely generated the knowledge related to histopathological changes and involved biochemical and molecular processes. In addition to the "weight-drop" method, other animal models of SCI include additional contusion models, clip or balloon compression, and surgical transection.

Table 2.1

Mechanical Forces Related to Primary Injury

Primary Mechanical Force	Illustrative Injury Mechanisms	Associated Spinal Column Injury[a]
Flexion	- Diving into shallow water - Being thrown off a motorcycle	- Bilateral facet dislocation - Simple wedge fracture - Anterior subluxation
Extension	- An elderly person sustaining a fall to the floor - Face hitting the windshield in a car accident	- Hyperextension fracture-dislocation - Laminar fracture - Traumatic spondylolistheis (hangman's fracture)
Flexion-rotation	- Rollover car accident	- Unilateral facet dislocation
Vertical compression	- Falling from a height onto head or feet	- Burst fracture - Jefferson fracture of atlas
Lateral flexion	- Fall - Car accident	- Uncinate process fracture
Distraction	- Car accident with seat belt incorrectly worn too high	- Transverse fracture through vertebra (Chance fracture)

[a]Not a comprehensive list, typical examples are listed.

The biological response to SCI has been temporally divided into several contiguous phases: acute, that occurs in the initial minutes to hours after injury; secondary or subacute, that occurs in days to weeks after injury; and chronic, that occurs months to years after injury. The latter phase can be further divided into an intermediate phase lasting up to 6 months, and a late/chronic phase after that period. Each phase includes distinct but overlapping processes and characteristics (Table 2.2).

A number of interrelated processes contribute to secondary damage after SCI. These include vascular perfusion abnormalities, edema, free radical generation, lipid peroxidation, excitotoxicity with alterations in local ionic concentrations and calcium influx, inflammation, and cell death (Table 2.3). There are several published reviews of the involved pathophysiology, including those by Kwon et al. (2004) and Rowland et al. (2008), included in the suggested reading at the end of this chapter, to refer for additional detail.

Figures 2.1 and 2.2 depict key steps in the cascade of events involved in the pathophysiology of SCI-related secondary damage. Some of the processes and feedback loops between the different steps in the pathophysiology of SCI are not shown in the figures, but it is important to understand that ischemia,

Table 2.2

Typical Sequence of Histopathological Changes in the Spinal Cord After Closed Trauma (Animal Model)

Acute Phase

- Petechial hemorrhages in central gray matter visible on microscopy within 15 mins of injury. Small white matter hemorrhages appear. Hemorrhages coalesce and become macroscopically visible in 1 hr
- Edema of the cord becomes evident within 2–4 hrs, with axonal swelling
- The area of hemorrhage and edema spreads in a centrifugal manner. Spreading edema at the level of injury obscures distinction between white and gray matter, and there is a spindle-shaped spread to adjacent rostral and caudal spinal cord segments
- Necrotic changes (involving neurons and glial cells) appear in the anterior horn earlier than the posterior horn
- Invasion by polymorphonuclear neutrophils (PMN) is seen in the first few hours, followed by mononuclear cells and then macrophages

Subacute and Intermediate Phases

- Partial resolution of edema
- Removal of necrotic debris by macrophages, hemosiderin-laden macrophages visible
- Vascular angiopathy with intimal proliferation
- As necrotic tissue is removed cystic cavity formation occurs in the central cord, which can extend centrifugally
- Disrupted axonal segments with demyelinated nerve fibers are present above and below the level of injury

Chronic Phase

- Connective scar tissue forms in the area of primary injury
- Wallerian degeneration of adjacent ascending and descending tracts
- Macroscopically the cord may become atrophic and sclerotic
- Scar tissue or cystic cavity filled with cerebrospinal fluid replaces lost spinal cord tissue

excitotoxicity, inflammation, free radical production, and lipid peroxidation are interrelated processes with several feedback loops between one another that propagate the progression of injury.

Mechanisms Behind Spontaneous Recovery After SCI

Following injury, the spinal cord can spontaneously recover to a varying extent through a number of biological mechanisms, but current understanding of the involved mechanisms is quite rudimentary. The possible mechanisms involved include: remyelination, recovery of conduction, strengthening of existing synapses, regrowth and sprouting of intact neurons to form new circuits, release of growth factors and guidance molecules, and shift of function to alternate circuits.

Table 2.3

Key Processes Involved in Pathophysiology of Secondary Damage After SCI

Ischemia and Microvascular Perfusion Alterations

- Hemorrhage
- Vasospasm and vasoconstriction
- Edema
- Intravascular thrombosis
- Loss of autoregulatory microvascular hemodynamic regulation
- Systemic effects of neurogenic shock/hypotension on vascular perfusion

Free Radical Generation and Lipid Peroxidation

- Free radicals are generated via several different processes (e.g., Ca++ activation of nitric oxide synthetase, lactate accumulation, activation of the arachidonic acid cascade, ischemia and reperfusion injury).
- Unpaired electrons of free radicals make them highly reactive; free radicals react with lipids in cell membrane and cause lipid peroxidation contributing to axonal disruption and cell death.
- Lipid peroxidation generates more free radicals, so can be self-propagating.

Excitotoxicity and Calcium Overload

- Excitotoxicity results from massive glutamate release that occurs in response to depolarization and ischemia.
- Excess glutamate stimulation of N-methyl-D-aspartate (NMDA) and non-NMDA receptors allows large amounts of calcium (and sodium) to move into the cell.
- Calcium accumulation due to this dyregulation has several deleterious effects, and is a central feature in cell death (Figure 2.2). These effects include:
  - Mitochondrial dysfunction → shift from aerobic to anaerobic metabolism → lactate accumulation
  - Activation of mitochondrial nitric oxide synthetase (NOS) → Free radical production (perioxynitrite) → Lipid peroxidation
  - Activation of phospholipase A2 and arachidonic acid (AA) cascade
    - AA is converted by cyclooxygenase to prostanoids → cause vasoconstriction → ischemia
    - Activated lipooxygenase pathway → accumulation of leukotrines → PMN and macrophage influx
  - Activation of calcium-dependent protease enzymes → degradation of cytoskeletal proteins → apoptotic cell death

Inflammatory and Immunological Response

- Some aspects of the inflammatory response in the central nervous system (CNS) are neuroprotective but others are neurotoxic.
- It has been suggested that the less pronounced macrophage response in CNS may contribute to poor regenerative capacity compared to the peripheral nervous system.
- Inflammatory cells produce cytokines, e.g., tumor necrosis factor (TNF-α) and interleukins that can contribute to additional tissue damage.

(continued)

Table 2.3

Key Processes Involved in Pathophysiology of Secondary Damage After SCI (*continued*)

Cell Death

- Both necrotic and apoptotic cell death may occur. Death of neurons occurs mostly through necrosis, while oligodendrocytes typically undergo apoptotic cell death.
- Necrotic cell death involves swelling of the cell and membrane lysis in response to a severe insult that overwhelms the cell's homeostatic mechanisms.
- Apoptosis is a form of programmed cell death, often seen in oligodendrocytes, in which extrinsic or intrinsic stressors initiate a cascade of intracellular pathways that results in orderly dismantling of the cell. After SCI, cells around the region of injury that are initially spared may experience sufficient biochemical insult to generate apoptotic self-destruction due to activation of capsases.

Figure 2.1

Pathophysiology of SCI-Related Secondary Injury—Part 1: Initial Sequence of Events Leading to Intracellular Calcium Overload

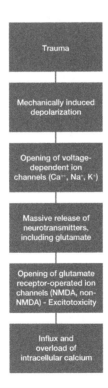

Abbreviation: NMDA, N-methyl-D-aspartate

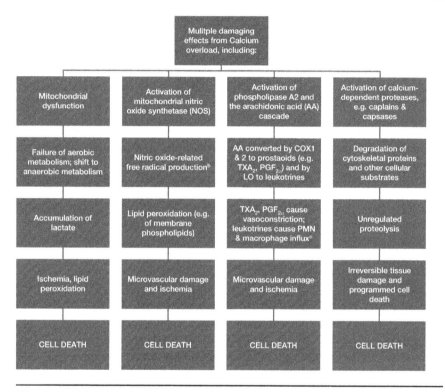

Figure 2.2

Pathophysiology of SCI-Related Secondary Injury—Part 2: Role of Intracellular Calcium Overload in Cell Death[a]

Abbreviations: COX, cyclooxygenase; LO, lipoxygenase; TXA2, thromboxane A2; PGF2α, Prostaglandin F2α; PMN, polymorphonuclear neutrophils.

[a]This is a partial representation of events. There are additional interrelations and positive feedback loops between these processes that are omitted from the figure for ease of illustration.
[b]Other free radicals may be generated by additional pathways and contribute to lipid peroxidation.
[c]Inflammatory response acts as a double-edged sword. Some aspects can be neuroprotective, but the secreted lytic enzymes and cytokines can also further damage local tissue.

Barriers to Axonal Regeneration

While the dogma that the central nervous system (CNS) cannot regenerate is no longer held to be true, it is recognized that the CNS neurons have a low intrinsic regenerative capacity and that the injured CNS is a relatively nonpermissive environment for growth.

Several factors have been identified that inhibit axonal regeneration after SCI. These include inhibitory factors in myelin such as myelin-associated glycoprotein (MAG), and Nogo-A. Downstream effects of these inhibitory pathways utilize the guanosine triphosphatase (GTPase) Rho.

An additional source of inhibition of regeneration is the glial scar that forms in the recovery process during the chronic phase of SCI. This can pose a physical as well as chemical barrier. Several proteoglycans in the glial scar have been found to be inhibitory to axonal regeneration, though a few have also been found to promote regeneration.

CLINICAL CONSIDERATIONS

An understanding of the pathophysiological processes occurring following SCI is critical for developing effective therapies to minimize or reverse the damage. These are further discussed in Chapter 3.

In addition to local pathophysiological processes at the site of injury that lead to secondary injury, systemic factors also contribute. Strategies such as prompt resuscitation, minimizing prolonged hypoxia, and prevention and management of neurogenic shock and hypotension during early acute management after SCI not only save lives but may also limit secondary damage to the spinal cord. It has been proposed that mean arterial pressure (MAP) be maintained at or above 90 mmHg after SCI, although further study is needed to define optimal MAP after SCI. Measures to prevent additional damage to the spinal cord, for example, from spinal instability and timely decompression when indicated, are of critical importance.

KNOWLEDGE GAPS AND EMERGING CONCEPTS

Much has been learned about the biochemical reactions and pathways that are involved in the progression of SCI, especially in the past two decades, but much remains to be understood. Knowledge about the molecular mechanisms that regulate formation and maintenance of the complex and intricate glial and neuronal neurological circuits, which control the function of the spinal cord, is continuing to evolve. Additional understanding of the molecular mechanisms that promote and inhibit axonal regeneration is needed.

SUGGESTED READING

Borgens RB, Liu-Snyder P. Understanding secondary injury. *Q Rev Biol.* 2012;87(2): 89-127.

Institute of Medicine. *Spinal Cord Injury: Progress, Promise, and Priorities.* Washington, DC: National Academies Press; 2005.

Kwon BK, Tetzlaff W, Grauer JN, Beiner J, Vaccaro AR. Pathophysiology and pharmacologic treatment of acute spinal cord injury. *Spine J.* July-August 2004;4(4):451-464.

Rowland JW, Hawryluk GW, Kwon B, Fehlings MG. Current status of acute spinal cord injury pathophysiology and emerging therapies: promise on the horizon. *Neurosurg Focus.* 2008;25(5):E2.

CHAPTER 3

Research in Neuroprotection, Regeneration, and Repair of the Injured Spinal Cord

GENERAL PRINCIPLES

Basic research in spinal cord protection and repair is promising. During the past few decades there has been a rapid expansion of discoveries in neuroscience and understanding of pathophysiological mechanisms associated with spinal cord injury (SCI), and an explosion of multiple avenues of research aimed at utilizing this knowledge to protect and restore spinal cord function after injury.

New discoveries have provided opportunities and hope for future therapies. At the same time enthusiasm for a "cure" for SCI has been tempered by difficulties and disappointments in translating animal research into strategies for clinical interventions. There has been an inability to demonstrate robust efficacy of various experimental interventions that would allow for widespread clinical acceptance.

What Constitutes a "Cure"?

Given that SCI involves multiple body systems, a pragmatic approach to defining a "cure" has been recommended, incorporating a broad definition of function rather than an "all or nothing" approach or a singular focus on restoration of walking.

It is also important to recognize that even small anatomical gains can lead to disproportionate functional benefits. An improvement of one or two neurological levels can be of great functional significance to an individual with SCI. Animal studies have suggested that even 10% retention of axonal white matter may be sufficient for functional recovery of locomotor function. In order to improve relevance of research in this area, it is crucial to target the priorities of individuals with SCI for functional recovery.

Research Strategies to Protect and Restore Function After SCI

There are multiple potential approaches and interventions to promote recovery from SCI (Table 3.1). These include: prevention of secondary injury (neuroprotection); promotion of axonal regeneration and repair; restoration of axonal transmission; replacement of destroyed spinal cord tissue; retraining the spinal cord; or strategies to bypass the injured segment. Neuroprotection strategies to prevent secondary damage are primarily applicable in the acute phase following injury, whereas several of the strategies for regeneration and repair are less time-specific.

Table 3.2 summarizes various neuroprotection research strategies to prevent secondary damage by countering the acute processes that are involved. The involved pathophysiological processes that are targets for experimental interventions are discussed in detail in Chapter 2. It may be helpful to refer to Figures 2.1 and 2.2 in conjunction with Table 3.2 to identify the sites of action of various neuroprotective agents in the secondary injury cascade.

Table 3.3 summarizes axonal repair and regeneration strategies after SCI, and potential cell replacement therapies that are currently being explored.

Strategies to retrain the spinal cord are important aspects of efforts to restore function and mobility after SCI. Another important avenue is ongoing research and advancement in technologies and methods to assist with or incorporate strategies to replace lost function. These aspects are discussed in further detail in the chapters in Section IV of this book.

CLINICAL CONSIDERATIONS

Despite the exponential growth of research avenues and opportunities, there has been a lack of any uniformly accepted or FDA-approved treatment for improving neurological function after SCI.

Methylprednisolone, administered intravenously within 8 hours of injury, was the only agent that was in widespread clinical use for a period of time following publication of positive studies in the 1990's that suggested improved outcomes (also see Chapter 8). However, that research has been subject of much debate

Table 3.1

Experimental Approaches to Promote Recovery After SCI

Neuroprotection from secondary injury (Table 3.2)

Promote axonal regeneration and repair; restore axonal transmission (Table 3.3)

Replace destroyed spinal cord tissue (Table 3.3)

Retrain the spinal cord (enhance purposeful function of remaining neural circuitry)

Substitute for or bypass the injured circuits (neural prostheses; epidural stimulation distal to injury site; brain-computer interface); Assist or replace function

Table 3.2

Neuroprotection Research Strategies to Target Acute Pathophysiological Processes After SCI

Pathophysiological Process*	Experimental Strategy/Agent
Excitotoxicity and calcium overload:	
■ Massive glutamate release and stimulation of receptors (e.g., N-methyl-D-aspartate [NMDA])	■ NMDA receptor blockers (e.g., gacyclidine, magnesium salts) and glutamate antagonists
■ Allows large influx of calcium (and sodium) into the cell	■ Prevent calcium overload with calcium channel blockers; reduce sodium influx with sodium channel blockers (e.g., riluzole)
Free radical formation	
■ E.g., by calcium-related activation of nitric oxide synthetase (NOS) in mitochondria	■ Antioxidants ■ NOS inhibitors, e.g., minocycline
Lipid peroxidation	
■ Leads to axonal disruption and cell death	■ Steroids ■ Erythropoietin
Activation of phospholipase A2 and arachidonic acid cascade	
■ Formation of vasoconstricting prostanoids through cyclooxygenase pathway	■ Phospholipase inhibition (e.g., steroids)
■ Generation of leukotrienes that increase polymorphonuclear neutrophils influx through lipooxygenase pathway	■ Modulation of mediators of cyclooxygenase and lipooxygenase pathways
Inflammatory and immunological response	
■ Microglial activation and/or inflammatory cytokines can increase cell damage	■ Agents that reduce inflammation, reduce microglial activation and/or block effects of cytokines, e.g., minocycline
■ Suboptimal macrophage response may decrease regenerative capacity	■ Transplantation of autologous macrophages
Ischemia	
■ Associated with microvascular perfusion abnormalities	■ Anti-vasospastic agents ■ Steroids
■ Metabolically overactive cells may be especially vulnerable to damage	■ Regional hypothermia
Activation of calcium-dependent proteases	
■ Activated capsases and caplains degrade cellular substrates	■ Capsase inhibitors ■ Caplain inhibitors
■ Leads to tissue damage and programmed tissue damage and programmed cell death	■ Block cytochrome *c* release, minocycline

(continued)

Table 3.2

Neuroprotection Research Strategies to Target Acute Pathophysiological Processes After SCI (*continued*)

Pathophysiological Process*	Experimental Strategy/Agent
Tissue damage and cell death	■ Prevent apoptosis (e.g., minocycline) and/or promote neural repair (e.g., ganglioside injection)
Multiple interrelated processes are involved	■ Use combination therapies

*Also see Figures 2.1 and 2.2 for pathophysiological processes in the injury cascade.

Table 3.3

Regeneration and Repair Strategies After SCI

Pathophysiological Process	Potential Intervention/Agent
Glial scar ■ May pose a physical as well as chemical barrier to axonal regeneration	■ Reduce glial scar, with enzymes such as chondroitinase ABC that degrade glial proteoglycans
Myelin-related inhibitory factors ■ These factors (e.g., nogo, myelin-associated glycoprotein or MAG) inhibit axonal growth through pathways that utilize the GTPase Rho	■ Receptor blockers or antibodies against inhibitory factors, e.g., anti-nogo antibodies or anti-MAG antibodies; ■ Rho antagonists to block its downstream inhibitory pathway (e.g., Cethrin)
Poor intrinsic regeneration capacity of the central nervous system (CNS) ■ Axonal growth is limited and incomplete	■ Up-regulate regeneration associated genes through gene therapy (e.g., introduce genes that code for growth factors into target cells)
Nonpermissive environment for axonal growth ■ The extrinsic environment of the CNS is much less conducive to regeneration than other tissues	■ Provide neurotrophic factors either directly, or indirectly by transplanting cells that produce these factors ■ Cyclic adenosine monophosphate (AMP) analogues to improve intracellular signaling to augment the effect of trophic factors ■ Facilitate nerve growth and sprouting e.g., through use of oscillating field stimulation
Axons grow haphazardly ■ Regenerating axons often don't reach their target	■ Guidance molecules to steer axons in a particular direction (netrins, ephrins) ■ Matrices and scaffolds as physical conduits

(continued)

Pathophysiological Process	Potential Intervention/Agent
Gaps in axonal connections	
■ Physical gaps interfere with axon connections	■ Use techniques to bridge axonal gaps e.g., through peripheral nerve bridges; biomaterials, scaffolds
Demyelinated axons conduct poorly	
■ Loss of myelin makes impulse conduction through exchange of ions much less effective	■ Agents to improve conduction in demyelinated axons, e.g., potassium channel blockers to decrease potassium leakage
	■ Enhance or inhibit specific subtypes of sodium channels
	■ Schwann cell transplant to facilitate remyelination
Loss of viable spinal cord tissue	
	■ Cellular transplant strategies, e.g., Schwann cells, olfactory ensheathing cells (OEC), bone marrow stem cells, genetically modified fibroblasts, human embryonic stem cells, adult stem cells
Multiple processes impair repair and regeneration	
	■ Combinational therapies

and consensus about its use is lacking. In fact, several professional organizations have increasingly recommended against its use, citing lack of consistent or compelling clinical evidence and demonstrated evidence of harmful side-effects. The American Association of Neurological Surgeons/Congress of Neurological Surgeons (AANS/CNS) guidelines for management of acute cervical spine and SCI, updated in 2013, now explicitly recommend against administration of methylprednisone for the treatment of SCI.

Only a small proportion of animal studies have been progressed to clinical trials, and none has shown convincingly demonstrated efficacy to date. Translational challenges relate to differences between the animal model and human subject, inadequate clinically meaningful objective outcome measures that lead to interpretational challenges, and issues with study design and implementation.

Measures to minimize systemic hypotension, systemic hypoxia, and spinal instability are important to prevent additional secondary insults to the spinal cord.

Rehabilitations strategies should be emphasized as crucial components to promote function in the clinical setting, in concert with other avenues of ongoing research to treat SCI. It is also important to prioritize further research to prevent the wide range of acute and chronic complications of SCI, such as pain, spasticity, bladder functions, and pressure ulcers.

Given the lack of proven, effective strategies, there is concern that patients may be willing to try nonvalidated experimental treatments for SCI that have not been adequately tested for safety and efficacy. Desperate patients may also be prone to victimization by individuals or organizations offering questionable treatments for material gain. Careful consideration and through study of therapies is necessary with full attention to patient safety. Clinicians should be prepared to offer advice or to direct patients to the appropriate source for guidance if they are considering experimental treatments. It is important to make sure that patients fully understand the risks involved and the extent of any potential benefits, and to steer them away from nonvalidated, unregulated interventions that don't meet the criteria for a well-designed clinical trial.

KNOWLEDGE GAPS AND EMERGING CONCEPTS

A continued focus on increased understanding of the biochemical and molecular mechanisms involved in SCI and potential targets for interventions is required. Several aspects of potential therapies such as cellular replacement therapies are still in their infancy.

Currently available outcome measures have limited sensitivity. More refined and meaningful outcome measures are needed to assess efficacy of future studies. Objective assessments that accurately predict recovery of function need to be established.

Given the multifaceted and interrelated pathophysiological processes involved in SCI, therapeutic approaches likely need to address multiple targets, making combination approaches especially attractive. Research to determine the particular therapies that can be combined safely and work in concert to provide maximum effectiveness is an important area of focus for the future.

SUGGESTED READING

Cadotte DW, Fehlings MG. Spinal cord injury: a systematic review of current treatment options. *Clin Orthop Relat Res.* 2011;469(3):732-741.

Curt A. The translational dialogue in spinal cord injury research. *Spinal Cord.* 2012;50(5):352-357.

Institute of Medicine. *Spinal Cord Injury: Progress, Promise, and Priorities.* Washington, DC National Academies Press; 2005.

Kwon BK, Okon E, Hillyer J, et al. A systematic review of non-invasive pharmacologic neuroprotective treatments for acute spinal cord injury. *J Neurotrauma.* 2011;28(8):1545-1588.

Kwon BK, Okon EB, Plunet W, et al. A systematic review of directly applied biologic therapies for acute spinal cord injury. *J Neurotrauma.* 2011;28(8):1589-1610.

Lammertse D, Tuszynski MH, Steeves JD, et al.; International Campaign for Cures of Spinal Cord Injury Paralysis. Guidelines for the conduct of clinical trials for spinal cord injury as developed by the ICCP panel: clinical trial design. *Spinal Cord.* 2007;45(3):232-242.

Lammertse DP. Clinical trials in spinal cord injury: lessons learned on the path to translation. The 2011 International Spinal Cord Society Sir Ludwig Guttmann Lecture. *Spinal Cord.* 2013;51(1):2-9.

Rowland JW, Hawryluk GW, Kwon B, Fehlings MG. Current status of acute spinal cord injury pathophysiology and emerging therapies: promise on the horizon. *Neurosurg Focus.* 2008;25(5):E2.

Tetzlaff W, Okon EB, Karimi-Abdolrezaee S, et al. A systematic review of cellular transplantation therapies for spinal cord injury. *J Neurotrauma.* 2011;28(8):1611-1682.

Tohda C, Kuboyama T. Current and future therapeutic strategies for functional repair of spinal cord injury. *Pharmacol Ther.* 2011;132(1):57-71.

II. Traumatic Spinal Cord Injury

CHAPTER 4

Epidemiology of Spinal Cord Injury

GENERAL PRINCIPLES

Much of the published data on epidemiology of traumatic spinal cord injury (SCI) for the Unites States (U.S.) comes from a few databases, primarily from the National Spinal Cord Injury Statistical Center (NSCISC). The NSCISC database is estimated to capture about 13% of new SCI cases in the U.S. (Table 4.1). Published reports from that database are the source of information for most of this chapter (except for estimated incidence, prevalence, and global data).

International registries and databases provide some information about global epidemiology of SCI, but are only collected in a systematic manner in a few countries. There is lack of standardization and much variation in data elements collected in existing data globally, so only limited broad generalizations about international comparisons can be made (Table 4.2).

Incidence

Incidence of traumatic SCI in the U.S. is estimated to be around 40 cases per million, but these estimates are based on old incidence studies, so it is not clear if these numbers are still accurate.

Interpretable global incidence data is only available for a few countries. The reported incidence in Australia and Western Europe at 15 to 16 per million is considerably lower than that in North America.

Prevalence

The number of people living with traumatic SCI in the U.S. is estimated to be around 273,000, with a range between 238,000 to 332,000. Some studies have suggested a significantly higher prevalence but the validity of that data is uncertain.

Sufficient data to derive a global prevalence for SCI is not available. The reported prevalence from different regions worldwide varies between 236 and

Table 4.1

Key Epidemiological Facts About Traumatic SCI in the U.S.[a,b]	
Age at injury (years)	- Most common age group—16 to 30 - Average age of injury since 2010—42
Gender	- 80% male
Etiology	- Vehicular—37% - Falls—29% - Violence—14% - Sports—9% - Other/unknown—11%
Neurological category at discharge	- Incomplete tetraplegia—41% - Incomplete paraplegia—19% - Complete paraplegia—18% - Complete tetraplegia—12% - Unknown ~ 10% - Complete recovery <1%

[a] Based on National Spinal Cord Injury Statistical Center (NSCISC) data, which captures an estimated 13% of new SCI cases in the U.S.
[b] Numbers rounded to the closest digit, may not add up to 100% due to rounding.

Table 4.2

Global Variations in the Etiology of SCI

- Falls from trees and rooftops are the leading reported cause of traumatic SCI in parts of South Asia

- Transportation-related SCI in South-east Asia is more likely to involve two-wheeled and nonstandard transportation than the four-wheeled motor vehicle accidents that are the commonest cause in the U.S. and other developed countries

- Sub-Saharan Africa has the highest reported violence-related SCI in the world. Rates are also high in North Africa, Middle East, and Latin America

- Western Europe and Australia have lower proportion of violence-related SCI than North America

- Nontraumatic SCI is most often related to degenerative conditions of the spine, followed by spinal tumors, in the U.S. and other developed countries

- Infections, including tuberculosis and HIV, are the predominant cause of nontraumatic SCI in many developing countries

over 1,000 per million, but prevalence data is missing for several major global populations.

Age at Injury

SCI continues to primarily affect young adults with highest incident rates in late teens and early twenties. However, the average age of injury in the U.S. has gone up steadily; it is reported to be 42.6 years since 2010. Possible contributors to this trend might include changes in age-specific incidence rates, age of the general population, survival rates of older individuals at injury, or changing referral patterns.

Gender

About 80% of traumatic SCI in the U.S. occurs in males, although there seems to be a slightly increasing percentage of SCI among women. A much smaller gender gap for SCI in the elderly may account for this trend.

Ethnicity/Race

Although whites continue to make up the majority of SCI in the U.S., NSCISC data seems to suggest that the proportion of injuries in black and Hispanic individuals in the database is steadily increasing. Possible reasons may be changes in the U.S. general population, changing location of model systems that contribute to the database, changing referral patterns, or changes in race-specific incidence rates.

Etiology of Injury

Motor vehicle crashes are the leading cause of SCI in the U.S. making up about 36.5% of cases in the database since 2010. Falls are the next most common cause, followed by violence, primarily due to gunshot wounds, and sports (Table 4.1).

Falls are the leading cause of SCI in the elderly, which likely accounts for the increased proportion of falls as a cause of injury. Violence as a cause of SCI, peaked in the 1990s, but has since declined. Sports injuries have decreased slightly, to 9.2% currently. Diving (especially into shallow water), football, and trampolines, that were the major causes of sports injuries, are still important, though these seem to have decreased in recent years in association with injury prevention initiatives. Winter sports-related injuries have increased concomitantly.

Globally, motor vehicle accidents are the most common cause of SCI in developed countries. Transportation-related injuries in several developing countries are more often related to accidents involving two-wheeled or nonstandard transportation. Falls from rooftops or trees are leading causes of traumatic SCI in parts of South Asia (Table 4.2).

Neurological Level and Completeness of Injury

The most frequent neurological category at discharge in the NSCISC database since 2010 is incomplete tetraplegia, and the least frequent is complete tetraplegia (Table 4.1).

There has been a slight increase in the proportion of cervical injuries over the years. The most common level of injury at discharge was C5 (15.3%), followed by C4 (14.7%), C6 (10.6%), T12 (6.4%), C7 (5.2%), and L1 (5.0%).

The proportion of incomplete injuries has been increasing. Possible reasons for this could include better acute treatment modalities, but trends in age and etiology of injury are at least part of the reason.

Thoracic injuries are more likely to neurologically complete. Lumbar and, especially, sacral injuries are often American Spinal Injury Association (ASIA) Impairment Scale (AIS) D. Cervical injuries are most often either AIS A or AIS D.

Etiology is associated with the neurological category of injury. For example, gun-shot wounds often result in paraplegia, while sport-related injuries, in the vast majority, result in tetraplegia.

Life Expectancy

Life expectancies remain substantially below normal, particularly for persons with tetraplegia and ventilator-dependency. Over the past few decades there has been a significant increase in life expectancy after SCI. It has been reported, however, that much of this increase in life expectancy can be contributed to a continued significant reduction in mortality rate during the first year after injury. After the first year or two of injury, progress in reducing annual mortality rates seems to have been much slower, with no additional demonstrable decrease in over two decades in that regard.

Mortality during the first year of injury is related to ventilator dependence, advanced age at injury, a higher level of injury, a neurologically complete injury, being male, and being injured by an act of violence.

These factors also affect mortality after the first year, though to a lesser extent. Other factors associated with higher long-term mortality rates are higher levels of dependence, poor general health, lower life satisfaction, poor adjustment to disability, poor community integration, and income level below the poverty line.

Causes of Death

Diseases of the respiratory system are the leading cause of death in people with SCI (over two-thirds of these were cases of pneumonia). Based on the 2012 annual NSCISC report, the second leading cause of death was infective and parasitic diseases. These were usually cases of septicemia (88.9%) and were usually associated with decubitus ulcers, urinary tract or respiratory infections. Cancer ranked third (lung cancer being the most prevalent), followed by hypertensive and ischemic heart disease.

Standardized mortality ratio (SMR) in SCI, that is, the ratio of observed death in those with SCI to expected deaths in the general population, is highest for deaths due to septicemia, pulmonary embolism, and pneumonia.

Diseases of the genito-urinary system as a cause of death have dramatically decreased in the last four decades associated with improvements in urological management.

Suicide accounts for about 3.5% of deaths. The suicide rate is reported to be about five times higher than the general population, with highest risk in the first 5 years. Higher rates are reported in those with neurologically complete paraplegia, and in whites compared to blacks.

Nontraumatic SCI

Data on nontraumatic SCI is not captured in NSCISC and has been collected systematically or comprehensively to a much lesser extent so only broad generalizations can be made.

Epidemiology of individual causes of nontraumatic SCI is covered in separate chapters in Section III of this book.

While epidemiological characteristics depend on the underlying etiology of nontraumatic SCI, overall as a group these are associated with older age, a higher percent of females, and a higher percent of paraplegia compared to tetraplegia (Table 4.3).

Table 4.3

Characteristics of Nontraumatic Versus Traumatic SCI (Also See Chapter 12)		
	Traumatic	**Nontraumatic**
Age of onset	Younger (although increasing incidence in older adults)	Depends on the underlying etiology, but older overall
Gender distribution	80% male, 20% females	Higher percent of females
Neurological level	Tetraplegia or paraplegia	More often paraplegia
Completeness of injury	Complete or incomplete	More often incomplete
Comorbidities	Fewer comorbidities with younger age	Higher prevalence of age-related comorbidities, may affect management and outcomes
Complications	Multiple complications, can affect all body systems	Many of the same complications as in traumatic but lesser prevalence of autonomic dysreflexia, orthostatic hypotension, venous thrombo-embolism, and pneumonia reported

Nontraumatic SCI in the U.S. and other developed countries is most often related to degenerative conditions of the spine, followed by spinal tumors. On the other hand, infections, including tuberculosis and HIV, are the predominant cause of nontraumatic SCI in many developing countries (Table 4.2).

CLINICAL CONSIDERATIONS

With the trend of an increasing proportion of injuries affecting those over age 60 years, there is a greater likelihood of encountering preexisting medical conditions and comorbidities that could adversely affect medical and functional outcomes, and complicate acute care and rehabilitation.

Given the especially great impact of pneumonia and septicemia on reduced life expectancy in people with SCI, measures to prevent, and expeditiously identify and treat these conditions are a critical component of care of people with SCI. While the greatest risk for pneumonia and septicemia is in the initial period after SCI when greatest vigilance is warranted, SMR for these conditions remains high in the longer-term so life-long attention to prevent and treat these complications is needed.

The SMR for cancer and ischemic heart disease is much lower in SCI compared to the general population than that for pneumonia and septicemia. However, given that those are the next commonest causes of death (with a trend suggesting continued increase), there is a need to ensure that people living with SCI get adequate prevention, screening, diagnostic measures, and management for those conditions.

Knowledge of the incidence and causes of SCI is needed to implement meaningful prevention initiatives.

KNOWLEDGE GAPS AND EMERGING CONCEPTS

Population-based incidence studies are needed to get accurate estimates.

Standardized data collection and reporting measures are needed, which will give the ability to combine and compare different epidemiological databases. The development of the International SCI Core Data Set and other International SCI Data Sets are an important step in the right direction.

More robust data collection and studies of nontraumatic SCI are required, again with standardized definition and data collection and reporting methods.

SUGGESTED READING

Chen Y, Tang Y, Vogel LC, Devivo MJ. Causes of spinal cord injury. *Top Spinal Cord Inj Rehabil.* 2013;19(1):1-8.

Cripps RA, Lee BB, Wing P, Weerts E, Mackay J, Brown D. A global map for traumatic spinal cord injury epidemiology: towards a living data repository for injury prevention. *Spinal Cord.* 2011;49(4):493-501.

Devivo MJ. Epidemiology of traumatic spinal cord injury: trends and future implications. *Spinal Cord.* 2012;50(5):365-372.

National Spinal Cord Injury Statistical Center. Spinal cord injury: facts and figures at a glance, Feb 2013. *J Spinal Cord Med.* 2013;36(4):394-395.

CHAPTER 5

Primary Prevention of Spinal Cord Injury

GENERAL PRINCIPLES

Prevention measures can be categorized as: primary prevention (i.e., measures to stop a disorder or injury from occurring), secondary prevention (i.e., measures to diagnose and treat the disorder or injury before it causes significant morbidity), and tertiary prevention (i.e., measures to reduce negative impact of the existent disorder or injury by restoring function and reducing disease-related complications). Various aspects of secondary and tertiary prevention of spinal cord injury (SCI) are covered in several other chapters in this book. The focus of this chapter is primary prevention of traumatic SCI.

A focus on primary prevention measures in health care is extremely important. Primary prevention programs are typically the most cost-effective type of prevention since they reduce the risk of catastrophic, high-cost injury. A challenge is to evaluate and demonstrate effectiveness and overall outcomes of prevention measures, but that is often not well documented.

Preventive measures can either be active, that is, targeting individual behavior, or passive, that is, the intervention does not require a conscious act on the part of the person to be protected. While passive measures, when feasible, are usually the more consistently effective ones, typically strategies involving both active and passive measures working in conjunction are the most effective.

As discussed in the previous chapter the most common causes of traumatic SCI are: vehicular accidents, fall-related injuries, violence (primarily firearm-related), and sports and recreational injuries. Preventive measures for each of these are discussed below and key measures for each etiological group are summarized in Tables 5.1 to 5.4.

Vehicular Crashes (Table 5.1)

As the leading cause of SCI, preventive measures targeting vehicular crashes are of greatest importance. Passive measures include incorporation of vehicular safety technology aimed at crash avoidance and at crash protection,

Table 5.1
Potential Measures to Prevent SCI Due to Vehicular Crashes

Safer road users	■ Decrease driving while impaired (DWI) – Education/ awareness initiatives about dangers of drinking (or drugs) and driving – Designated driver programs – Legislation and enforcement of DWI laws (e.g., expanded sobriety checks, minimum legal drinking age, zero tolerance laws, ignition interlocks for convicted DWI offenders) ■ Decrease distracted driving – Banning and enforcement of laws regarding texting and driving – Restricting cell phone use while driving – Education/awareness initiatives about texting and other forms of distracted driving ■ Special attention to high risk groups, e.g., teens – Teen driving laws, graduated driver licensing systems (designed to delay full licensure while allowing teens to get initial driving experience under low-risk conditions) – Special focus on teen driving safety (e.g., initiatives to reduce teen alcohol access, eliminate teen texting while driving, increase seatbelt use) ■ Avoiding drowsy driving – Preventive measures e.g., adequate sleep, scheduled breaks, avoiding sedating medications and alcohol – Countermeasures (stop driving, take a nap, drink a caffeinated beverage)
Safer vehicles	■ Deploying, enforcing, and complying with road safety laws (e.g., "Click it or Ticket") ■ Safety technology for crash avoidance – Electronic stability control – Lane departure warnings – Anti-lock brakes ■ Safety technology for crash protection – Advanced head-restraints (reduce head, neck injuries in crashes) – Advanced air bags (protect head, neck, chest in crashes) – Seat belts, seat-belt pretensioners to restrain occupants, eliminating lap-only or improperly worn seat belts to reduce distraction injuries – Child safety seats, booster seats (recommended till 8 yrs of age or taller than 4 ft., 9 in.) related laws, education, and distribution programs ■ Conducting and disseminating car crash safety ratings ■ Proper vehicle maintenance (including brakes, tires)
Safer roads	■ Planning and safety conscious design of roads and road networks – minimum lane and shoulder widths, proper stoppage sight distance, road hazard markings, traffic signals, speed controls ■ Identifying and addressing accident black-spots ■ Well lighted roads

Table 5.2

Potential Measures to Prevent SCI Due to Falls

Home/environment modifications	■ Grab bars in showers and bathtubs
	■ Removing tripping hazards (electric cords, throw rugs, uneven surfaces)
	■ Nonslip mats in bathrooms and tub/showers
	■ Handrails for stairs
	■ Proper lighting
	■ Window guards, safety gates for children
Reducing personal fall risk	■ Review and adjustment of medications that contribute to fall risk, dizziness, or balance problems
	■ Therapeutic exercise to improve strength and balance
	■ Timely diagnosis and correction of visual impairment
	■ Taking care to avoid situations that increase fall risk e.g., using a sturdy step stool to reach higher areas instead of climbing on a chair
	■ Wearing nonslip shoes

Table 5.3

Potential Measures to Prevent SCI Due to Gunshot Wounds and Violence

Personal behaviors	■ Keeping guns unloaded and locked up, with bullets locked and stored in a separate location.
	■ Educating children about dangers of guns and about not touching them
	■ Prevention-oriented program to reduce interpersonal and gang-related violence
	■ Initiatives to educate youth and teens about resolution of arguments and conflicts without resorting to guns or violence
Firearm safety regulations	■ Consensus-based development, implementation, and enforcement of regulations to assure safe and responsible gun use
Product design	■ Incorporating technology to make guns safer e.g., safety locks, measures to prevent unauthorized or unintentional use

as well as safe roadway planning and design. Active measures target the road user and include interventions to reduce distracted driving including, especially, texting while driving which is considered one of the most dangerous forms of distracted driving since it involves all three forms of distraction concomitantly: manual, visual, and cognitive. According to the National Highway Traffic Safety Administration (NHTSA), studies have shown a 23 times greater likelihood of crashing if the driver is texting while driving. Other active measures target drunk driving or driving while impaired (DWI), aggressive driving, drowsy driving, and compliance with road safety and seat

Table 5.4

Potential Measures to Prevent SCI Due to Sports and Recreational Activities	
Personal behaviors	■ Avoiding head-first dive into pools or other recreational water source without being certain water depth is at least 8–10 ft.
	■ Abstaining from alcohol while swimming/diving
	■ Avoiding tackling head-first in football (spearing) or sliding head-first onto bases in baseball
	■ Avoiding trampoline use without competent supervision, avoiding risky or acrobatic maneuvers without supervision of a trained professional
	■ Following safe skiing and snow-boarding practices, avoiding high-risk jumps
	■ Improving all-terrain vehicle (ATV) safety awareness
	■ Educational initiatives that address personal vulnerability and risk taking (e.g., THINK FIRST)
Regulations	■ Development, adoption, and consistent enforcement of regulations to reduce sports-related injuries
	– Banning of spearing in football, regulating scrummage in rugby, penalizing hard slams in wrestling, penalizing push or check from behind on to the boards in ice hockey
	■ Ensuring that players of matched skill levels, size, and maturity play with each other
	■ Ensuring that players have training in proper and safe techniques, and adequate strength and conditioning required for that activity
Equipment/ facilities	■ Wearing appropriate and properly secured and fitted protective gear and/or helmet as recommended for the sport or activity
	■ Clearly marked depth indictors for swimming pools; trampolines should be placed at ground level to prevent falls off the side

belt regulations. A special focus on teen drivers is indicated, since they are an especially high-risk group.

Fall Prevention (Table 5.2)

Falls are an especially important cause of SCI in older individuals. Prevention measures include environmental and home modification to reduce fall risk by minimizing fall hazards and providing safety measures, as well as measures that are aimed at the individual person making them less likely to fall. Young children are at risk for falls from windows and stairs, so appropriate prevention measures for those are needed.

Violence and Firearm Related Prevention Measures (Table 5.3)

While violence-related SCI has decreased from its peak in the 1990's it is still an important cause of injury. The vast majority of violence-related SCI in the United States is related to gun-shot wounds. Measures to reduce firearm-related injuries target personal behaviors, firearm safety regulations, and incorporation of safety measures in firearm product design.

Preventing Sports and Recreational Activity-Related Injuries (Table 5.4)

Diving is still the most common of these causes and typically involves diving head-first into shallow water. Alcohol is often involved in such diving-related injuries. Football and trampoline injuries were traditionally the other most common causes of sports-related injuries but have been declining, with water and snow-sports becoming increasingly common more recently. Sport or activity-related measures target individual behaviors, enforcement of rules to protect from injury (e.g., banning of head-first tackling or "spearing" in football that has significantly reduced the incidence of football-related SCI), and appropriate protective gear and equipment.

CLINICAL CONSIDERATIONS

Physicians and allied health professionals are natural spokespeople for prevention of SCI by virtue of their role in treating people who have sustained traumatic injuries. It has been shown in other contexts that, if properly done, physician-provided education and counseling can be especially effective in facilitating behavior change. Partnering with people who have sustained a SCI to provide prevention-related awareness and education can be particularly powerful. It is, therefore imperative for professionals who treat SCI to be aware of the contributors to risk of sustaining and injury and the related counter-measures, and to get involved in SCI prevention efforts as individuals and as professional organizations.

KNOWLEDGE GAPS AND EMERGING CONCEPTS

There is a lack of published data on the effectiveness of various SCI primary prevention initiatives and programs. More evidence-based studies are needed. Prevention programs should publish not only their program designs and underlying rationale, but also their successes, failures, and outcomes so that others can apply those findings as they develop and implement preventive services and programs.

SUGGESTED READING

Bellon K, Kolakowsky-Hayner SA, Chen D, McDowell S, Bitterman B, Klaas SJ. Evidence-based practice in primary prevention of spinal cord injury. *Top Spinal Cord Inj Rehabil.* 2013;19(1):25-30.

Center for Disease Control (CDC). Motor Vehicle Safety Website. http://www.cdc.gov/motorvehiclesafety/index.html. Accessed June 22, 2013.

Center for Disease Control (CDC). National Center for Injury Prevention and Control Website. http://www.cdc.gov/injury/index.html. Accessed June 22, 2013.

National Highway Traffic Safety Administration (NHSTA) website. http://www.nhtsa.gov. Accessed June 22, 2013.

Sandin KJ, Klaas SJ. Assessment and evaluation of primary prevention in spinal cord injury. *Top Spinal Cord Inj Rehabil.* 2013;19(1):9-14.

Think first foundation website. http://www.thinkfirst.org/home.asp. Accessed June 22, 2013.

CHAPTER 6

Prehospital Management of Spinal Cord Injury

GENERAL PRINCIPLES

Proper care for patients with spinal injuries at the scene of the accident includes immobilization, extrication, initial resuscitation, evaluation, and early transport of the patient to a medical center with the capability for diagnosis and treatment.

Development and advances of emergency medical services (EMS) have significantly improved prehospital management of spinal cord injury (SCI). The establishment of EMS is credited to be responsible, at least in part, for the observed improvement in neurological category, with a significantly higher proportion of incomplete injuries in those arriving to the emergency department with SCI, compared to the 1970s.

Expeditious and careful transport of patients with acute cervical spine or spinal cord injuries is recommended from the site of injury by the most appropriate mode of transportation available to the nearest capable definitive care medical facility.

Delayed transportation of spinal injury patients to a definitive treatment center has been associated with less favorable outcomes. Whenever possible, the transport of patients with acute cervical spine or spinal cord injuries to specialized acute SCI treatment centers has been recommended.

The goal is to expedite safe and effective transportation without an unfavorable impact on patient outcome. Cervical spinal cord injuries have a high incidence of airway compromise and pulmonary dysfunction, and respiratory support measures should be available during transport.

CLINICAL CONSIDERATIONS

Key aspects of prehospital management that are especially pertinent in the setting of spine and spinal cord injuries are summarized in Table 6.1.

Table 6.1

Key Aspects of Prehospital Management for Suspected SCI	
Immobilization	■ Rigid cervical collar and supportive blocks on a backboard with straps to maintain neutral spine position ● Backboard with occipital recess (or padding under the shoulder and upper back to raise torso in relation to the head) in children <8 yrs ● Leave helmet and shoulder pads on for athletic injuries
Airway	■ If intubation is needed, use manual in-line stabilization
Circulation	■ Maintain mean arterial pressure (MAP) >85 mmHg, avoid systolic blood pressure <90 mmHg, avoid fluid overload, treat severe or symptomatic bradycardia
Transportation	■ Expeditious transportation to the closest capable trauma center

Resuscitation Including Airway, Breathing, and Circulation

As with all trauma patients, addressing airway, breathing, and circulation are the highest priorities.

Supplemental oxygen is administered in all patients. Urgent intubation may be needed in the presence of hypoventilation, and patients with high cervical injuries may even be apneic. Airway management of patients with suspected SCI, who require intubation in the prehospital setting, should include the use of manual in-line stabilization (MILS) of the cervical spine. MILS is provided by an assistant during airway assessment and intubation who immobilizes the cervical spine in a neutral position. The goal is to secure the airway with as little movement of the cervical spine as possible. If paramedics have the ability and approval to perform rapid sequence induction (RSI), the recommended technique is RSI with an inducing agent (e.g., etomidate) followed by oro-tracheal intubation with cricoid pressure and manual in-line immobilization of the head and neck. Fiberoptic tracheal intubation, although an appropriate alternative, is not usually available in the prehospital setting.

Hypotension in the prehospital setting is treated with fluid resuscitation after ensuring adequate intravenous access. As needed, bleeding is controlled with direct manual pressure and pressure dressings. The goal is to maintain optimal tissue perfusion and resolve shock. In acutely injured patients with cervical or high-thoracic SCI, often both hypovolemic and neurogenic shock are present (Table 6.2). Neurogenic shock is due to disruption of sympathetic output to the heart and peripheral vasculature. The spine-immobilized patient may be placed in the Trendelenburg position to decrease pooling of blood in the lower extremity. On arrival to the medical center, additional evaluation is needed to determine the need for ongoing fluid resuscitation while avoiding fluid over-load, and the need for vasopressor management. The recommended goal is to keep mean arterial pressure (MAP) greater than 85 mmHg, although further study is needed in that regard. Systolic blood pressure less than 90 mmHg should be avoided.

Table 6.2

Characteristics of Neurogenic and Hypovolemic Shock[a]	
Hypovolemic Shock	**Neurogenic Shock**
Cold, clammy extremities	Warm, flushed extremities
Tachycardia	Bradycardia
Decreased urine volume	Urine volume often maintained

[a]Hypovolemic and neurogenic shock often co-exist in acute cervical or high thoracic SCI.

Table 6.3

Suggested Guidelines for Cervical Spine Clearance in the Field[a]
No neck pain, tenderness, or discomfort
No altered sensorium
No intoxication
No motor or sensory deficit
No distracting injuries

[a]Spinal immobilization not needed if patient meets all the above criteria.

Bradycardia is frequent in those with complete cervical injuries, and, if severe, may need to be treated with atropine or vasopressors.

Patients with cervical or high thoracic injury may be poikilothermic and it is important to monitor and regulate temperature, and avoid prolonged exposure to extremes of temperature.

Immobilization and Handling

A major concern during the initial management of patients with potential cervical spinal injuries is that neurologic function may be impaired as a result of an unstable spine with pathologic motion of the injured vertebrae. With an unstable spine, SCI may occur after the initial traumatic insult, either during transit or early in the course of management, so proper handling during this period is most important. Depending on the urgency of the situation and presence of life-threatening hazards such as a fire, either an extrication device or manual-in line stabilization may be used to get the patients out of the vehicle safely.

Triage for Immobilization

Spinal immobilization is recommended for all trauma patients with a cervical spine injury or SCI, or with a mechanism of injury having the potential to cause cervical spinal injury. Triage of patients with potential spinal injury at the scene by trained and experienced EMS personnel to determine the need for immobilization during transport is recommended (Table 6.3).

The use of spinal immobilization particularly for those patients with a low likelihood of traumatic cervical spinal injury has been questioned. Immobilization of trauma patients is not needed if they meet all the following conditions:

- Awake and alert;
- Not intoxicated;
- Without neck pain or tenderness;
- Do not have an abnormal motor or sensory examination; and
- Do not have any significant associated injury that might detract from their general evaluation

Spinal immobilization in patients with penetrating trauma (gunshot or knife-stab) is not recommended since they rarely have spinal instability and because delayed resuscitation from applying immobilization devices has been associated with increased mortality and morbidity in that group.

Method of Immobilization
A combination of a rigid cervical collar and supportive blocks on a backboard with straps is effective in limiting motion of the cervical spine and is recommended. Attempted spinal immobilization with sandbags and tape is insufficient and is not recommended. Since spinal injuries may involve multiple noncontinuous vertebral levels, complete spinal immobilization has been used in prehospital spinal care to limit motion until injury has been ruled out.

Children younger than 8 years have a relatively large head compared to their torso. To avoid excessive neck flexion, child-specific spine boards with an occiput cut-out or recess should be used, or the torso raised 2 to 3 cm with padding under the shoulders and chest leaving the head at the board level. On the other hand, in the presence of a kyphotic spine, for example, in older adults, a folded sheepskin under the head or neck should be placed to avoid excessive neck extension during immobilization on the board.

Transfer From Immobilization Device
Immobilization devices are effective but can result in morbidity including discomfort, pressure ulcers, and increased risk of aspiration. Spinal immobilization devices should be used to achieve the goals of spinal stability for safe extrication and transport. They should be removed as soon as a definitive evaluation is completed and/or definitive management is initiated.

The patient with a potential spinal injury should be transferred as soon as possible off the backboard onto a firm padded surface while maintaining spinal alignment. Measures to prevent skin breakdown should be initiated if prolonged time on a backboard is anticipated. In cases of confirmed spinal injury or SCI, spine immobilization should be maintained until definitive treatment. An adequate number of personnel should be employed during patient transfers and for repositioning to maintain the alignment of a potentially unstable spine and avoid shearing of the skin. Patients with a potentially unstable spine should be logrolled as a unit when repositioning, turning, or preparing for transfers.

Prehospital Care of Athletes With a Potential Spine Injury

It is recommended that the helmet and shoulder pads should be left in place as the injured athlete is immobilized and transported on a rigid backboard. If needed, only the face mask may be carefully removed to assess and secure the airway. A properly fitted football helmet with shoulder pads holds the head in a position of neutral spinal alignment, and field removal of these devices is not recommended. Immobilizing the player with only the helmet or only the shoulder pads in place has been shown to cause significant misalignment of the cervical spine, and should be avoided.

Simultaneous removal of the helmet and shoulder pads should be done after clinical assessment at the hospital. Removal of football shoulder pads and helmet requires at least four individuals to maintain spinal alignment. All straps and laces that secure the pads to the torso and arms are cut, not unbuckled or unsnapped.

SCI in the Setting of Polytrauma

Injury to the spine must always be considered in the polytrauma patient and managed with the principles outlined above. Injuries such as limb or pelvic fractures, traumatic brain injury, vascular injuries, chest and abdomen injuries can complicate assessment and management of SCI.

When performing an injury survey in a person with trauma, the presence of certain injuries can alert the examiner to the possibility of associated spinal injury. For example, facial trauma may suggest the possibility of an injury to the cervical spine. An abrasion under the strap of a restraint can be associated with injuries to the cervical spine. Lap belt contusions should heighten suspicion for flexion–distraction injuries to the thoracolumbar spine. Calcaneal fractures (e.g., falls, motor vehicle crashes) may be associated with fractures of the thoracolumbar and lumbar spines due to axial loading.

Clues to the presence of SCI in a patient with multi-trauma and impaired consciousness may include response to pain above but not below a level, flaccid areflexic extremities, loss of anal sphincter tone, presence of paradoxical breathing (i.e., chest goes in as abdomen goes out), unexplained bradycardia, inappropriate vasodilation with warm flushed extremities in the presence of hypotension, and priapism (Table 6.4).

Table 6.4

Clues to the Presence of SCI in a Multi-Trauma Setting
Response to pain above but not below a level
Flaccid areflexic extremities
No anal sphincter tone
Paradoxical breathing
Warm flushed extremities in the presence of hypotension
Unexplained bradycardia
Priapism

KNOWLEDGE GAPS AND EMERGING CONCEPTS

Development and refinement of transportation protocols for patients with cervical spine and SCI should be undertaken and could be accomplished with a large prospectively collected data set. The optimal device for immobilization of the cervical spine after traumatic vertebral injury should be studied in a prospective fashion.

SUGGESTED READING

Ahn H, Singh J, Nathens A, et al. Pre-hospital care management of a potential spinal cord injured patient: a systematic review of the literature and evidence-based guidelines. *J Neurotrauma.* 2011;28(8):1341-1361.

Boden BP, Jarvis CG. Spinal injuries in sports. *Neurol Clin.* 2008;26(1):63-78.

U.S. Department of Health and Human Services Program Support Center, Visual Communications Branch. *Model Trauma System Planning and Evaluation.* Rockville, MD: Health Resources and Services Administration; 2006.

U.S. Department of Health and Human Services Program Support Center, Visual Communications Branch. *Resources for Optimal Care of the Injured Patient.* Rockville, MD: Health Resources and Services Administration; 2006.

CHAPTER 7

Imaging of the Injured Spine and Spinal Cord

GENERAL PRINCIPLES

Criteria for Spinal Imaging After Trauma

Spine or spinal cord injury (SCI) should be considered in anyone with an appropriate traumatic mechanism of injury. Concerns about cost and radiation exposure require thoughtful selection of patients who truly are at risk and need imaging after potential trauma. Validated guidelines have been developed to identify low risk criteria when cervical spine imaging is not indicated. These include the National Emergency X-Radiography Utilization Study (NEXUS) criteria that were validated in a large study published in 2000 (Table 7.1), and the Canadian C-Spine Rule (CCR) that was created following evaluation of multiple criteria in a multicenter study of Canadian medical centers and is applicable to alert and stable trauma patients (Table 7.2). A 2003 study comparing CCR and NEXUS criteria found that CCR had somewhat higher sensitivity and specificity.

The American Association of Neurological Surgeons and the Congress of Neurological Surgeons (AANS/CNS) Joint Guidelines Committee *Guidelines for the Management of Acute Cervical Spine and Spinal Cord Injury*, updated in 2013, include the following recommendation regarding radiographic assessment for the awake, asymptomatic patient:

- In the awake, asymptomatic patient who is without neck pain or tenderness, has a normal neurological examination, is without an injury detracting from an accurate evaluation, and who is able to complete a functional range of motion examination; radiographic evaluation of the cervical spine is *not* recommended. Discontinuance of cervical immobilization for these patients is recommended without cervical spinal imaging.

Trauma patients who are symptomatic, that is complain of neck pain, have cervical spine tenderness, have symptoms or signs of a neurological deficit, and those who cannot be assessed for symptoms or signs (those who are unconscious, uncooperative, incoherent, intoxicated, or who have associated traumatic injuries that distract from their assessment) require radiographic study of the cervical spine prior to the discontinuation of cervical spine immobilization.

Table 7.1

National Emergency X-Radiography Utilization Study (NEXUS) Criteria[a]

Absence of midline tenderness

Normal level of alertness and consciousness

No evidence of intoxication

Absence of focal neurological deficit

Absence of painful injury that may detract from an accurate evaluation

[a]Cervical spine imaging is unnecessary if the patient meets all five criteria.

Table 7.2

Canadian C-Spine Rule (CCR) for Alert and Stable Trauma Patients[a]

Criteria or Assessment	Definitions
There are no high-risk factors that mandate radiography	High risk factors include any of the following: - Age 65 yrs or older - Dangerous mechanism of injury (fall from height >3 ft., axial loading injury, high-speed motor vehicle crash, rollover, or ejection, motorized recreational vehicle or bicycle collision) or - Paresthesias in the extremities
There is a low-risk factor that allows safe assessment of neck range of motion	Low risk factor includes any of the following: - Simple rear-end motor vehicle collision, - Sitting up in the Emergency Dept. - Ambulatory at any time following injury - Delayed onset of neck pain, or - Absence of midline cervical spine tenderness
The patient is able to actively rotate their neck	- Can rotate neck 45° to the right and to the left

[a]Cervical spine imaging is unnecessary if patients meet all three criteria.

Similar criteria are applied for thoracic and lumbar spine imaging, though those have been less formally specified or evaluated. Thoracolumbar spine injuries are often multiple and frequently missed in patients with multiple injuries. Indications of imaging include high-risk mechanisms of injury (e.g., gunshot, high energy motor vehicle accident with rollover or ejection, fall from a significant height, or a pedestrian hit by a car), clinical findings of midline back pain and/or tenderness or evidence of neurological deficit consistent with spinal cord or nerve root involvement, or significant associated injuries (e.g., cervical fracture, rib fracture, aortic or hollow viscus injuries).

Recommended Imaging Modalities

Initial Imaging Study
Cervical Spine Imaging
For patients in whom imaging is indicated based on the criteria outlined above (i.e., in the awake, symptomatic patient, and in the obtunded or not evaluable patient):

- High-quality computed tomography (CT) imaging of the cervical spine is recommended as the initial imaging study of choice.
- If high-quality CT imaging is not available, a three-view cervical spine series (anteroposterior [AP], lateral, and odontoid views) is recommended. This should be supplemented with CT (when it becomes available) if necessary to further define areas that are suspicious or not well visualized on the plain cervical x-rays. Oblique or pillar views are not recommended in this setting since they add time, expense, and radiation without providing definitive answers (that may be obtained by CT as needed). If the C7 and T1 vertebrae are obscured by soft tissue of the shoulder in the lateral view, a swimmer's view may be performed or a CT scan obtained if/when available to adequately visualize the cervico-thoracic junction.

While the choice of initial imaging may depend on the available resources, several studies have demonstrated that CT is significantly superior to plain film radiography for the initial evaluation of cervical spinal injuries following trauma and should be the imaging modality of choice. CT scans using thin axial cuts with saggital and coronal reconstruction are highly sensitive in detecting injuries. Technical advances in multi-detector CT (MDCT) have significantly improved the quality of imaging allowing for both high slice resolution and coverage. In addition to CT's superior sensitivity and specificity in fracture detection, authors have reported on other advantages of CT over plain radiography in the acute trauma setting. Average time involved to obtain a cervical CT scan was 11 to 12 minutes, approximately half the time required to obtain a full radiographic series of the cervical spine. A cost-effectiveness analysis for high risk subjects concluded that the higher short-term cost of CT would be offset by the increased sensitivity of CT for fracture detection, the shortened time required for the evaluation, and a decreased need for additional imaging.

Thoracolumbar Spine Imaging
Although less well-defined, similar considerations apply to choice of initial imaging in thoracolumbar spine injuries. In the patient with neurological deficit or strong suspicion of spinal injury it is often advisable to move directly to CT, if it is available. If plain films are obtained as the initial imaging method, those should include AP and lateral views. Oblique views add little in the setting of acute trauma and are typically not indicated.

Imaging Patients With Ankylosing Spondylitis and Stiff Spine
Patients with a stiff spine, for example, with ankylosing spondylitis or diffuse interstitial skeletal hyperostosis (DISH) are at higher than normal risk of getting spine fractures, but fractures may be un-displaced initially, leading to delayed cord damage. CT or magnetic resonance imaging (MRI) should be strongly considered in such cases in the presence of midline tenderness, even if radiographs are negative and even with minor trauma.

Penetrating Injuries
In gunshot injuries, plain films may be useful initially to assess location of bullet fragments. Once level of injury is determined, CT is helpful to evaluate the precise nature of the bone injuries and possible involvement of the spinal canal. After it is clear that there is no contraindication (i.e., metal in the spinal canal), MRI can be used to visualize the spinal cord.

Imaging of the Entire Spine
Spine injury often involves multiple levels, and noncontiguous fractures are estimated to occur in about 16% of cases after identification of a fracture, so survey of the entire spine is indicated if one fracture is detected.

The Role of MRI in Spine and Spinal Cord Trauma
MRI has a very important role in imaging after spine and spinal cord trauma but is more often performed later in the course, though often within hours. It is typically not the initial imaging performed after spine trauma because of several reasons. These include relative insensitivity to detection and detail of fractures (since cortical bone appears dark), challenges with patient monitoring during the procedure, and longer imaging time than CT or plain radiographs.

MRI in Suspected or Known SCI
MRI of known or suspected areas of SCI should be performed. MRI has several advantages over other imaging modalities. It provides excellent visualization of the spinal cord and of soft-tissues, hematomas, ligaments, and intervertebral disks. It characterizes the cause and severity of myelopathy, and may be used to guide surgical intervention.

MRI in SCI Without Radiological Abnormality
SCI may sometimes occur with negative bony imaging of the spinal column (i.e., SCI Without Radiological Abnormality [SCIWORA]). It is important to be alert to that possibility, especially in children and adolescents. MRI will almost always show some abnormalities (e.g., evidence of ligamentous and soft

tissue damage) in the presence of neurological deficits, so MRI of the region of suspected neurological injury is recommended in such instances.

MRI Consideration in Patients With Normal CT and Plain Radiographs

MRI has been recommended by some as an imaging to consider for patients with normal CT and radiographic evaluation if they are either unconscious/obtunded but there is high suspicion of injury, or if they are awake but continue to have neck pain or tenderness. However, evidence for use of MRI in these settings (vs. just continuing cervical immobilization until asymptomatic or until it is discontinued at the discretion of the treating physician), is less compelling and its role not well defined or consistently recommended. Some studies have found that routine MRI screening of both conscious and unconscious patients was only cost-effective in the setting of neurological deficits.

Dynamic flexion/extension radiographs prior to discontinuing immobilization in the awake, symptomatic patient with continued neck pain and tenderness and normal CT and/or plain radiographs are sometimes considered an option, but their utility in the acute setting is limited. Limitations of flexion-extension radiographs in the acute setting include risk of worsening spinal cord compromise if the spine is, in fact, unstable (motion should be stopped immediately as soon as subluxation or abnormal motion is visualized), and a high incidence of muscle spasm or guarding that limits adequate neck movement to assess stability. Their use is not recommended in obtunded patients. Delayed studies, several weeks after trauma and after muscle spasm has subsided, with the patient co-operative and in control of neck motion, are when dynamic flexion-extension radiographs are typically performed, if needed, for evaluating stability of the cervical spine.

With the availability of MRI, there is now little role for myelography in the evaluation of spinal trauma.

Technical Considerations Regarding MRI

MRI utilizes the interaction between the magnetic spin property of hydrogen protons in biological tissue, a static magnetic field provided by an external magnet, and radiofrequency waves introduced by coils. The elicited data is processed by a computer to provide images. Differences between density of hydrogen protons within tissues, and differences in relaxation times of hydrogen protons between different tissues, create different signal intensities and provide tissue contrast in the images. The rate of return to equilibrium of perturbed protons is called the relaxation rate.

Two relaxation rates, T1 and T2, influence the signal intensity of the image. The terms T1 and T2 refer to the time constants for proton relaxation; these may be altered to highlight certain features of tissue structure.

- Structures containing more water, such as cerebrospinal fluid (CSF) and edema have long T1 and T2 relaxation rates, resulting in relatively

lower signal intensity (dark) on T1-weighted images (T1W) and higher
signal intensity (white) on T2-weighted images (T2W).

▦ The spinal cord has intermediate signal intensity in both T1W and
T2W but appears relatively lower in signal intensity on T2W, being surrounded by CSF that is hyperintense.

▦ Structures with little water content (i.e., hydrogen protons) for example,
air or dense cortical bone, appear dark on both T1W and T2W.

▦ Appearance of spinal cord pathology on MRI is discussed below and
summarized in Table 7.3.

Short inversion recovery (STIR) imaging is a technique that suppresses fat to
improve visualization of adjacent edema and other abnormalities on MRI. A fat
saturation pulse can be added to fast spin-echo imaging sequences to achieve
the same result.

CLINICAL CONSIDERATIONS

Imaging Findings

Spinal Cord Pathology on MRI (Table 7.3)
The spectrum of spinal cord-related findings that may be seen on MRI after
SCI is summarized in Table 7.3. Findings include extrinsic cord compression
for example, by bone, disk, and/or epidural hematoma and identification of
intrinsic spinal cord pathology including cord swelling, edema, and hemorrhage in the acute stage. Myelomalacia may be evident in the subacute stage,
and if posttraumatic syrinx or cyst develops in the chronic stage, that will be
evident on MRI. Cord atrophy may be evident after several years postinjury.

Assessing Severity of Injury by MRI
While the precise role of MRI findings in determining prognosis after SCI is
not fully established, certain generalizations have been demonstrated. The
length of spinal cord affected by edema has been shown to relate to the extent
of neurological deficits. Extensive intramedullary hemorrhage has been associated with severe injuries and poor neurological recovery. Hemorrhage location
typically correlates with the neurological level of injury.

Fracture Patterns and Ligamentous Disruption
The primary initial considerations in evaluation of patients with suspected spinal injury include identification of fractures and assessment of spinal stability.
Plain radiographs, CT, and MRI show pathology related to vertebral column
injury, including fractures, abnormalities of alignment, and ligamentous disruption. Ligamentous disruption is seen on MRI as loss of the usual low signal
from the anterior and posterior longitudinal ligaments, with increased signal
on T2-weighted images in the adjacent tissues. Fat-suppression MRI sequences
are useful to distinguish ligament damage from normal fat signal since both
have similar signal characteristics on T2W images. CT is better than MRI for
visualization and characterization of fractures.

Table 7.3
MRI Appearance of Spinal Cord Pathology After Traumatic SCI

Pathology	Appearance
Acute:	
Extrinsic compression of the spinal cord	- Presence and cause of cord compression (i.e., due to bone/bone fragments, extruded disk or disk material, or epidural hematoma) can be determined
Cord swelling	- Smooth enlargement of the cord contour
Edema	- High intensity signal on T2W - Low intensity (intermediate between cord and CSF) signal on T1W
Hemorrhage	- Acute hemorrhage within the spinal cord most reliably seen as a hypointense signal on T2W (often as a lens shaped hypointensity surrounded by rim of hyperintense edema) - The signal intensity of hemorrhage on T1W and T2W varies based on stage of hemoglobin breakdown (transitioning from deoxyhemoglobin in the acute stage to methemoglobin in the next few days and hemosiderin after 2 wks)
Ligamentous injury/tear	- Bright signal on T2W images - Fat-suppression MRI sequences are needed to distinguish ligament damage from normal fat signal since both have similar signal characteristics
Bony fracture	- Bony fragments have decreased signal on T1W images against high signal of marrow fat (though better visualized on CT)
Subacute:	
Myelomalacia	- Ill-defined signal alteration similar to edema (High intensity signal on T2W, and T1W signal intensity intermediate between cord and CSF)
Chronic:	
Posttraumatic cyst or syrinx	- Well-demarcated, isointense with CSF (dark on T1W, white on T2W),
Cord atrophy	- Antero-posterior (AP) dimension of ≤7 mm in cervical cord and ≤6 mm in thoracic cord

Abbreviations: CSF, cerebrospinal fluid; T1W, T1-weighted image; T2W, T2-weighted image.

Fracture patterns based on the primary mechanism/force of injury, and related imaging findings are summarized in Table 7.4.

Findings on Plain Radiographs

Though CT has supplanted plain radiographs as the initial imaging of choice (as mentioned above), a three-view cervical spine series (AP, lateral, and odontoid views) is still often done and is recommended in settings where high-quality CT imaging is not available. Most anatomic features of the spine are identifiable on plain radiographs including vertebral bodies, facet joints, disk spaces, pedicles, laminae, transverse processes and spinous processes.

(text continues on page 50)

Table 7.4

Spinal Injuries and Imaging Findings Based on Mechanism of Injury

Primary Mechanical Force (Typical Mechanisms)	Spinal Injury
Flexion injury (e.g., diving into shallow water, being thrown off a motorcycle)	Bilateral facet dislocation - *Inferior articular facets either come to rest on top of superior facet of the vertebra below ("perched facets") or leapfrog over them ("locked facets")* - *A 50% shift of one vertebral body over another suggests bilateral facet dislocation* - *Implies disruption of anterior longitudinal ligament, posterior longitudinal ligament, and facet capsules* Anterior wedge fracture - *Often stable* - *>50% vertebral body compression is associated with posterior ligamentous injury and flexion instability* Anterior subluxation Flexion teardrop fracture - *Involves the anterior inferior corner of vertebral body, most often C5* - *Unstable injury indicative of severe ligamentous disruption and associated with severe SCI due to retropulsion of the entire posterior fragment of the vertebral body into spinal canal* Clay-shoveler's fracture - *Avulsion fracture of spinous process in the lower cervical spine, stable*
Extension injury (e.g., an elderly person sustaining a fall to the floor, head hitting the windshield in a car accident)	Hyperextension dislocation/hyperextension fracture-dislocation - *Cord is pinched between the dislocated vertebral body and the buckled ligamentum flavum and lamina* - *Variable neurological damage, may result in central cord syndrome* Traumatic spondylolisthesis (Hangman's fracture) - *Bilateral fractures of the pars interarticularis of C2 (may extend obliquely into body of C2)* - *Variable cord damage due to wide canal diameter at this level* Laminar fractures (without facet dislocation) Widening of the anterior disk space

(continued)

Primary Mechanical Force (Typical Mechanisms)	Spinal Injury
	Extension teardrop fracture
	- *Differentiated from flexion teardrop fracture by involving upper (usually C2) rather than lower cervical vertebra, and location at the superior aspect of the vertebral body*
Flexion-rotation injury (e.g., rollover car accident)	Unilateral facet dislocation
	- *Lateral radiograph shows abrupt change from the usual lateral appearance below the injury to an appearance of oblique projection above the dislocation, often stable with incomplete SCI or nerve root injury*
Axial compression (e.g., falling from a height on to feet, direct blow to top of the head)	Jefferson fracture
	- *Burst fracture of C1 vertebra with disruption of anterior and posterior arches*
	- *Usually no neurodeficit or instability if transverse ligament remains intact. Greater than or equal to 7 mm transverse separation of lateral masses of C1 on C2 in open mouth view or CT suggests disrupted transverse ligament which can be visualized on MRI*
	Burst fracture
	- *Sagittally oriented fracture line through vertebral body on axial CT*
	- *In the thoracolumbar spine, T12-L1 fractures are the commonest; in the subaxial C-spine C5 is commonest*
	- *Neurological deficit is variable depending on displacement of fragments into spinal canal*
Lateral flexion (e.g., car accident, fall)	Uncinate process fracture
Flexion-distraction (e.g., car accident while wearing lap seatbelt vs. a three-point seatbelt with shoulder harness)	Chance or Chance-equivalent fracture
	- *Horizontal fracture through the vertebral body that extends through pedicles and supporting ligaments*
	- *Typically affects L1 or L2 vertebra, usually unstable*
	- *May have significant associated intraabdominal injury*
Diverse injury mechanisms	Odontoid fracture
	- *Three types: involve tip (type I) or base (type II) of the odontoid process, or extend into the body of C2 (type III)*
	- *Of these, type II is most unstable and most prone to nonunion*
	Atlanto-axial instability
	- *The ADI, measured from the posterior arch of C1 to anterior margin of the odontoid should not exceed 3 mm in adults and 5 mm in children*

(continued)

Table 7.4

Spinal Injuries and Imaging Findings Based on Mechanism of Injury (*continued*)

Primary Mechanical Force (Typical Mechanisms)	Spinal Injury
	Cranio-cervical junction injury - *Occipital condyle fracture* - *Atlanto-occipital dislocation (often fatal)*

Table 7.5

Key Points in Evaluating Lateral View Plain Radiographs of the Cervical Spine for Spinal Injury

All seven cervical vertebral bodies are seen

Alignment of four imaginary lines
    Anterior spinal line (along the anterior aspect of the vertebral body)
    Posterior spinal line (along the posterior aspect of the vertebral body)
    Spinolaminar line (along the junction of the lamina and spinous processes)
    Spinous process line (joining tips of the spinous processes)

Predental space or atlanto-dens interval (ADI)

Each vertebra examined for fractures

Intervertebral angulation

Fanning of spinous processes (ruptured inter-spinous ligament, suggests flexion injury)

Prevertebral soft tissue (normally <5 mm at C3)

Findings suggestive of cervical spine instability
- ADI >3 mm in adults and >5 mm in children
- Anterior or posterior translation of vertebral bodies >3.5 mm
- Angulation between adjacent vertebrae 11° more than contiguous cervical vertebrae
- Flexion tear-drop fracture (see Table 7.4)

Table 7.5 summarizes key features to look for in evaluation of the lateral view in evaluation of cervical trauma. Ligamentous damage is implied, though not directly visualized, on plain radiographs. In the upper cervical spine, an atlanto-dens interval (ADI) greater than 3 mm in adults and greater than 5 mm in children suggests atlanto-axial instability due to ligamentous insufficiency or disruption. In the subaxial cervical spine, anterior or posterior translation of vertebral bodies greater than 3.5 mm implies instability. A 50% shift of one vertebral body over another is suggestive of bilateral facet dislocation. Angulation between two adjacent vertebrae of 11° more than contiguous cervical vertebrae also suggests instability. The open-mouth view facilitates visualization of the atlanto-axial (C1-2) articulation and provides additional views to examine the occipital condyles, lateral masses of C1 and C2, and the dens.

Thoracolumbar spine injury and stability can be assessed by the Denis' Three-Column Spine Concept (Table 7.6). Findings that suggest instability of

Table 7.6

Denis' Three-Column Spine Concept to Assess Stability of the Thoracolumbar (T-L) Spine[a]

The spine is divided into three columns:
- *Anterior column:* anterior longitudinal ligament, anterior half of the vertebral body, and anterior half of the intervertebral disk
- *Middle column:* posterior half of the vertebral body, posterior half of the intervertebral disk, posterior longitudinal ligament
- *Posterior column:* pedicles, facets, ligamentum flavum, lamina, spinous processes, interspinous and supraspinous ligaments

Thoracolumbar injuries that only involve one column are stable; those involving two or three columns are unstable. The middle column is the most critical for thoracolumbar stability

[a]Though originally described for T-L injuries, it is also applied to cervical spine injuries (as such or adapted to a two-column model combining anterior & middle columns into one).

the thoraco-lumbar spine include: displacement of the vertebral body >2mm indicating possible ligamentous disruption, widening of the interspinous space, widening of the facet joints, disruption of the posterior vertebral body line, or loss of vertebral body height by >50%.

Vascular Injuries
CT angiography can demonstrate carotid and vertebral injury. In some institutions, it has become part of imaging protocol if a cervical spine fracture is evident by noncontrast CT. Magnetic resonance angiography (MRA) is another option.

Practice Pearls

It is important to make sure that the entire cervical spine is visible on imaging including the junction with the thoracic spine and skull. Example in plain radiographs, soft tissue of the shoulders may obscure the C7-T1 junction on lateral radiographs and may be missed unless a swimmer's view or CT is done to view the obscured area.

KNOWLEDGE GAPS AND EMERGING CONCEPTS

The issue of discontinuing cervical spinal immobilization after blunt trauma remains an area of controversy in both the symptomatic patient with negative initial imaging, and in the obtunded or unevaluable patient with normal cervical spinal imaging. An appropriately designed and conducted prospective multicenter trial has the potential to define the optimum methodology to accurately exclude a significant cervical spinal injury in these patients prior to discontinuing immobilization. While limited and conflicting medical evidence suggests that MRI is recommended to further study these patients, this has yet to be definitely proven. The question of whether there is any role for dynamic imaging in this setting should be determined.

New and evolving techniques have potential in improving assessment of SCI in the future. Diffusion tensor imaging may demonstrate more extensive axonal injury than otherwise evident. Magnetic resonance (MR) spectroscopy has potential for studying chemical changes reflective of ischemia of the spinal cord. Functional MRI may have a role in identifying residual neurological pathways in injuries that otherwise seem complete (e.g., by demonstrating brain activation in response to anorectal stimulation).

SUGGESTED READING

Daffner RH, Deeb ZL, Goldberg AL, Kandabarow A, Rothfus WE. The radiologic assessment of post-traumatic vertebral stability. Skeletal Radiol. 1990;19(2):103-108.

Daffner RH, Weissman BN, Wippold FJ II, et al. *ACR Appropriateness Criteria® suspected spine trauma.* [Online publication.] Reston, VA: American College of Radiology (ACR); 2012.

Fehlings MG, Rao SC, Tator CH, et al. The optimal radiologic method for assessing spinal canal compromise and cord compression in patients with cervical spinal cord injury. Part II: Results of a multicenter study. Spine (Phila Pa 1976). 1999 Mar 15;24(6):605-613.

Hadley MN, Walters BC. Introduction to the guidelines for the management of acute cervical spine and spinal cord injuries. *Neurosurgery.* 2013;72(Suppl 2):5-16.

Lammertse D, Dungan D, Dreisbach J, et al. Neuroimaging in traumatic spinal cord injury: an evidence-based review for clinical practice and research. *J Spinal Cord Med.* 2007;30(3):205-214.

Quencer RM, Bunge RP. The injured spinal cord: imaging, histopathologic clinical correlates, and basic science approaches to enhancing neural function after spinal cord injury. Spine (Phila Pa 1976). 1996 Sep 15;21(18):2064-2066.

Stiell IG, Clement CM, McKnight RD, et al. The Canadian C-spine rule versus the NEXUS low-risk criteria in patients with trauma. *N Engl J Med.* 2003;349:2510-2518.

CHAPTER 8

Early Hospital Care Following SCI: Medical, Surgical, and Rehabilitation

GENERAL PRINCIPLES

The basic principles regarding attention to airway, breathing, and circulation and spinal protection, including proper handling and immobilization, that are applied during prehospital care (as described in Chapter 6) carry over to emergency department and early hospital management of traumatic spinal cord injury (SCI).

In addition to these aspects, early hospital care includes diagnostic assessments for definitive care and surgical decision making, assessment and management of associated injuries, surgical interventions as/when indicated, assessment of prognosis, nutritional support, assessment and management of pain, and prevention and management of complications such as skin breakdown, venous thromboembolism (VTE), respiratory, genitourinary, and gastrointestinal issues. It is important to initiate early rehabilitation interventions and measures to address psychosocial and family issues and to maintain these throughout the acute care stay.

Published guidelines on various aspects of early management following acute SCI are available and have been used to inform this chapter. These include the Consortium for Spinal Cord Medicine clinical practice guidelines on *Early Acute Management in Adults with Spinal Cord Injury* and the American Association of Neurological Surgeons/Central Nervous System (AANS/CNS) *Guidelines for Management of Acute Cervical Spine and Spinal Cord Injury*, which were updated in 2013.

CLINICAL CONSIDERATIONS

Acute Cardiopulmonary Monitoring and Management

Patients with an acute SCI, especially those with complete or severe cervical SCI, should be managed in an intensive care unit or similarly monitored setting, with use of cardiac, hemodynamic, and respiratory monitoring devices to detect cardiovascular dysfunction and respiratory insufficiency. These patients frequently develop hypotension, hypoxemia, pulmonary dysfunction, thermoregulatory abnormalities, and cardiovascular instability, even after initial stable cardiac and pulmonary function.

Prevention and treatment of hypotension as soon as possible is recommended, with efforts to maintain mean arterial blood pressure (MAP) greater than or equal to 85 mmHg for the first 7 days following an acute SCI (although ideal MAP to optimize outcomes is not definitively known). Bradycardia is common in the acute phase in people with complete cervical SCI; symptomatic bradycardia needs monitoring and treatment (see Chapter 33A).

Patients should be monitored closely for respiratory failure in the first few days following SCI. Baseline respiratory parameters, including vital capacity, forced expiratory volume in 1 second (FEV1), and arterial blood gases, should be obtained when patients are first evaluated and at intervals until stable. Mechanical ventilation should be considered for patients with tetraplegia (see Chapter 32 and 32B). Measures to prevent ventilator-associated pneumonia in patients with acute SCI who require mechanical ventilation for respiratory failure are of critical importance.

Retained secretions due to expiratory muscle weakness should be treated with manually assisted coughing ("quad coughing"), pulmonary hygiene, mechanical insufflation-exsufflation, or similar expiratory aids in addition to suctioning (see Chapter 32). Tracheal suctioning alone is often insufficient for secretion mobilization; suction catheters often don't adequately reach into the left main bronchus due to bronchial anatomy.

Neuroprotection

For several years over the past two decades, following publication of positive studies in the 1990's, methylprednisolone, administered intravenously as a 30mg/kg bolus within 8 hours of injury and continued at a rate of 5.4 mg/kg/hr for 24 to 48 hours by intravenous infusion, was in relatively widespread clinical use. While it still remains an option in individual cases, that research has been subject of much debate, and several professional organizations have increasingly recommended against its use, citing lack of consistent or compelling clinical evidence and demonstrated evidence of significant harmful side-effects (e.g., increased incidence of pneumonia, sepsis, and gastrointestinal hemorrhage).

The Consortium for Spinal Cord Medicine clinical practice guidelines on *Early Acute Management in Adults with Spinal Cord Injury* state that no clinical evidence exists to definitively recommend the use of any neuroprotective pharmacologic agent, including steroids, in the treatment of acute SCI to improve functional recovery. The 2013 AANS/CNS *Guidelines for Management of Acute*

Cervical Spine and Spinal Cord Injury explicitly recommend against administration of methylprednisolone for the treatment of SCI.

Diagnostic Assessments for Definitive Care

Clinical Neurological Assessment
A baseline neurological assessment should be completed on any patient with suspected spinal injury or SCI to document the presence of SCI. If neurologic deficits are consistent with SCI, a neurological level and the completeness of injury is determined in accordance with the International Standards for Neurological Classification of SCI (ISNCSCI) as discussed in Chapter 10. Serial examinations should be performed as indicated to detect neurological deterioration or improvement.

After the first 48–72 hours, the clinical neurological assessment as described by the ISNCSCI can also be used to determine the preliminary prognosis for neurological recovery.

Diagnostic Imaging
Radiographic evaluation of patients following SCI is central to diagnostic assessment for definitive care and surgical decision making, as detailed in Chapter 7.

Associated Injuries

A comprehensive tertiary trauma survey to identify associated injuries should be completed on anyone with suspected or confirmed SCI.

Patients with SCI have a high incidence of extra-spinal fractures. Most common sites of extra-spinal fractures associated with SCI include chest, lower extremity, upper extremity, head, and pelvis. Loss of sensation due to SCI and/or altered sensorium due to associated traumatic brain injury (TBI) increases the likelihood of missed fractures in this setting. Early stabilization of extra-spinal fractures is indicated.

Individuals with SCI, especially those with high cervical injury, have a high incidence of TBI. In addition to the Glasgow Coma Scale assessed in the acute setting, evaluation of posttraumatic amnesia with a reliable test such as the Galveston Orientation and Amnesia Test (GOAT) is indicated, keeping in mind that, in addition to TBI, medications or hypoxia could influence test results in the acute setting. Additional discussion about the dual diagnosis of TBI and SCI is included in Chapter 41.

Chest and abdominal injuries are common especially in those with thoracolumbar spinal injuries. Clinical examination may not be reliable in the setting of impaired sensorium or sensory loss, and additional diagnostic measures are needed, for example, diagnostic ultrasound and/or computerized tomography (CT) scan of the abdomen.

Patients with cervical SCI may have concomitant injury to the carotid or vertebral circulation and screening with CT or magnetic resonance (MR) angiography should be considered as part of evaluation of cervical SCI.

Surgical Decision Making and Intervention

Surgical intervention involves reducing or realigning the spinal elements, decompressing compromised neural tissue, and/or stabilizing the spine.

Initial Closed Reduction

Closed or open reduction should be performed as soon as permissible on patients with bilateral cervical facet dislocation, especially in the setting of an incomplete SCI. If traction reduction is not preferred or possible, open reduction should be performed. Decompression of the spinal cord and restoration of the spinal canal is the goal.

Closed reduction of fracture/dislocation injuries of the cervical spine by traction-reduction appears to be generally safe and effective for the reduction of acute traumatic spinal deformity in alert patients, if carried out by trained personnel. Closed traction is safer than manipulation under anesthesia. The procedure is generally performed using Gardner-Wells tongs or Halo rings (which are now also available in MRI-compatible versions). Patients must be examined after each increase in added weight. Traction typically begins with small weight that is gradually increased. There is a small risk of neurological deterioration, which is usually transient but could very rarely be permanent. Causes of neurological deterioration include inadequate immobilization, unrecognized rostral injuries, over-distraction, or loss of reduction. Patients who fail attempted closed reduction of cervical fracture injuries have a higher incidence of anatomic obstacles to reduction, including facet fractures and disk herniation, and should undergo more detailed radiographic study before attempts at open reduction. Tong or halo traction is avoided in the presence of skull fractures.

Role and Timing of Surgery

The role that timing of surgical intervention plays in SCI management remains a controversial topic although there is accumulating evidence to suggest that early surgical decompression is safe and is possibly associated with better neurological outcomes. A recent prospective multicenter study comparing early (designated as within 24 hours of injury) versus delayed decompression for traumatic cervical SCI (Surgical Timing in Acute Spinal Cord Injury Study— STASCIS) concluded that decompression prior to 24 hours after SCI can be performed safely and is associated with improved neurologic outcome. However, there were inherent limitations of the cohort study design used in the STASCIS study. For example, the early surgery group included patients with a slightly lower mean age and contained a significantly greater proportion of patients with a more severe degree of initial injury as compared to the late group. Therefore, further study is necessary to more accurately define which patients with SCI benefit the most from early surgical intervention.

Choice of Surgical Approach
The decision to proceed with surgery and the chosen surgical approach should be determined on a case by case basis with full consideration of surgical benefits versus risks and the specific treatment goals. The choice of surgical intervention is often a function of severity of injury, level of injury, mechanism of injury, and the extent of compression. In patients with complete SCI, the primary goal of surgery is spinal stabilization, which reduces pain and facilitates participation in rehabilitation. For incomplete SCI, especially in the setting of deteriorating neurological function, surgery may also improve neurological recovery, though conclusive literature regarding that is relatively limited.

Table 8.1 outlines key aspects of management approach to specific cervical spine fractures. While there are no universally accepted treatment algorithms, surgical indications for thoraco-lumbar injuries include >50% loss of vertebral height with posterior ligamentous disruption or a three-column injury (Chapter 7). Decompression with laminectomy alone can lead to kyphotic deformity and further neurological deterioration, and is not recommended in the setting of SCI.

Table 8.1

Key Aspects of Management and Surgical Considerations in Specific Cervical Spine Injuries[a]	
Cervical Spine Injury	**Management Approach**
Occipital Condylar Fractures (OCF)	External cervical immobilization is recommended for all types of occipital condyle fractures. More rigid external immobilization in a halo vest device should be considered for bilateral OCF. Halo vest immobilization or occipitocervical stabilization and fusion are recommended for injuries with associated atlanto-occipital ligamentous injury or evidence of instability
Atlanto-Occipital Dislocation (AOD)	AOD is often fatal. If patients survive the injury, treatment with internal fixation and fusion is recommended. Traction is not recommended in management of patients with AOD, since it is associated with a high risk of neurological deterioration
Atlas Fractures	Treatment is based on specific fracture type and integrity of the transverse ligament. For an isolated fracture of the atlas with an intact transverse atlantal ligament, cervical immobilization is recommended. For fractures of the atlas with disruption of the transverse atlantal ligament, either cervical immobilization alone or surgical fixation and fusion is recommended.

(continued)

Table 8.1

Key Aspects of Management and Surgical Considerations in Specific Cervical Spine Injuries[a] (*continued*)

Cervical Spine Injury	Management Approach
Axis Fractures: Odontoid	Consideration of surgical stabilization and fusion for type II odontoid fractures in patients ≥50 yrs of age is recommended (since risk of nonunion is significantly greater than in younger patients). Initial management of nondisplaced odontoid fractures with external cervical immobilization is recommended, recognizing that a decreased rate of union (healing) has been reported with type II odontoid fractures. Surgical stabilization and fusion of type II and type III odontoid fractures with dens displacement ≥5 mm, comminuted odontoid fracture, and/or inability to achieve or maintain fracture alignment with external immobilization are recommended
Axis Fractures: Hangman	The initial management of Hangman fractures has typically been nonsurgical, and high success rates have been reported. External immobilization is recommended. Surgery is recommended if there is angulation or instability.
Axis Fractures: Body	In the presence of comminuted fracture of the axis body, evaluation for vertebral artery injury is recommended.
Atlas/Axis Combination Fractures	Treatment is based on characteristics of axis fracture. External immobilization of most C1-C2 combination fractures is recommended. C1-type II odontoid combination fractures with an atlanto-dental ratio of ≥5 mm and C1-Hangman combination fractures with C2-C3 angulation of ≥11° should be considered for surgical stabilization and fusion.
Subaxial Cervical Spine Injuries	Closed or open reduction of subaxial cervical fractures or dislocations is recommended. Decompression of the neural elements and the restoration of sufficient spinal stability to allow early mobilization and rehabilitation remain basic treatment tenets. Treatment must be individualized on the basis of the specific characteristics of each particular injury. Stable immobilization by either internal fixation or external immobilization to allow for early patient mobilization and rehabilitation is recommended. If surgical treatment is considered, both anterior or posterior fixation and fusion are acceptable as long as the goals of treatment can be accomplished.
Spinal Cord Injury Without Radiographic Abnormality (SCIWORA)	External immobilization of the spinal segment of injury is recommended for up to 12 weeks. Early discontinuation of external immobilization is recommended for patients who become asymptomatic and in whom spinal stability is confirmed with flexion and extension radiographs.

[a]See Chapter 7 and Table 7.4 for imaging findings that influence surgical decision making.

Spinal Orthoses

Details of spinal orthoses, including indications and choice of orthoses after acute SCI and/or postoperatively, are discussed in Chapter 9

Prevention and Management of Secondary Complications

Pain
Pain may be under-recognized and undertreated in the acute setting. Patients with SCI may experience distressing pain immediately or very soon after injury, including both at-level and below-level neuropathic pain, and at-level musculoskeletal pain. Allodynia, that is, hypersensitivity to touch, is often seen in cervical SCI, especially with incomplete injuries, although it typically diminishes over weeks or months. Taking care to avoid contact with the oversensitive region and minimizing evoked pain through thoughtful patient handling is helpful. Pharmacological management of the pain (see Chapter 38C) may be needed, balanced with risk of side effects such as over-sedation or respiratory depression.

Skin Protection
See Chapter 37 for details regarding skin protection and prevention of pressure ulcers. At-risk areas such as bony prominences should be assessed for skin breakdown frequently. Patients should be placed on a pressure reduction mattress or a mattress overlay, as appropriate. A pressure reducing cushion should be used when the patient is mobilized out of bed to a sitting position. Meticulous skin care is crucial and includes repositioning to provide pressure relief or turn at least every 2 hours while maintaining spinal precautions, keeping the area under the patient clean and dry, and inspecting the skin under pressure garments and splints.

Venous Thromboembolism (VTE)
Mechanical and chemical prophylaxis should be started early. There is a high incidence of VTE associated with substantial morbidity and mortality in untreated patients after acute SCI and prophylactic treatment has been shown to be effective.

Pathophysiology and Risk of VTE after SCI
Contributing factors to pathophysiology of VTE in acute SCI include venous stasis due to muscle paralysis and immobility, hypercoagulability due to transient clotting factor and platelet aggregation abnormalities, and intimal injury (Virchow's triad). Motor complete SCI, older age, smoking, obesity, associated injuries such as lower limb fracture, prior history of thromboembolism coexisting coagulopathies, and comorbidities such as heart failure or cancer further increase VTE risk.

Diagnosis of VTE

Clinical findings may include unilateral leg edema, increased calf diameter, localized tenderness, and/or low grade fever, although deep venous thrombosis (DVT) may be present without any of these findings. Sudden onset of shortness of breath, hypotension, tachycardia, pleuritic chest pain, or unexplained hypoxia in individuals with acute SCI warrant prompt consideration of pulmonary embolism (PE). Diagnostic testing or screening for DVT typically includes duplex ultrasound. Diagnostic tests for PE include ventilation-perfusion scan, electrocardiogram (characterized by a right ventricular strain pattern), and spiral CT of the lungs. Testing for D-dimer levels has poor specificity, although good negative predictive value for VTE. Venogram and pulmonary angiogram are gold standards but are only done if clinical suspicion remains strong but other tests are indeterminate or negative.

Prophylaxis of VTE

Mechanical compression: Mechanical compression devices should be applied early after injury. If trauma to the lower extremities prevents the application of stockings or devices, use of a foot pump may be considered. If initiation of VTE prophylaxis is delayed by more than 3 days, a duplex scan of the leg may be indicated to exclude deep vein thrombosis prior to placing compression devices.

Chemical prophylaxis: Low molecular weight heparin (LMWH), should be started in all patients, as soon as feasible, when primary hemostasis becomes evident. Low dose heparin therapy alone is not recommended as a prophylactic treatment strategy and oral anticoagulation alone is not recommended for prophylaxis. Intracranial bleeding, spinal hematoma, or hemothorax are contraindications to the initial administration of anticoagulants, but anticoagulants may be appropriate when bleeding has stabilized. Chemical prophylaxis is often held 1 day before and 1 day following surgical intervention to minimize bleeding risk. Prophylactic treatment should be continued for 8 to 12 weeks after SCI in patients without other major risk factors for VTE, since risk decreases substantially after that time. Prophylactic treatment may be discontinued earlier in patients with useful motor function in the lower extremities, as these patients appear to be at less risk for VTE.

Vena cava filters: Vena cava filters are not recommended as a routine prophylactic measure, but are recommended for select patients who fail anticoagulation or who are not candidates for anticoagulation and/or mechanical devices. An inferior vena cava filter (IVC) should be considered with active bleeding only if it is anticipated to persist for more than 72 hours and anticoagulants should be started as soon as feasible once bleeding has stabilized. IVC filters can be associated with complications such as distal migration, intra-peritoneal erosion, and symptomatic IVC occlusion. It has been suggested that loss of abdominal muscle tone and use of the "quad cough" maneuver may increase risk of IVC complications in people with SCI.

Early mobilization: Early mobilization and passive exercise should be initiated as soon as the patient is medically and surgically stable in coordination with other prophylactic measures. With documented DVT, mobilization of the involved lower extremity should be withheld for 48 hours till appropriate medical therapy is implemented.

Reinstitution of prophylactic measures should be considered in people with SCI if they are immobilized with bed rest for a long time, readmitted for medical illnesses or altered medical conditions, or undergo surgical procedures.

Treatment of VTE
In patients with established VTE anticoagulant treatment should be promptly initiated either with LMWH (usually preferred due to safety and comparable effectiveness as unfractionated heparin) or unfractionated heparin. Warfarin is started at an initial dosage of 5-10 mg/day at the same time, with overlap in heparin and warfarin treatment for 4-5 days after which heparin is discontinued. Warfarin dosage is adjusted with frequent testing of the International Normalized Ratio (INR) to maintain the INR in the recommended therapeutic range of 2 to 3. Although optimal duration of treatment is not certain, anticoagulation is often continued for 3 to 6 months for a known DVT and 6 months for established PE.

Genitourinary Management
Urinary retention is common in the immediate aftermath of SCI. An indwelling urinary catheter should be placed as part of the initial patient assessment unless contraindicated, and left in place at least until the patient is hemodynamically stable and strict attention to fluid status is no longer needed. If contraindicated, for example due to urethral injury (suspected in those with pelvic fractures, hematuria, blood at the meatus, or high-riding prostate on rectal exam), urgent urological consultation should be sought and emergent suprapubic drainage initiated.

Priapism is usually self-limited in acute SCI and does not require treatment. Urethral catheter can still be place in the presence of priapism secondary to acute SCI.

Gastrointestinal and Bowel Management
Stress Ulcer Prophylaxis
Patients with acute SCI are at high risk of bleeding from stress ulcers in the first 4 weeks, and stress ulcer prophylaxis should be initiated. Proton pump inhibitors (PPI) or histamine H2-receptor antagonists are used for prophylaxis. While these agents have been shown to be safe and effective, they should not be continue indiscriminately and should be stopped after 4 weeks since the risk greatly diminishes, unless there are other risk factors. Prolonged PPI use has been associated with increased *Clostridium difficile* infection.

Swallowing
Patients with cervical SCI, halo fixation, cervical spine surgery (especially anterior discectomy and fusion), prolonged intubation, tracheotomy, or concomitant TBI, are at increased risk of dysphagia after acute SCI, and swallowing function should be evaluated prior to oral feeding in these patients. If a feeding tube must be placed for long-term enteral feeding, risk of aspiration may be lower with a jejunostomy tube than a gastrostomy tube.

Bowel Management
Reduced gut motility and even ileus are common after acute SCI. Bowel distention and inadequate evacuation can lead to nausea and vomiting, high gastric residuals, anorexia, decreased respiratory excursion. A bowel program should be initiated early during hospitalization to ensure regular scheduled evacuations. In the early stages, patients are often areflexic and have a lower motor neuron bowel; return of bulbocavernosus reflex often indicates concomitant return of reflex bowel function in those with supra-sacral injuries and the bowel program should be modified accordingly (See Chapter 36A).

Nutrition

Appropriate nutritional support is important in the acute phase after SCI. Severely injured patients are at risk for prolonged nitrogen losses and advanced malnutrition within 2 to 3 weeks following injury with resultant increased susceptibility for infection, impaired wound healing, and difficulty weaning from mechanical ventilation. These factors added to the inherent immobility, denervation, and muscle atrophy associated with SCI provide the rationale for targeted nutritional support of spinal cord injured patients following trauma.

The actual caloric needs are lower after SCI than predicted by conventional assessment, although these differences are less pronounced in the acute phase. Equation estimates of energy expenditure in SCI are inaccurate, and the use of indirect calorimetry (with a metabolic cart) has been recommended as the technique to assess energy expenditure in both the acute and chronic settings among patients with SCI (Chapter 39A). Protein catabolism does occur after acute, severe SCI, and marked losses in lean body mass due to muscle atrophy result in huge nitrogen losses, prolonged negative nitrogen balance, and rapid weight loss.

Nutritional support of patients with SCI and early enteral nutrition to meet caloric and nitrogen needs is safe and may reduce the deleterious effects of the catabolic, nitrogen wasting process that occurs after acute SCI. Enteral nutrition rather than parenteral nutrition is recommended whenever feasible. A standard, polymeric enteral formula can be initiated, using the semi-recumbent position when possible to prevent aspiration (balancing with the need to prevent shear and risk of skin breakdown which is increased in the semi-recumbent position). It has been suggested that high-fat/low-carbohydrate enteral nutrition has favorable physiologic effects on CO_2 production and respiratory quotient, rendering this type of nutrition potentially useful in patients with impaired ventilatory reserve, but there are no definitive recommendations regarding that due to lack of conclusive evidence about the outcomes on duration of ventilation and weaning success. Hyperglycemia has been associated with worse medical outcomes in critically ill and/or mechanically ventilated patients, so care should be taken to maintain normoglycemia.

Rehabilitation Interventions in the Acute Stage

Rehabilitation specialists should be involved early in the management of persons with SCI, immediately following injury during the acute hospitalization phase. They can prescribe interventions that will assist in recovery, including preventive measures against potential secondary complications, and facilitate discharge to the next level of care.

Rehabilitation consultation and interventions in an acute setting should address range of motion (to prevent painful and functionally limiting contractures, for example, of the heel cords, shoulders, elbows, and hip flexors), positioning, early mobilization following medical and spinal stability, bowel and bladder management programs, clearance of respiratory secretions, prevention of pressure ulcers, input about functional implications of options for surgery and spinal orthosis, and education of the patient and family. Orthostatic hypotension may need to be addressed as patients start assuming the upright position (see Chapter 33B). Assessment and management of swallowing, communication, and cognitive deficits due to concomitant TBI need to be addressed.

Psychosocial Concerns and Issues in the Acute Setting

Assessment
Mental health concerns and possible risk for psychosocial problems should be addressed after admission and throughout acute care stay. Particular attention should be paid to current or past history of major depression, acute stress disorder/posttraumatic stress disorder (PTSD), or substance intoxication and withdrawal, availability or lack of a social support network, cognitive functioning and learning style, preferences in coping style, and concurrent life stressors.

Requests to Withdraw Life-Sustaining Treatment or Suicidal Ideation
Suicidal ideation, requests for assisted suicide, treatment refusals, and requests for withdrawal of treatment should be taken very seriously. Although suicidal ideation and completed suicide are more prevalent among people with SCI than the general population, these are still infrequent occurrences and should not be considered a normal response to SCI. In the case of high tetraplegia, and there is evidence to suggest that acute medical and emergency personnel may significantly underestimate the potential quality of life for these patients. Therefore, any decision to withdraw life support soon after SCI needs to be scrutinized carefully.

An honest and sincere response, acknowledging the patient's suffering, is appropriate if such requests are expressed. An ongoing dialogue about the recovery process and the likelihood of returning to a meaningful life after SCI should be maintained. A number of factors must be balanced when considering an overt refusal or a request for withdrawal of treatment. This includes balancing the patient's right to self-determination and the health care provider's duty to benefit the patient and prevent harm (see Chapter 48). Underlying depression should be assessed and treated. The patient's decision-making capacity should be assessed. For competent patients who express an explicit unwavering request to withdraw life-sustaining treatment such as a ventilator, negotiating a time-limited trial (TLT) has been suggested as an option. This is a mutual agreement between the physician/treatment team and the patient to revisit goals of treatment and the potential for treatment cessation after a predefined period. It allows opportunity for patient reflection, adaptation to life with SCI, palliation of symptoms and suffering, time to build trust, goal setting, evaluation of trends and progress, recruitment of supportive resources, and rehabilitation and functional improvement. The institution's ethics committee should be consulted when appropriate, and legal counsel consult may be needed if conflict continues or if there is any uncertainty regarding the patient's request (See Chapter 48).

Coping Strategies
Effective coping strategies, health promotion behaviors, and independence can be fostered through a variety of interventions including use of assistive devices. Breaking the news about SCI, and answering questions and providing information about prognosis can be challenging but very important communication (see Chapter 48). It is often best to provide medical and prognostic information matter-of-factly, yet at the same time leave room for hope. Expressions of hope should be respected and direct confrontations of denial concerning probable implications of the injury should be avoided. Feelings of hope have been shown to assist with a future orientation and help patients move forward through the recovery process. Over time, the hope becomes more realistic, though the time frame differs among individuals. Helping patients and family identify effective coping strategies that have aided them in the past is useful. Efforts to develop a partnership of patient, family, and health care team help promote involvement in the treatment plan and optimize patient outcomes.

KNOWLEDGE GAPS AND EMERGING CONCEPTS

While significant progress is continuing to be made in the early, acute, management of people with SCI, there are many areas of controversy and lack of consistent evidence for which further systemic study is needed.

For example, the issue of whether or not blood pressure augmentation has an impact on outcome following SCI is important and deserves to be further investigated. If augmentation of MAP is determined to be of potential benefit, the most appropriate threshold levels of MAP and the length of augmentation therapy need further definition. Further study regarding timing of surgery to examine efficacy within specific SCI subgroups, and evaluating for synergistic effects of decompression with other SCI therapies, would be helpful in developing best practice guidelines.

SUGGESTED READING

Consortium for Spinal Cord Medicine. *Early Acute Management in Adults with Spinal Cord Injury. Clinical Practice Guidelines for Health Care Professionals.* Washington, DC: Paralyzed Veterans of America; 2008.

Consortium for Spinal Cord Medicine. *Prevention of Thromboembolism in Spinal Cord Injury.* 2nd ed. Washington, DC: Paralyzed Veterans of America; 1999.

Dhall SS, Hadley MN, Aarabi B, et al. Deep venous thrombosis and thromboembolism in patients with cervical spinal cord injuries. *Neurosurgery.* 2013;72(suppl 2):244-254.

Dhall SS, Hadley MN, Aarabi B, et al. Nutritional support after spinal cord injury. *Neurosurgery.* 2013;72(suppl 2):255-259.

Fehlings MG, Vaccaro A, Wilson JR, et al. Early versus delayed decompression for traumatic cervical spinal cord injury: results of the Surgical Timing in Acute Spinal Cord Injury Study (STASCIS). *PLoS One.* 2012;7(2):e32037.

Hadley MN, Walters BC. Introduction to the guidelines for the management of acute cervical spine and spinal cord injuries. *Neurosurgery.* 2013;72(suppl 2):5-16.

Hadley MN, Walters BC, Aarabi B, et al. Clinical assessment following acute cervical spinal cord injury. *Neurosurgery.* 2013;72(suppl 2):40-53.

Hurlbert RJ, Hadley MN, Walters BC, et al. Pharmacological therapy for acute spinal cord injury. *Neurosurgery.* 2013;72(suppl 2):93-105.

Kirshblum S, Fichtenbaum J. Breaking the news in spinal cord injury. *J Spinal Cord Med.* 2008;31(1):7-12.

Liu JC, Patel A, Vaccaro AR, Lammertse DP, Chen D. Methylprednisolone after traumatic spinal cord injury: yes or no? *PM R.* 2009;1(7):669-673.

McMahon D, Tutt M, Cook AM. Pharmacological management of hemodynamic complications following spinal cord injury. *Orthopedics.* 2009;32(5):331.

Ryken TC, Hurlbert RJ, Hadley MN, et al. The acute cardiopulmonary management of patients with cervical spinal cord injuries. *Neurosurgery.* 2013;72(suppl 2):84-92.

CHAPTER 9

Spinal Orthoses

GENERAL PRINCIPLES

Orthoses are external devices applied to the body to restrict motion in that particular body segment.

Categories of Spinal Orthoses

Spinal orthoses are broadly categorized based on the regions or body segments that they are intended to restrict. These include: cervical orthoses (CO), cervicothoracic orthoses (CTO), cervicothoracolumbosacral orthoses (CTLSO), thoracolumbosacral orthoses (TLSO), lumbosacral orthoses (LSO), and sacral orthoses (SO).

Spinal orthoses can be rigid or soft. In general, soft spinal orthoses have very limited role in management of spinal cord injury (SCI) and will not be discussed further. For example, while soft (foam) cervical collars may serve as a kinesthetic reminder to restrict motion, they offer no significant restriction of motion themselves. The same applies to soft LSO or corsets that are primarily used for low back pain but have little utility in SCI.

The primary example of a CTLSO is the Milwaukee brace, which is indicated for management of progressive and significant (25°–35°) idiopathic thoraco-lumbar scoliosis in the immature skeleton and is not used in the setting of SCI, and will also not be discussed further.

The remainder of this chapter focuses primarily on the spinal orthoses that are used in the setting of SCI (Table 9.1).

Mechanism of Action of Spinal Orthoses

One or more three-point pressure systems providing counteractive forces (i.e., a force in one direction acting in equilibrium with two forces in a different direction) is a primary principle involved in motion control by spinal orthoses. General containment, increased intra-abdominal forces with load transfer from the vertebral disks to surrounding soft tissue, traction distraction forces are other mechanisms in play with some types of orthoses.

Table 9.1

Spinal Orthoses in Management of SCI			
Type	Examples	Indications	Considerations
Cervical orthoses (CO)	Philadelphia, Aspen, Miami J collar	Stable mid cervical injuries; Following mid or low cervical spine surgery/instrumentation; as an interim measure while awaiting surgery or HCTO immobilization	Primarily restrict flexion-extension, less effective in restricting rotation or lateral bending
Cervicothoracic orthoses (CTO)	SOMI, Yale, Four poster	Stable cervical fractures; Atlanto-axial instability or C2 arch fractures (where restriction of flexion-extension is the primary objective)	Not adequate for highly unstable injuries (those require additional incorporation of head restriction)
Head cervicothoracic orthoses (HCTO)	Halo, Minerva	Unstable injuries of the cervical or upper thoracic spine	Halo is especially effective at limiting C1-C2 movement; Custom-molded Minerva jacket can provide as good or better restriction for most cervical spine movements (except lateral bending) as halo; potential for segmental movement (snaking) despite overall limited of cervical spine motion with halo
Thoracolumbosacral orthoses (TLSO)	Custom-molded body jacket, CASH, Jewett extension brace	Custom-molded TLSO is used as an adjunct to surgical treatment for T6-L1 fractures, or by itself with relatively stable vertebral injury; Prophylactic bracing with a TLSO may delay need for scoliosis in pediatric SCI surgery when curve <20°; CASH or Jewett brace can be used for stable vertebral compression fracture	Not effective at controlling lower lumbar motion, or for highly unstable injury involving two- or three-columns

(*continued*)

Table 9.1

Spinal Orthoses in Management of SCI (*Continued*)

Type	Examples	Indications	Considerations
Lumbosacral orthoses (LSO)	Chair-back, Williams Flexion	Role in SCI is limited; Williams brace can be used to restrict lumbar extension in traumatic spondylolysis or spondylolisthesis; Chair-back brace used postoperatively for lumbar laminectomies/ fusion	Limited effect on restricting segmental motion even if overall spinal motion is restricted with LSO; can cause deconditioning of trunk muscles with prolonged use
Sacral orthoses (SO)	Sacral corset, Trochan- teric belt	Pelvic or pubic symphysis injury	Little role in SCI

Table 9.2

Spine Biomechanics Considerations in Role of Spinal Orthoses

C1-2 (atlantoaxial) joint provides almost 50% of cervical spine axial rotation

C2-3, C3-4, and C4-5 have the main contribution to lateral bending of the cervical spine

C5-6 is the segment where the most flexion occurs in the cervical spine

T1-T10 motion is significantly limited naturally by the rib cage. The lower thoracic segments that lack rib attachments are considerably more mobile

T12-L1 and T11-T12 are the primary contributors to flexion and extension of the thoracic spine. T12-L1 acts as a fulcrum between the immobile thoracic and sacral spine.

T1-T2 is the part of the thoracic spine with the most axial rotation, with a gradual decrease going lower down the thoracic spine

An understanding of some aspects of spinal biomechanics is useful when considering appropriateness and effectiveness of spinal orthoses (Table 9.2).

CLINICAL CONSIDERATIONS

Indications for Orthoses in SCI

Spinal orthoses are used to limit spinal motion, stabilize, support and realign the spine, and/or to protect it after acute trauma or surgery.

The duration of use varies with the nature and stability of the spinal injury, evidence of healing, and concomitant use of definitive measures such as spinal surgery and instrumentation. In general, spinal orthoses are worn for 10 to 12 weeks after spine surgery or spine fracture to allow for healing. There may be concomitant restrictions placed on certain activities and movements to avoid compromising spinal stability during this period.

Specific Orthoses Used in SCI (Table 9.1)

CO

The Philadelphia and Miami J collars provide some restriction of flexion and extension, but are much less effective at controlling lateral bending and cervical rotation. These orthoses are prefabricated and consist of two pieces that are secured with Velcro straps. They are used for stable cervical fractures or ligamentous injuries, to restrict motion following mid or low cervical spine surgery or instrumentation, and as an interim measure (in conjunction with other restrictions) while awaiting surgery or head cervicothoracic orthoses (HCTO) immobilization. A thoracic extension can be incorporated with these orthoses which converts them to CTO.

CTO

Examples of these include the Sternal Occipital Mandibular Immobilizer (SOMI), Yale, and Four Poster orthoses. These are used for stable cervical fractures but are not adequate for highly unstable injuries, for which additional incorporation of head restriction is needed. The SOMI orthoses can be donned in the supine position and used for people who are restricted to bed. The Yale orthoses extend a little higher in posterior region.

Head CTO

These provide the most restriction of cervical spine motion and include the Halo orthoses and the Minerva jacket. These are indicated for more unstable cervical injuries and can also be used postoperatively when significant restriction of cervical motion is desired.

Halo Orthosis

This includes a prefabricated halo ring (which comes in different sizes), uprights, vest, and pins. In adults typically four pins are used with 6 to 8 in/lb torque setting. The anterior pins are placed less than an inch above the lateral third of the eyebrow to avoid sinuses and cranial nerves, and the posterior pins are placed less than an inch above and just posterior to the ear. When lesser torque forces are desired (e.g., in young children and infants or those with skull fractures), the number of pins is increased. Pins should be checked to confirm tightness 1 to 2 days after placement, and pin sites should be cleaned twice daily. Studies have shown potential movement (snaking) between individual cervical spine segments despite overall limited of cervical spine motion with halo.

Custom Molded Minerva Orthosis

A properly fitted, thermoplastic custom molded Minerva can provide comparable or better restriction of most cervical movements than a Halo, without the need for pin insertion. Unlike older plaster-versions of the Minerva, the light weight thermoplastic jacket allows for better hygiene and self-care abilities.

TLSO

A rigid custom-molded TLSO can be used for management of traumatic or pathological fractures of the mid to lower thoracic or upper lumbar spine, but may not provide adequate restriction of lower lumbar spine injuries or highly unstable injuries. TLSO is also available in a prefabricated off-the-shelf version. The Cruciform Anterior Spinal Hyperextension (CASH) or Jewett orthoses are used primarily for stable compression fractures of the lower thoracic and thoracolumbar spine, but are not appropriate for unstable or burst fractures.

LSO and SO
These have a very limited role in SCI. The Williams Flexion brace can be used to restrict lumbar extension in traumatic spondylolysis or spondylolisthesis. The Chair-back brace may be used postoperatively for lumbar laminectomies and fusion.

Cautions and Complications in Use of Spinal Orthoses

While some discomfort is to be expected with the use of restrictive orthoses that often need to be snug fitting to be effective, the edges should not dig into the skin and there should be little persistent redness 10 to 15 minutes after removal of orthosis. The orthoses may restrict certain movements and activities but should ideally allow the patient to sit comfortably while wearing it, and should not restrict breathing, digestion, or chewing. Superior mesenteric artery syndrome (see Chapter 36) is a rare complication with use of an overly restrictive TLSO. It is important to be vigilant to the possibility of skin breakdown. Excess perspiration may occur with inability to adequately dissipate body heat. Prolonged use may exacerbate trunk muscle weakness. While the orthoses may be effective in restricting total motion of a particular region or body segment, there may still be segmental motion resulting in "snaking" of spinal alignment.

KNOWLEDGE GAPS AND EMERGING CONCEPTS

Improvements in materials available for manufacture of spinal orthoses have led to significant enhancements in design.

The use of computer-aided design (CAD) and computer-aided manufacturing (CAM) can improve efficiency in design and fabrication of spinal orthoses.

SUGGESTED READING

Consortium for Spinal Cord Medicine. *Early Acute Management in Adults with Spinal Cord Injury. Clinical Practice Guidelines for Health Care Professionals.* Washington, DC: Paralyzed Veterans of America; 2008.

German JW, Hart BL, Benzel EC. Nonoperative management of vertical C2 body fractures. *Neurosurgery.* 2005;56(3):516-521.

Hadley MN, Walters BC. Introduction to the guidelines for the management of acute cervical spine and spinal cord injuries. *Neurosurgery.* 2013;72(suppl 2):5-16.

Hrodyski MB, DiPaoloa CP, Rechtine GR. Cervical collars are insufficient for immobilizing an unstable cervical spine injury. *J Emerg Med.* 2011;41(5):513-519.

Rechtine GR. Nonsurgical treatment of thoracic and lumbar fractures. *Instr Course Lect.* 1999;48:413-416.

CHAPTER 10

Neurological Assessment for Classification of Traumatic Spinal Cord Injury

This chapter focuses on the International Standards for Neurological Classification of Spinal Cord Injury (ISNCSCI) published by the American Spinal Injury Association (ASIA), which include motor and sensory assessments.

The International Standards to Document Remaining Autonomic Function after Spinal Cord Injury (ISAFSCI) are discussed elsewhere (Chapter 33).

GENERAL PRINCIPLES

Definitions

Tetraplegia and Paraplegia
Cervical spinal cord injury (SCI) results in tetraplegia. The term *tetraplegia* (preferred to quadriplegia) refers to impairment or loss of motor or sensory function in the cervical segments of the spinal cord due to damage of neural elements within the spinal canal. The result is impairment of function in the arms as well as in the trunk, legs, and pelvic organs.

The term *paraplegia* refers to impairment or loss of motor or sensory function in the thoracic, lumbar, or sacral segments of the spinal cord, secondary to damage of neural elements within the spinal canal. With this level of injury, arm functioning is spared, but the trunk, legs, and pelvic organs may be involved.

A couple of points are important to note in the above definitions.

* These terms refer only to damage of neural elements *within* the spinal canal. Impairment of sensorimotor involvement outside the spinal canal, such as plexus lesions or injury to peripheral nerves, should not be referred to as tetraplegia. Similarly while the term paraplegia is

appropriate to use in referring to conus medullaris and cauda equina injuries (since these are within the spinal canal), it should not be used to refer to lumbosacral plexus lesions or injury to peripheral nerves where the neural involvement is outside the spinal canal.

▓ The terms tetraplegia or paraplegia are appropriate to use regardless of the severity of the impairment or loss of motor or sensory function in the segments of the spinal cord due to damage of neural elements within the spinal canal. Use of the terms "tetraparesis" and "paraparesis" is discouraged, as they describe incomplete lesions imprecisely, and incorrectly imply that tetraplegia and paraplegia should only be used for neurologically complete injuries. Instead, the ASIA Impairment Scale (AIS) provides a more precise approach to description of severity (completeness) of the SCI.

Dermatomes and Myotomes
The neurologic exam is conducted by systematic examination of the dermatomes and myotomes. The term *dermatome* refers to the area of skin innervated by the sensory axons within each spinal nerve root/segment. The term *myotome* refers to the collection of muscle fibers innervated by the motor axons of each nerve root. Most muscles are innervated by more than one root, and most nerve roots innervate more than one muscle. By convention if a muscle has a grade of at least 3, it is considered to have intact innervation by the more rostral of the innervating segments.

Measures/Descriptors of Neurological Damage (Table 10.1)
The International Standards examination is used to determine the sensory, motor, and neurological levels, to generate motor and sensory scores, and to determine completeness of the injury. Thorough understanding and correct use of definitions of these measures of neurological damage generated from ISNCSCI is crucial for accuracy and consistency in communication. These measures, including Sensory Level, Motor Level, Neurological Level of Injury (NLI), Sensory Scores, Motor Scores, Incomplete Injury, Complete Injury, and Zone of Partial Preservation (ZPP), are defined in Table 10.1.

CLINICAL CONSIDERATIONS

Neurological Examination

The International Standards examination used for neurological classification of SCI has sensory and motor components. A neurological rectal examination is part of these components.

The examination can be performed with minimal equipment (safety pin and cotton wisp) in almost all clinical settings and phases of care. It should be performed with the patient in the supine position (except for the rectal examination

Table 10.1

Measures/Descriptors of Neurological Damage, Generated From ISNCSCI

Measure	Definition
Sensory level	The most caudal, normally innervated dermatome for both Pin-Prick (sharp/dull discrimination) and Light Touch sensations
Motor level	The lowest key muscle function that has a grade of at least 3/5 on manual muscle testing in the supine position, providing the key muscle functions represented by segments above that level are judged to be intact (graded as a 5/5)
Neurological level of injury (NLI)	The most caudal segment of the spinal cord with normal sensory and antigravity motor function on both sides of the body, provided that there is normal (intact) sensory and motor function rostrally
Sensory scores	Refers to a numerical summary score of sensory function. There is a maximum total score of 56 (key sensory points for 28 dermatomes, each graded from 0 to 2) each for Light Touch and Pin-Prick (sharp/dull discrimination) modalities, for a total of 112 points per side of the body.
Motor scores	Refers to a numerical summary score of motor function. There is a maximum score of 25 for each extremity (five key muscles in each extremity graded from 0 to 5), totaling 50 for the upper limbs (Upper Extremity Motor Score, UEMS) and 50 for the lower limbs (Lower Extremity Motor Score, LEMS)
Incomplete injury	Preservation of any sensory and/or motor function below the neurological level that includes the lowest sacral segments S4-S5 (i.e., "sacral sparing")
Complete injury	Absence of sensory and motor function in the lowest sacral segments (S4-S5)
Zone of partial preservation (ZPP)	Used only with complete injuries, the term refers to those dermatomes and myotomes caudal to the sensory and motor levels that remain partially innervated. The most caudal segment with some sensory and/or motor function defines the extent of the sensory and motor ZPP respectively

Abbreviation: ISNCSCI, International Standards for Neurological Classification of Spinal Cord Injury.

that can be performed side-lying) to allow for a valid comparison of scores between serial exams.

The examination can be recorded on a standardized worksheet (Figure 10.1). The worksheet may be freely downloaded and photocopied (but not altered) from the ASIA website (www.asia-spinalinjury.org). The ASIA website also provides web-based instructional modules (InSTeP) about conducting and scoring the exam and additional training material with details about the examination.

Sensory Examination
The sensory examination has both required and optional elements. The required elements are the ones necessary for classification based on the standards.

Required Elements
The required portion of the sensory examination is completed through the testing of a key point in each of the 28 dermatomes (from C2 to S4-5) bilaterally that can be easily located in relation to bony anatomical landmarks. Key points for each dermatome are specified in Table 10.2 and illustrated in Figure 10.1.

At each of these key points, two aspects of sensation are examined: light touch (LT) and pin-prick (PP) (sharp-dull discrimination).

LT and PP sensation at each key point is separately scored on a three-point scale (with comparison to the sensation on the patient's cheek as a frame of reference for normal):

0 = absent
1= altered (impaired or partial appreciation, including hyperesthesia)
2 = normal or intact (same as on the cheek)
NT = not testable

LT sensation is tested with a tapered wisp of cotton stroked once across an area not to exceed 1 cm of skin (for consistency of sensory input) with the eyes closed or vision blocked. PP sensation (sharp/dull discrimination) is performed with a disposable safety pin that is stretched to allow testing on both ends; using the pointed end to test for sharp and the rounded end of the pin for dull.

Deep Anal Pressure (DAP): DAP awareness is examined through insertion of the index finger and applying gentle pressure to the anorectal wall. Alternatively, pressure can be applied by using the thumb to gently squeeze the anus against the inserted index finger. Consistently perceived pressure is graded as being present or absent. Any reproducible pressure sensation felt in the anal area during this part of the exam signifies that the patient has a sensory incomplete lesion.
(text continues on page 78)

Table 10.2
Key Sensory Points (Tested Bilaterally) (see Figure 10.1)

Level	Key Sensory Point
C2	At least 1 cm lateral to the occipital protuberance (alternatively 3 cm behind the ear)
C3	Supraclavicular fossa (posterior to the clavicle) and at the midclavicular line
C4	Over the acromioclavicular (AC) joint
C5	Lateral (radial) side of the antecubital fossa (just proximal to elbow crease)
C6	Thumb, dorsal surface, proximal phalanx
C7	Middle finger, dorsal surface, proximal phalanx
C8	Little finger, dorsal surface, proximal phalanx
T1	Medial (ulnar) side of the antecubital fossa, just proximal to the medial epicondyle of the humerus
T2	Apex of the axilla
T3	Midclavicular line and the third intercostal space (IS) found by palpating the anterior chest to locate the third rib and the corresponding IS below it
T4	Fourth IS (nipple line) at the midclavicular line
T5	Midclavicular line and the fifth IS (midway between T4 and T6)
T6	Midclavicular line and the sixth IS (level of xiphisternum)
T7	Midclavicular line and the seventh IS (midway between T6 and T8)
T8	Midclavicular line and the eighth IS (midway between T6 and TI0)
T9	Midclavicular line and the ninth IS (midway between T8 and T10)
T10	Midclavicular line and the tenth IS (umbilicus)
T11	Midclavicular line and the eleventh IS (midway between T10 and TI2)
T12	Midclavicular line and the mid-point of the inguinal ligament
L1	Midway distance between the key sensory points for TI2 and L2
L2	On the anterior-medial thigh at the midpoint drawn connecting the midpoint of inguinal ligament (T12) and the medial femoral condyle
L3	Medial femoral condyle above the knee
L4	Medial malleolus
L5	Dorsum of the foot at the third metatarsal phalangeal joint
S1	Lateral heel (calcaneus)
S2	Mid-point of the popliteal fossa
S3	Ischial tuberosity or infra-gluteal fold
S4–5	Perianal area <1 cm lateral to the mucocutaneous junction (taken as one level)

Figure 10.1

International Standards for Neurological Classification of SCI Exam Worksheet

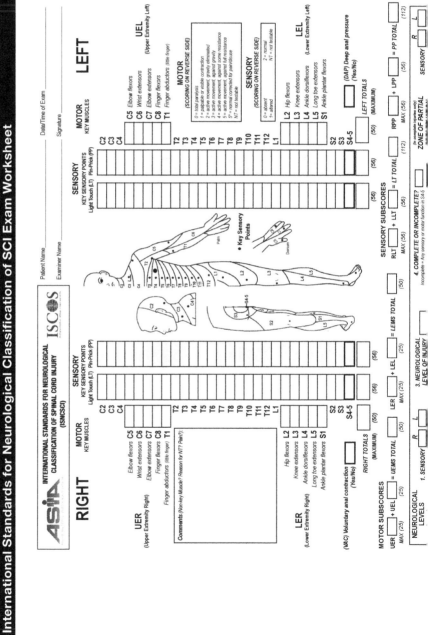

Muscle Function Grading

0 = total paralysis

1 = palpable or visible contraction

2 = active movement, full range of motion (ROM) with gravity eliminated

3 = active movement, full ROM against gravity

4 = active movement, full ROM against gravity and moderate resistance in a muscle specific position

5 = (normal) active movement, full ROM against gravity and full resistance in a functional muscle position expected from an otherwise unimpaired person

5* = (normal) active movement, full ROM against gravity and sufficient resistance to be considered normal if identified inhibiting factors (i.e. pain, disuse) were not present

NT = not testable (i.e. due to immobilization, severe pain such that the patient cannot be graded, amputation of limb, or contracture of > 50% of the normal range of motion)

Sensory Grading

0 = Absent

1 = Altered, either decreased/impaired sensation or hypersensitivity

2 = Normal

NT = Not testable

Non Key Muscle Functions (optional)

May be used to assign a motor level to differentiate AIS B vs. C

Movement	Root level
Shoulder: Flexion, extension, abduction, adduction, internal and external rotation **Elbow:** Supination	C5
Elbow: Pronation **Wrist:** Flexion	C6
Finger: Flexion at proximal joint, extension. **Thumb:** Flexion, extension and abduction in plane of thumb	C7
Finger: Flexion at MCP joint **Thumb:** Opposition, adduction and abduction perpendicular to palm	C8
Finger: Abduction of the index finger	T1
Hip: Adduction	L2
Hip: External rotation	L3
Hip: Extension, abduction, internal rotation **Knee:** Flexion **Ankle:** Inversion and eversion **Toe:** MP and IP extension	L4
Hallux and Toe: DIP and PIP flexion and abduction	L5
Hallux: Adduction	S1

ASIA Impairment Scale (AIS)

A = Complete No sensory or motor function is preserved in the sacral segments S4-5

B = Sensory Incomplete Sensory but not motor function is preserved below the neurological level and includes the sacral segments S4-5 (light touch or pin-prick at S4-5 or deep anal pressure) AND no motor function is preserved more than three levels below the motor level on either side of the body

C = Motor Incomplete Motor function is preserved below the neurological level**, and more than half of key muscle functions below the neurological level of injury (NLI) have a muscle grade less than 3 (Grades 0-2)

D = Motor Incomplete Motor function is preserved below the neurological level**, and at least half (half or more) of key muscle functions below the NLI have a muscle grade ≥ 3

E = Normal If sensation and motor function as tested with the ISNCSCI are graded as normal in all segments, and the patient had prior deficits, then the AIS grade is E. Someone without an initial SCI does not receive an AIS grade

** For an individual to receive a grade of C or D, i.e. motor incomplete status, they must have either (1) voluntary anal sphincter contraction or (2) sacral sensory sparing with sparing of motor function more than three levels below the motor level for that side of the body. The International Standards at this time allows even non-key muscle function more than 3 levels below the motor level to be used in determining motor incomplete status (AIS B versus C)

NOTE: When assessing the extent of motor sparing below the level for distinguishing between AIS B and C, the *motor level* on each side is used; whereas to differentiate between AIS C and D (based on proportion of key muscle functions with strength grade 3 or greater) the *neurological level of injury* is used)

Steps in Classification

The following order is recommended for determining the classification of individuals with SCI.

1. Determine sensory levels for right and left sides.
The sensory level is the most caudal, intact dermatome for both pin-prick and light touch sensation

2. Determine motor levels for right and left sides.
Defined by the lowest key muscle function that has a grade of at least 3 (on supine testing), providing the key muscle functions represented by segments above that level are judged to be intact (graded as a 5)
Note: In regions where there is no myotome to test, the motor level is presumed to be the same as the sensory level, if testable motor function above that level is also normal

3. Determine the neurological level of injury (NLI)
This refers to the most caudal segment of the cord with intact sensation and antigravity (3 or more) muscle function strength, provided that there is normal (intact) sensory and motor function rostrally respectively.
The NLI is the most cephalad of the sensory and motor levels determined in steps 1 and 2

4. Determine whether the injury is Complete or Incomplete.
(i.e. absence or presence of sacral sparing)
If voluntary anal contraction = *No* AND all S4-5 sensory scores = 0 AND deep anal pressure = *No*, then injury is *Complete*.
Otherwise, injury is *Incomplete*.

5. Determine ASIA Impairment Scale (AIS) Grade:

Is injury Complete?   If YES, **AIS=A** and can record ZPP (lowest dermatome or myotome on each side with some preservation)

NO ↓

Is injury Motor Complete?   If YES, **AIS=B**
(No=voluntary anal contraction OR motor function more than three levels below the motor level on a given side, if the patient has sensory incomplete classification)

NO ↓

Are at least half (half or more) of the key muscles below the neurological level of injury graded 3 or better?

NO ↓   YES ↓

AIS=C   **AIS=D**

If sensation and motor function is normal in all segments, AIS=E
Note: AIS E is used in follow-up testing when an individual with a documented SCI has recovered normal function. If at initial testing no deficits are found, the individual is neurologically intact; the ASIA Impairment Scale does not apply

INTERNATIONAL STANDARDS FOR NEUROLOGICAL CLASSIFICATION OF SPINAL CORD INJURY

ISCOS
INTERNATIONAL SPINAL CORD SOCIETY

Examination for DAP is not required in patients who have LT or PP sensation at S4–S5.

Optional Elements
Optional sensory elements include:

1. Joint movement appreciation and position sense: joints that can be tested include the inter-phalangeal (IP) joint of the thumb, the proximal IP joint of the little finger, the wrist, the IP joint of the great toe, the ankle, and the knee, and
2. Awareness of deep pressure/deep pain: tested by applying firm pressure to the skin for 3 to 5 seconds at different locations of the wrist, fingers, ankles, and toes

Motor Examination
The motor examination also has required and optional elements.

Required Elements
The required portion of the motor examination is completed through the testing of key muscle groups corresponding to 10 paired myotomes (C5-T1 and L2-S1). The key muscles were each chosen since they can be tested for all grades of strength in the supine position and represent one myotome in each extremity (Tables 10.3 and 10.4).

There are several ways in which muscle testing as part of ISNCSCI differs from traditional manual muscle testing (MMT) (Table 10.5).

Table 10.3

Key Muscle Groups for the Upper Extremities[a]

Level	Muscle Group	Positions for Testing Key Muscles for Grades 4 or 5
C5	Elbow flexors (biceps, brachialis)	Elbow flexed at 90°, arm at patient's side, forearm supinated
C6	Wrist extensors (extensor carpi radialis longus and brevis)	Wrist in full extension
C7	Elbow extensors (triceps)	Shoulder in neutral rotation, adducted, and in 90° of flexion, with elbow in 45° of flexion
C8	Finger flexors (flexor digitorum profundus) to the middle finger	Full-flexed position of the distal phalanx with the proximal finger joint stabilized in extended position
T1	Small finger abductors (abductor digiti minimi)	Full-abducted position of the fifth digit of the hand

[a]For those myotomes that are not clinically testable by manual muscle examination (e.g., C1 to C4), the motor level is presumed to be the same as the sensory level.

Table 10.4

Key Muscle Groups for the Lower Extremities		
Level	Muscle Group	Position for Testing Grade 4 or 5 Strength
L2	Hip flexors (iliopsoas)	Hip flexed to 90°
L3	Knee extensors (quadriceps)	Knee flexed to 15°
L4	Ankle dorsiflexors (tibialis anterior)	Full-dorsiflexed position of the ankle
L5	Long toe extensors (extensor hallucis longus)	First toe fully extended
S1	Ankle plantar flexors (gastrocnemius, soleus)	Hip in neutral rotation, knee fully extended, and ankle in full planter flexion

Table 10.5

How Muscle Strength Testing for the International Standards Examination Differs From Traditional MMT
All MMT for classification of SCI is conducted in the supine position
Use of + and – is not recommended when grading muscle strength from 0 to 5
Use of "NT" (Not Testable) when unable to test (e.g., due to immobilization of extremity)
Use of 5* (when muscle is felt to be normally innervated by the examiner despite weakness on MMT, which is attributed to nonneurogenic causes e.g., disuse or pain)

Abbreviation: MMT, Manual muscle testing.

The strength of each muscle function is graded on a six-point scale from 0 to 6.
  0 = total paralysis.
  1 = palpable or visible contraction.
  2 = active movement, full range of motion (ROM) with gravity eliminated.
  3 = active movement, full ROM against gravity.
  4 = active movement, full ROM against gravity and moderate resistance in a muscle specific position.
  5 = (normal) active movement, full ROM against gravity and full resistance in a muscle specific position expected from an otherwise unimpaired person.
  5* = (normal) active movement, full ROM against gravity and sufficient resistance to be considered normal if identified inhibiting factors (i.e., pain, disuse) were not present.
  NT = not testable (i.e., due to immobilization, severe pain such that the patient cannot be graded, amputation of limb, or contracture of greater than 50% of the range of motion).

Voluntary anal contraction (VAC): The external anal sphincter is tested for reproducible voluntary contractions around the examiner's finger and graded as being present or absent. The suggested instruction to the patient is "squeeze my finger as if to hold back a bowel movement." If there is VAC present, then the patient has a motor incomplete injury. VAC should be distinguished from reflex anal contraction.

Optional Elements
For purposes of the SCI evaluation, other non-key muscles may be evaluated; for example, the diaphragm, deltoid, finger extension, hip adductors, and hamstrings. While these muscle functions are not used in determining motor levels or scores or in the determination of AIS C versus D, at this time the International Standards allows non-key muscles to determine motor incomplete status; i.e. AIS B versus C. Suggested non-key muscle functions included on the examination worksheet are listed in Table 10.6.

Pitfalls in Neurological Examination: (Table 10.7)
Commonly encountered pitfalls in assessment of the sensory and motor components of the standards examination are summarized in Table 10.7.

It is important to properly stabilize and position the joints being tested during MMT to prevent confusion from substitutions by other muscles that may give

Table 10.6

Non-Key Muscle Functional (Optional) May be Used to Assign a Motor Level to Differentiate AIS B vs. C

Movement	Root Level
Shoulder: Flexion, extension, abduction, adduction, internal and external rotation **Elbow:** Supination	C5
Elbow: Pronation **Wrist:** Flexion	C6
Finger: Flexion at proximal joint, extension **Thumb:** Flexion, extension and abduction in plane of thumb	C7
Finger: Flexion at MCP joint **Thumb:** Opposition, adduction and abduction perpendicular to palm	C8
Finger: Abduction of the index finger	T1
Hip: Adduction	L2
Hip: External rotation	L3
Hip: Extension, abduction, internal rotation **Knee:** Flexion **Ankle:** Inversion and eversion **Toe:** MP and IP extension	L4
Hallux and Toe: DIP and PIP flexion and abduction	L5
Hallux: Adduction	S1

Abbreviations: MCP, metacarpophalangeal; MP, metatarsophalangeal; IP, interphalangeal; DIP, distal interphalangeal; PIP, proximal interphalangeal.

the erroneous perception of intact muscle function in the muscle being tested (Table 10.8).

Table 10.7

Common Testing Pitfalls in the International Standards Neurological Exam

Sensory Exam

- In grading PP sensation, inability to distinguish the sharp end from the dull end should be graded as PP=0 (absent) even if the patient is able to feel the pin. PP is graded as 1 if the patient can distinguish between sharp and dull at least 80% of the time but the sharpness feels different (less or more intense) than the face
- Sensory preservation in the T3 dermatome with absent sensation in T1, T2, and T4 dermatomes should be scored as absent since it likely represents C4 sensation (from supraclavicular nerves that can extend down the anterior chest wall to a variable level up to the third intercostal space)

Motor Exam

- Improper positioning and stabilization of the extremity being tested may lead to muscle substitution. Consistency and accuracy in placing stabilizing and resisting hands as recommended is important
- Trace function may be overlooked if not palpating correctly
- Passive ROM should be checked prior to MMT to detect any contracture, otherwise it can lead to under-grading strength since the patient will not be able to complete movement across the full ROM (even though not necessarily due to muscle weakness, but due to contracture)
- Reflex withdrawal or spasticity may mimic voluntary muscle contraction. Patients should be able to isolate and voluntarily be able to repeat movement
- Muscle substitutions causing joint movement may lead to erroneous perception of muscle function that is absent (Table 10.8)

Table 10.8

Muscle Substitutions That Can Lead to Erroneous Interpretation of Muscle Function[a]

Wrist extension mimicked by forearm supination (and the use of gravity)

Elbow extension mimicked by external rotation of the shoulder

Elbow extension mimicked by quickly flexing and relaxing the elbow

Long finger flexion mimicked by wrist extension (due to tenodesis)

Long finger flexion (flexor digitorum profundus) mimicked by hand intrinsic or flexor digitorum superficialis contraction

Finger abduction mimicked by finger extension

Hip flexion mimicked by adductor or abdominal contraction

Ankle dorsiflexion mimicked by long toe extensors

Great toe extension mimicked by active flexion followed by relaxation of the toe

Ankle plantar flexion mimicked by hip flexion

---

[a]Proper technique, including positioning and stabilization of the limb being tested, will avoid these muscle substitutions during testing of muscle function.

Reliability of Examination
In general, the elements of the motor and sensory examination have been demonstrated to have good inter-rater and test-retest reliability when conducted by trained examiners. PP scores had slightly lower reliability than LT scores in one study. Inter-rater reliability of motor and sensory has been shown to be better for complete than for incomplete injuries. Studies have demonstrated that while it is not uncommon to have variation in single dermatome and myotome scores (usually within one muscle grade) between skilled examiners, summed motor and sensory scores are much more reliable. Follow-up examination should be done to clarify discrepancies. As mentioned in the next paragraph, certain circumstances can affect the reliability of the examination.

Circumstances that Impact Conduct and Interpretation of the Examination (Table 10.9)
Several circumstances, for example, young children, potentially unstable spine, presence of contractures, and associated conditions or complications, may affect the ability to complete and interpret the classification standards examination. Specific guidance about these circumstances is summarized in Table 10.9.

Neurological Classification

Steps in classification of SCI (Table 10.10 and Figure 10.1)
The following order is recommended for determining the classification of individuals with SCI:

1. *Determine sensory levels* for right and left sides (i.e., the most caudal, intact dermatome for both PP and LT sensation)
2. *Determine motor levels* for right and left sides (i.e., the lowest key muscle function that has a grade of at least 3, providing the key muscle functions represented by segments above that level are judged to be intact [graded as a 5])
   Note: In regions where there is no myotome to test, the motor level is presumed to be the same as the sensory level, if testable motor function above that level is also normal
3. *Determine the NLI* (i.e., the most caudal segment of the cord with intact sensation and antigravity [≥3] muscle function strength, provided that there is normal [intact] sensory and motor function rostrally respectively). The NLI is the most cephalad of the sensory and motor levels determined in steps 1 and 2
4. *Determine whether the injury is Complete or Incomplete* (i.e., absence or presence of sacral sparing)
   - If VAC = No AND all S4-5 sensory scores = 0 AND DAP = No, then injury is Complete
   - Otherwise, injury is Incomplete
5. *Determine AIS Grade* (Table 10.10):
   - Is injury Complete? If YES, AIS=A
   - Is injury Motor Complete? If YES, AIS=B

Table 10.9

Particular Circumstances That Impact Conduct and Interpretation of the International Standards Examination

Condition	Resolution
Young children	- Neurological exam based on ISNCSCI is not useful and should not be attempted for children <4 yrs; - Can attempt for older than 5 yrs though individual components (e.g., anorectal exam, pin-prick testing) may be difficult to complete and interpret reliably in children <10 yrs
Contractures	- If the patient exhibits ≥50% of the normal range, then the muscle function can be graded through its available range with the usual 0–5 scale - If the ROM is limited to <50% of the normal ROM, a numerical grade cannot be provided and "NT" (Not Testable) should be documented
Potentially unstable spine	- When examining a patient with a suspected acute traumatic injury below the T8 level, the hip should not be allowed to flex beyond 90° due to the increased kyphotic stress placed on the lumbar spine. Examination should be performed isometrically and unilaterally, so that the contralateral hip remains extended to stabilize the pelvis - In the presence of potential cervical spine instability, shoulder flexion or abduction >90° or resistance to shoulder movement should be avoided - To complete the anorectal exam, if there is spinal instability without adequate orthotic stabilization, the patient should be log-rolled (so there is no twisting of the spinal column) on their side, or alternatively an abbreviated exam can be performed in the supine position
Associated injuries in the acute stage (e.g., traumatic brain injury, brachial plexus injury, limb fracture)	- When associated injuries interfere with completion of the examination; the neurological level should still be determined as accurately as possible. However, obtaining the sensory/motor scores and impairment grades should be deferred to later examinations

Abbreviation: ROM, range of motion.

▨ If NO, AIS=C or D (No=VAC OR motor function more than three levels below the motor level on a given side, if the patient has sensory incomplete classification)

  ● Are at least half (half or more) of the key muscles below the NLI graded 3 or better? If NO, AIS=C; If YES, AIS=D

(NOTE: When assessing the extent of motor sparing below the level for distinguishing between AIS B and C, the motor level on each side is used; whereas to differentiate between AIS C and D [based on proportion of key muscle functions with strength grade three or greater below the injury level] the single NLI is used).

▨ If sensation and motor function is normal in all segments, AIS=E

Table 10.10

American Spinal Injury Association (ASIA) Impairment Scale		
Grade	Category	Description
A	Complete	No sensory or motor function is preserved in the sacral segments S4-5.
B	Sensory incomplete	Sensory but no motor function is preserved below the neurologic level including the sacral segments S4-5, and no motor function is preserved more than three levels below the motor level on either side of the body.
C	Motor incomplete[a]	Motor function is preserved below the neurologic level, and more than half of key muscles below the neurologic level have a muscle grade <3.
D	Motor incomplete[a]	Motor function is preserved below the neurologic level, and at least half of key muscles below the neurologic level of injury have a muscle grade ≥3.
E	Normal	Sensory function and motor function are normal, and the patient had prior deficits.

[a]For an individual to receive a grade of C or D, that is, motor incomplete status, they must have either (1) voluntary anal sphincter contraction or (2) sacral sensory sparing (at S4/5 or DAP) with sparing of motor function more than three levels below the motor level for that side of the body. Even nonkey muscle function more than three levels below the motor level can be used in determining motor incomplete status (AIS B versus C).
NOTE: When assessing the extent of motor sparing below the level for distinguishing between AIS B and C, the *motor level* on each side is used; whereas to differentiate between AIS C and D (based on proportion of key muscle functions with strength grade 3 or greater) the single *NLI* is used.

(Note: AIS E is used in follow-up testing when an individual with a documented SCI has recovered normal function. If at initial testing no deficits are found, the individual is neurologically intact; the AIS does not apply).

KNOWLEDGE GAPS AND EMERGING CONCEPTS

The stated purpose of the SCI classification standards since inception has been to facilitate accurate communication between clinicians and researchers working with patients with SCI, and this has remained unchanged. However, the classification standards have not been a static document and there have been several adjustments, revisions, and additional clarifications over the years.

At the time of this writing, the available standards were most recently revised in 2011. In 2013, a new version of the worksheet for ISNCSCI was made available. The new worksheet now lists non-key muscle functions as optional elements that may be used to assign a motor level to differentiate AIS B vs C (Figure 10.1 and Table 10.6). Table 10.11 summarizes the main changes in the 2011 revision of the standards and the 2013 changes in the worksheet.

It is anticipated that there will continue to be additional changes and refinements in the standards with future revisions and updates.

Table 10.11
Recent Revisions and Updates in ISNCSCI and Related Exam Worksheet

- The term deep anal sensation has been replaced by deep anal pressure (DAP). It was felt that the new terminology would reinforce the technique of applying pressure to the anorectal wall with the examiners distal thumb and index finger as opposed to more vigorous techniques

- It has been specified that if sensation is abnormal at C2 and intact on the face, the level should be designated as C1 (for consistency amongst clinicians and researchers)

- It has been clarified that in patients who have light touch or pin-prick sensation at S4–S5, examination for DAP is not required

- The definition for ZPP in patients with a neurologically complete injury (AIS A) has been revised. Specifically, the method used to determine the levels of the ZPP has been changed to include the 'dermatomes and myotomes caudal to the sensory and motor levels on each side of the body that remain partially innervated' in a neurologically complete injury. In the previous edition of the ISNCSCI, the ZPP was determined from the NLI. This distinction is important when discussing the levels of sparing for the ZPP

- The motor and sensory examination is described in greater detail, including specific positions to be used when testing for grade 4 or 5 strength (Tables 10.3 and 10.4)

- Some of the figures on the worksheet have been updated, and the worksheet has been adjusted for ease of use. For example, the 2013 worksheet has both the motor and sensory functions from the right side of the body on one half and motor and sensory functions from the left side on the other half of the worksheet (instead of motor from both sides of the body being on one half and sensory on the other)

- Non-key muscle functions for C5 to T1 and L2 to S1 root levels are now listed on the back of the 2013 version of the worksheet as optional elements that may be used to assign a motor level to differentiate AIS B vs. C (Figure 10.1)

Abbreviations: AIS, ASIA Impairment Scale; ISNCSCI, International Standards for Neurological Classification of Spinal Cord Injury; ZPP, zone of partial preservation.

SUGGESTED READING

American Spinal Injury Association: *International Standards for Neurological and Functional Classification of Spinal Cord Injury, Revised 2011.* Atlanta, GA.

Marino RJ, Jones L, Kirshblum S, Tal J, Dasgupta A. Reliability and repeatability of the motor and sensory examination of the international standards for neurological classification of spinal cord injury. *J Spinal Cord Med.* 2008;31:166-170.

Zariffa J, Kramer JL, Jones LA, et al. Sacral sparing in SCI: beyond the S4-S5 and anorectal examination. *Spine J.* 2012;12(5):389-400.

CHAPTER 11

Traumatic Spinal Cord Injury in Children

GENERAL PRINCIPLES

The primary focus of this chapter is to highlight the unique aspects of traumatic spinal cord injury (SCI) in children. Other disorders of the spinal cord in children, for example, developmental disorders including myelomeningocele (Chapter 22), are discussed elsewhere.

Many aspects of SCI in children and adolescents are similar to adults. However, there are also many unique differences that impact the assessment and management of pediatric SCI (Table 11.1).

Etiology

Motor vehicle accidents are the most common cause of SCI in children as in adults, followed by violence and sports. Violent etiology increases during adolescence, especially among Hispanics and black youth. Behavioral differences and risk exposure account for some of the differences in etiology of spinal injuries between children and adults. Specific measures for prevention of SCI, including those that are particularly applicable to children, are discussed in Chapter 5.

There are some unique etiologies of SCI in children. These include:

Lap-belt injury: This is most common in children between 40 and 60 pounds. The lap seat belt can act as a fulcrum during impact, causing flexion-distraction forces on the mid-lumbar spine. This is typically related to absence of booster seat use in a child who is too short to be sitting without it and an improperly fitted seat belt. SCI may be accompanied by abdominal bruising or intra-abdominal bleeding. Vertebral injury most commonly occurs between L2 and L4, and the typical injury is a transverse fracture going through the vertebral body and posterior elements (Chance fracture). Twenty-five percent to 30% have SCI without radiological abnormalities (SCIWORA). Preventive measures include properly secured booster seats for ages 4 to 8 years (and for height up to 4ft., 9 in.), and proper placement of seat belts.

Table 11.1

Unique Aspects of SCI in Children Compared to Adults

Etiology	■ Though vehicular crashes are the most common cause as in adults, there are also some unique causes of injury, e.g., lap-belt injury, birth injuries, child abuse
Gender distribution	■ Equal in males and females up to age 3 yrs; progressively increasing male preponderance after that (unlike adults where ~80% are male)
Neurological category of injury	■ Complete paraplegia is more common in children under 10 yrs of age (~2/3rd have paraplegia, 2/3rd have complete SCI) ■ High cervical injury more common in infants from 0–2 yrs of age (relatively large heads, poorly developed neck muscles)
Pathophysiology	■ Children have increased elasticity of the spine, a less flexible spinal cord, and vertebral anatomical differences that result in greater resistance being shifted to ligaments; these factors contribute to increased proportion of SCIWORA ■ Delayed neurological abnormalities may be more common in children
Clinical assessment	■ Eliciting history of neck discomfort in young children may be difficult; neurological exam may be less reliable; these factors contribute to challenges in clearance of the cervical spine
Imaging	■ Higher incidence of SCIWORA (although abnormalities can often be seen on MRI) ■ Normal findings in children (e.g., normally anteriorly wedged configuration of the vertebral body, absent anterior ossification of the atlas, 3–4.5 mm atlanto-dental interval) that may be considered pathological in adults, can lead to misinterpretation of plain radiographs
Transportation/ immobilization	■ Backboard with occipital recess (or padding under shoulder to raise torso) needed for neutral spine alignment in view of proportionately larger head size in children <8 yrs of age ■ Halo fixation in young children done with more pins to allow for lesser torque and pin pressure in view of thinner skull bones
Complications	■ Scoliosis, hip instability, and limb growth problems are common following SCI occurring at <8–10 yrs of age, before skeletal maturity ■ Immobilization hypercalcemia in first 3 months postinjury is especially common in adolescents males ■ Latex allergy is common, probably related to young age of initial exposure and longer exposure ■ Venous thrombo-embolism is less common in children <12 yrs of age
Psychosocial considerations	■ Unique issues related to each developmental stage e.g., schooling, adolescence, transition to adulthood
Rehabilitation	■ Developmentally based goals needed; dynamic, responsive to changing needs at each developmental stage ■ Particular involvement of family and school in the rehabilitation team ■ Incorporation of recreation and play into rehabilitation program is especially important

Abbreviation: SCIWORA, spinal cord injury without radiological abnormalities.

Birth injuries: Neonatal SCI occurs in 1 per 60,000 births. Upper cervical injury occurs with torsional injury during delivery (e.g., during difficult forceps delivery), while lower cervical/upper thoracic injuries occur with breech delivery. May have associated injuries (brachial plexus, hypoxic brain injury).

Child abuse: Spinal injuries related to nonaccidental trauma are usually the result of shaking of the infant or young child. Spine injuries may be overlooked if they are not associated with clinical findings. There is a propensity for vertebral body and anterior end plate injury, consistent with hyper-flexion injury.

Other conditions associated with SCI in children include Down syndrome with atlanto-axial instability juvenile rheumatoid arthritis, and skeletal dysplasia.

Epidemiology

Three percent to 5% of SCI in the United States occurs in children less than 15 years. Up to 3 years of age, SCI occurs equally in males and females, with an increasing male preponderance as age increases.

Children under 8 to 10 years are more likely to have paraplegia and complete lesions than adults.

Infants and younger children ages 0 to 2 years have a greater proportion of high cervical injuries from C1 to C4, probably related to disproportionately large heads and underdeveloped neck muscles (see below).

Pathophysiology

There is a relative cephalo-cervical disproportion in young children. The average weight of a baby's head is 25% of body mass compared to 10% in adults. This, combined with poorly developed cervical musculature, puts the infants' cervical spine at a mechanical disadvantage and accounts for the relatively high incidence of high cervical injury in infants.

Children have increased elasticity of the spine, a less flexible spinal cord, and vertebral anatomical differences (e.g., anteriorly wedged orientation of vertebral bodies, horizontal orientation of facets, and absence of uncinate processes on the vertebral bodies) that result in greater resistance being shifted to ligaments rather than to the bones. This helps explain the high incidence of SCIWORA in children; reported to be over 60% of SCI in children less than 5 years of age. SCIWORA usually occurs in the cervical cord, most commonly at C5–C8 levels.

Delayed neurological abnormalities are more common in children, including those with SCIWORA. Possible factors may include occult injury with repeated trauma, cord swelling, or post-traumatic radicular artery occlusion.

Associated Conditions and Complications in Pediatric SCI

SCI affects each body system in children as in adults, including bladder and bowel dysfunction, autonomic and cardiovascular dysfunction, respiratory problems, metabolic problems, pressure ulcers, and spasticity.

Certain complications occur more frequently in children. Scoliosis, hip-instability, and impaired growth of the paralyzed limb are common after SCI sustained at less than 8 to 10 years of age prior to development of skeletal maturity. Young children and infants with tetraplegia and related thermoregulatory problems are especially vulnerable to environmental temperature extremes due to relatively large surface area and decreased ability to communicate and problem solve. Latex allergy may occur and is probably due to frequent exposure to latex containing medical equipment/supplies. Young age at initial exposure and longer duration of exposure are risk factors. Hypercalcemia in the first 3 months postinjury is especially common in adolescent males due to high bone turnover (Chapter 39B, Table 39B.1).

CLINICAL CONSIDERATIONS

Assessment

History and Physical Exam
Clinical assessment of spinal injury in children can offer special challenges. Eliciting history of neck discomfort in young children may be difficult.

Neurological assessment and classification of SCI should be done in accordance with the International Standards for Neurological Classification of SCI, but the neurological exam may be less reliable and difficult to interpret in children, and is not useful in children younger than 4 years. Certain elements of the exam (anorectal exam, pin-prick testing) are often difficult to complete and interpret in children younger than 10 years. When assessing motor function, it is important to take into account that normal motor strength in a young child is different from that in older teens or adults.

Cervical spine clearance can be particularly difficult to do in children because of these reasons.

Imaging
Some special considerations are needed when assessing spinal radiographs of children. Normal findings in children (e.g., normally anteriorly wedged configuration of the vertebral body, absent anterior ossification of the atlas, 3–4.5 mm atlanto-dental interval) that may be considered pathological in adults, can lead to misinterpretation of plain radiographs by physicians not used to reading these films in young children.

As mentioned previously, there is a high incidence of SCIWORA in children, although abnormalities can usually be seen on magnetic resonance imaging (MRI) in cases where the plain radiographs look normal.

Management
The basic principles of management of SCI in children parallel those in adults, although there are some important differences.

Initial Management
In prehospital care, priorities are centered around resuscitation, airway, breathing, and circulation, evaluation, immobilization, and safe and expeditious transportation to the definitive medical care facility. For spinal stabilization in children less than 8 years of age, child-specific spine boards with a cut-out recess for the occiput should be used. Immobilization on a standard spine board can cause excessive neck flexion because of proportionately larger head size compared with the rest of the body. If a standard spine board is used, raising the torso 2 to 4 cm above the head with a mattress pad under the shoulder and chest will avoid excessive neck flexion.

Surgical Management
As in adults, the main considerations in surgical treatment are to decompress the neural elements and stabilize the spine to prevent further injury. Certain anatomic and developmental factors are important to consider in planning surgery. Spinal fusion and related growth arrest can have a significant impact on the developing spine so trying to limit the number of levels fused is appropriate. It is important to consider the effect of an isolated fusion on subsequent development of excessive kyphosis. Because of the relatively better recuperative capacity in children, some injuries that would require surgical stabilization in adults may only need immobilizing in children.

Halo traction is possible even in young children. The primary concern is to avoid excessive pressure and skull erosion from the pins. For halo use in infants and younger children 8 to 10 pins, instead of four pins as in adults, are used and lower torque force is applied. A more frequently used option to stabilize the spine currently is custom construction of an orthosis using thermoplastic material.

Rehabilitation
In addition to the rehabilitation principles that apply to adults with SCI, there are some unique aspects to rehabilitation of children with SCI. It is important to be aware of the special needs of the child at various levels of development and to incorporate development-based goals (Table 11.2).

The specialized needs of the individual vary from infancy through childhood to teen years and continue into transition to adulthood. Responsiveness to changing needs at different development stages is crucial. Equipment needs also change because of change in size and needs as children grow. Growth spurt during adolescence increases the tendency to develop scoliosis.

The role of the family in rehabilitation of SCI is vital, and is even more significant in children. It is important to remain sensitive to the impact of the child's

Table 11.2

Developmental Age-Related Functional Goals	
Functional Goal/Skill	Starting Age
Assistive devices for standing (e.g., parapodium)	1–1.5 yrs
Ambulatory assistive devices	2–3 yrs
Independent wheelchair mobility	2–3 yrs
Establishment of bowel program	2–4 yrs
Ability to self-catheterize	5–6 yrs
Independence in bowel program	5–7 yrs
Adult level basic activities of daily living skills	7 yrs

SCI on the family, and to support parents through the process and engage their involvement and cooperation in rehabilitation.

In addition to the various participants and disciplines that provide multidisciplinary rehabilitation of individuals with SCI at any age, teachers and child life specialists are important additional members of the rehabilitation team for children. An important part of rehabilitation is to return the child to the most appropriate school setting. Therapy and support is provided at the school as needed. Ongoing communication with the school is very important especially during the transition phase.

Bowel and bladder training can begin in preschool years when children normally become toilet trained. At development age of 5 to 6 years, those with good hand function and adequate sitting balance can become independent in self-catheterization, and can soon after learn to insert a suppository if needed for bowel care. Surgical options are sometimes considered in children for bladder or bowel care. The Mitrofanoff procedure creates a stoma on the abdominal wall, typically through the umbilicus, to allow accessibility for bladder catheterization. A surgical option for bowel evacuation in children is the Malone procedure or antegrade continence enema (ACE), which creates a stoma (catheterizable appendicostomy) to allow antegrade use of enemas for bowel evacuation.

Rehabilitation of children typically incorporates recreation and play as important components. Adaptive sports can be very beneficial.

Psychosocial Considerations

Decreased ability to explore environment in a developmentally appropriate manner due to limited mobility after SCI can have a significant psychosocial, educational, or vocational impact. The influence of peers becomes especially significant in school years. Adolescence can be particularly tumultuous. Anger or rebelliousness may surface. Physical appearance and relationship issues may arise. Support groups and sexual counseling are important at this stage.

Ongoing Medical Management and Continuing Care
General pediatric and wellness care is important to incorporate in management. In addition to the general immunization schedule, pneumococcus and influenza vaccination is indicated to decrease the risk of chest infections. Attention to nutrition is vital, avoiding both malnutrition and obesity.

Prevention, expeditious identification, and management of complications is an essential part of ongoing management and is similar to adults with SCI in many aspects.

Autonomic dysreflexia (AD) in children can occur with SCI above T6 neurological level, as in adults with similar etiology and pathophysiology. Young children may not be able to readily communicate symptoms of headache. It is important to use appropriate sized cuff to measure blood pressure in children (width of cuff ~ 40% of arm circumference); too large cuffs tend to underestimate and small cuffs tend to overestimate blood pressure. Developmental variations in baseline blood pressure in children are important to keep in mind. Systolic blood pressure greater than 15 to 20 mmHg above baseline in adolescents and greater than 15 mmHg in children may be a sign of AD.

Latex allergy is probably due to frequent exposure to latex containing medical equipment/supplies. Young age at initial exposure and longer duration of exposure are risk factors. Clinical features include urticaria, angioedema, wheezing, and anaphylaxis. Intra-operative (e.g., latex glove contact) reaction may be missed due to skin coverage by surgical drapes and may manifest with anaphylactic reaction, unexplained hypotension, and tachycardia. History (e.g., rash with latex balloon, allergies to certain fruits) may provide a clue. Skin tests can be helpful in establishing diagnosis. Preventive measures include maintenance of a latex free environment, medical alert identification, and ready access to auto-injectable epinephrine (EpiPen) for emergency use.

Scoliosis is extremely common if SCI occurs before skeletal maturity, with a large proportion requiring surgical correction. Spine radiographs to monitor for scoliosis are recommended every 6 months prior to puberty and annually after that. Problems include pelvic obliquity and seated posture with reduced upper extremity function, pressure ulcers, pain, gastrointestinal, and cardiovascular dysfunction.

- Prophylactic bracing with thoracolumbosacral orthosis (TLSO) may delay need for surgery for curves less than 20° (though may interfere with mobility and self-care)
- Surgical correction indicated for curves greater than 40° in children over 10. Younger children can be managed conservatively for curves up to 80° if flexible and decrease in a TLSO, otherwise surgery is indicated

Hip instability (sublaxation, dislocation, contractures) is common with SCI less than 8 to 10 years of age, and may require surgical correction for improving function or if associated with complications (pressure ulcers, spasticity, AD). Preventive measures include soft tissue stretching, spasticity management, and prophylactic (abduction) bracing.

Transition to adulthood requires multidimensional planning and integration including attention to independent living, employment, financial independence, social participation, and continuing health care into adulthood.

KNOWLEDGE GAPS AND EMERGING CONCEPTS

Additional prospective studies are needed to better delineate optimal timing and indications of surgical decompression of SCI in children. Further research is needed on etiology and treatment options for SCIWORA. Longitudinal studies will be helpful to determine the natural history of neurological recovery in children.

Transition of children with SCI into adulthood is an area where research is relatively sparse and additional study is needed.

SUGGESTED READING

Calhoun CL, Schottler J, Vogel LC. Recommendations for mobility in children with spinal cord injury. *Top Spinal Cord Inj Rehabil.* 2013;19(2):142-151.

Mulcahey MJ, Gaughan JP, Betz RR, Samdani AF, Barakat N, Hunter LN. Neuromuscular scoliosis in children with spinal cord injury. *Top Spinal Cord Inj Rehabil.* 2013;19(2):96-103.

Parent S, Dimar J, Dekutoski M, Roy-Beaudry M. Unique features of pediatric spinal cord injury. *Spine (Phila Pa 1976).* 2010;35(21 suppl):S202-S208.

ParentS, Mac-Thiong JM, Roy-Beaudry M, Sosa JF, Labelle H. Spinal cord injury in the pediatric population: a systematic review of the literature. *J Neurotrauma.* 2011;28(8):1515-1524.

Rozzelle CJ, Aarabi B, Dhall SS, et al. Management of pediatric cervical spine and spinal cord injuries. *Neurosurgery.* 2013;72(suppl 2):205-226.

Vogel L, Samdani A, Chafetz R, Gaughan J, Betz R, Mulcahey MJ. Intra rater agreement of the anorectal exam and classification of injury severity in children with spinal cord injury. *Spinal Cord.* 2009;47:687-691.

Vogel LC, Betz RR, Mulcahey MJ. Spinal cord injuries in children and adolescents. *Handb Clin Neurol.* 2012;109:131-148.

III. Nontraumatic Myelopathies

CHAPTER 12

Nontraumatic Myelopathies: Overview and Approach

GENERAL PRINCIPLES

A variety of nontraumatic conditions can involve the spinal cord (Table 12.1). Nontraumatic spinal cord involvement in the United States and other developed countries is most often related to degenerative conditions of the spine, followed by spinal tumors. On the other hand, infections, including tuberculosis and HIV, are the predominant cause of nontraumatic myelopathy in many developing countries.

While systems of care for people with traumatic spinal cord injury (SCI) have evolved over the past few decades, barring a few exceptions, systems of care for the assessment and management of nontraumatic myelopathies are less well defined and these disorders have been less well studied, despite their relative overall high prevalence.

However, SCI centers are now reporting increasing proportions of admissions for nontraumatic spinal cord injuries over the last several years, and a more thorough understanding and study of these disorders is warranted.

There is much in common between the presentation, consequences, complications, and management of traumatic and nontraumatic myelopathies. However, there are also some significant differences (Table 12.2).

CLINICAL CONSIDERATIONS

Assessment

Approach to assessment depends on the presentation and context.

Often the first priority is to exclude a treatable compression of the spinal cord (Table 12.3). Neck or back pain, bladder dysfunction, and sensory symptoms

Table 12.1

Causes of Nontraumatic Myelopathy

1. Spondylotic/degenerative
   a. Cervical spondylotic myelopathy
   b. Lumbar stenosis or disk-related cauda equina syndrome
2. Neoplastic
   a. Spinal metastases
   b. Primary spinal tumors
3. Vascular
   a. Ischemic
   b. Hemorrhagic
4. Infectious (bacterial, viral, mycoplasma, parasitic)
5. Inflammatory
   a. Multiple sclerosis
   b. Acute transverse myelitis, acute disseminated encephalomyelitis (ADEM)
   c. Neuromyelitis optica
   d. Connective tissue disorders
      i. Systemic lupus erythematosus
      ii. Sjögren-related
      iii. Sarcoidosis
      iv. Vasculitis
   e. Arachnoiditis
6. Metabolic/nutritional
   a. Vitamin B12 deficiency (subacute combined degeneration)
   b. Copper deficiency
7. Toxic/environmental
   a. Chemical
   b. Radiation
   c. Electrical
   d. Lightning
   e. Decompression sickness
8. Developmental and hereditary conditions
   a. Syringomyelia (often with Chiari malformation)
   b. Myelomeningocele
   c. Tethered cord syndrome
   d. Inherited disorders of metabolism
   e. Spinocerebellar degeneration
   f. Hereditary spastic paraplegia
   g. Spinal muscular atrophy
9. Motor neuron disease/amyotrophic lateral sclerosis

Table 12.2

Characteristics of Nontraumatic Versus Traumatic Myelopathies

	Traumatic	Nontraumatic
Age of onset	Younger (although increasing incidence in older adults)	Depends on the underlying etiology, but older overall
Gender distribution	80% male, 20% females	Higher percent of females
Neurological level	Tetraplegia or paraplegia	More often paraplegia
Completeness of injury	Complete or incomplete	More often incomplete
Neurological examination and classification	Based on the International Standards for Neurological Classification of Spinal Cord Injury (ISNCSCI)	While examination based on ISNCSCI can also apply to several nontraumatic myelopathies, it is inappropriate for others, e.g., multiple sclerosis (with the exception of transverse myelitis) or amyotrophic lateral sclerosis
Comorbidities	Fewer comorbidities with younger age	Higher prevalence of age-related comorbidities, may affect management and outcomes
Complications	Multiple complications, can affect all body systems	Many of the same complications as in traumatic but less prevalence of autonomic dysreflexia, orthostatic hypotension, venous thrombo-embolism, and pneumonia reported

Abbreviation: ISNCSCI, International Standards for Neurological Classification of Spinal Cord Injury.

Table 12.3

Causes of Compressive Myelopathy

Posttraumatic

Epidural, intradural, or intramedullary tumor

Epidural abscess

Hemorrhage

Cervical spondylosis, spinal stenosis

Midline disk herniation, subluxation, or dislocation

often accompany or precede the paralysis caused by epidural compression. Magnetic resonance imaging (MRI) with gadolinium infusion, focused on the clinically suspected area, is often the initial test of choice.

Once spinal cord compression is excluded, additional investigation is often required to establish the cause of acute myelopathy including laboratory studies and often a lumbar puncture (Table 12.4).

While assessment and classification based on the International Standards for Neurological Classification of SCI can be applied to several types of nontraumatic myelopathies that present with a neurological level, it is not applicable to disorders such as multiple sclerosis (MS) (except when there is a distinct sensory level as in transverse myelitis) or amyotrophic lateral sclerosis (ALS).

Management

Management depends on the underlying cause, associated impairments, and functional limitations.

Several of the same complications may occur with nontraumatic myelopathies as with traumatic SCI, including skin, bowel, and bladder dysfunction. However, some complications are reported to be significantly less common including

Table 12.4

Evaluation of Acute Transverse Myelopathy

Rationale/Etiology Being Evaluated	Tests
Compressive causes (Table 12.3)	Spinal imaging, MRI with and without contrast
Intrathecal inflammation or infection	Cerebrospinal fluid studies, including: Cell count, protein, glucose, IgG index/synthesis rate, oligoclonal bands, VDRL; Gram's stain, acid-fast bacilli, and India ink stains; PCR viral studies; antibody for Borrelia, Mycoplasma, and Chlamydia; viral, bacterial, mycobacterial, and fungal cultures
Infectious causes	Blood studies for infection: e.g., HIV; RPR; enterovirus antibody; mumps, measles, rubella, antibodies
Immune-mediated etiology	ESR; ANA; dsDNA; rheumatoid factor; complement levels; antiphospholipid and anticardiolipin antibodies Sjögren syndrome suspected: Schirmer test, salivary gland scintography, and salivary/lacrimal gland biopsy Sarcoidosis: Serum angiotensin-converting enzyme; serum Ca; 24-h urine Ca; chest x-ray; chest CT; total body gallium scan; lymph node biopsy
Demyelinating disease	Brain MRI, evoked potentials, oligoclonal bands
Vascular causes	CT myelogram, spinal angiogram

Abbreviations: ANA, antinuclear antibodies; CT, computerized tomography; dsDNA, double-stranded DNA; ESR, erythrocyte sedimentation rate; PCR, polymerase chain reaction; RPR, rapid plasma reagin (test); VDRL, Venereal Disease Research Laboratory.

autonomic dysreflexia, orthostatic hypotension, venous thrombo-embolism, and pneumonia. Lower neurological level of injury and greater incompleteness of injury likely contribute to these differences.

KNOWLEDGE GAPS AND EMERGING CONCEPTS

Systems of care for the assessment and management of nontraumatic myelopathies are less well defined than those for traumatic SCI, and these disorders have not been as well studied.

SUGGESTED READING

McKinley WO. Nontraumatic spinal cord injury/disease: etiologies and outcomes. *Top Spinal Cord Inj Rehabil.* 2008;14(2):1-9.
McKinley WO, Seel RT, Hardman JT. Nontraumatic spinal cord injury: incidence, epidemiology, and functional outcome. *Arch Phys Med Rehabil.* 1999;80(6):619-623.
New PW, Cripps RA, Bonne Lee B. Global maps of non-traumatic spinal cord injury epidemiology: towards a living data repository. *Spinal Cord.* 2013 Jan 15. Epub 2013 Jan 15.

CHAPTER 13

Cervical Spondylotic Myelopathy

GENERAL PRINCIPLES

Cervical spondylotic myelopathy (CSM) is a condition in which the spinal cord is damaged, either directly by traumatic compression and abnormal movement, or indirectly by ischemia due to arterial compression, venous stasis, or other consequences of the degenerative changes that characterize cervical spondylosis.

The average anteroposterior (AP) diameter of the canal measures ~17 mm from C3–C7. The space required by the spinal cord averages 10 mm. An absolute spinal canal stenosis exists with a sagittal diameter of less than 10 mm. The stenosis is relative if the diameter is 10 to 13 mm.

Etiology

CSM results from degenerative changes that occur in the cervical spine, including the joints, intervertebral discs, ligaments, and connective tissue.

A congenitally narrow canal lowers the threshold by which trivial trauma or early degenerative changes may cause myelopathy.

Less common etiologies include ossification of the posterior longitudinal ligament, which has a particularly high incidence in the Asian/Japanese population.

Epidemiology

CSM is the most common cause of spinal cord dysfunction in persons more than 55 years of age in North America. Men are affected more than women.

The most frequently involved levels are the more mobile segments: C5-C6, C6-C7, and C4-C5.

Patients older than age 60 often have multi-segmental disease.

Pathophysiology

Both static and dynamic factors contribute to the development of CSM.

Static Factors
Static factors include narrowing of the spinal canal from: decreased height of the degenerating inter-vertebral disk leading to increased sagittal diameter and bulging of the disk, reactive hypertrophy and osteophyte formation at the vertebral end plates, projection of osteophytes from the uncovertebral and facet joints, and hypertrophy of facet capsules and ligamentum flavum.

Dynamic Factors
Dynamic factors may also affect spinal canal dimensions. With hyperextension, the ligamentum flavum buckles into the canal and the degenerated disk may bulge posteriorly, which decreases the space available for the cord. In those with a kyphotic sagittal alignment, the cord can become tethered over spondylotic anterior elements during flexion even though the canal diameter is increased. As spinal segments are stiffened by spondylotic change, adjacent segments may develop relative hypermobility or even subluxation, which contributes to cord impingement.

Pathological Changes
Pathological cord findings in cervical myelopathy include gray as well as white matter destruction, with ascending and descending demyelination. There is relative sparing of anterior columns.

The extent to which direct mechanical compression of neural elements and neuroischemia contribute to pathological changes is unclear. With progressive compression, blood flow through the terminal branches of the anterior spinal artery within the spinal cord maybe interrupted.

Secondary spinal cord injury (SCI) in CSM is likely related to a variety of mechanisms such as glutamate toxicity, free radical mediated cell injury, and apoptosis.

Disease Course

Natural history of CSM is highly variable and still not well defined. Onset is typically insidious but may be acute, for example, with a hyperextension injury after a fall.

Some patients experience a benign clinical course with neurological improvement, though complete resolution is infrequent. The majority, however, do not experience spontaneous improvement and may experience neurological deterioration over time. Stepwise neurological worsening with interspersed periods of quiescent stability is common; less commonly patients may experience slow, steady progression.

Prognostic Indicators
Favorable prognostic indicators include symptoms of less than 1 year duration, mild myelopathic symptoms at presentation, and younger age at initial presentation. Motor symptoms tend to be more progressive and less likely to improve than sensory abnormalities.

Associated Conditions and Complications
CSM often occurs concomitantly with cervical radiculopathy. Over 5% of patients with CSM are estimated to have coexisting lumbar stenosis, which may complicate assessment and diagnosis. Patients with CSM may develop acute cord compression with central cord syndrome even with relatively minor hyperextension trauma, for example, after a fall.

CLINICAL CONSIDERATIONS

Assessment

History
Depending on the magnitude and chronicity of the spinal cord dysfunction, patients may be asymptomatic or severely disabled. Patients with CSM present with a broad spectrum of signs and symptoms.

Early symptoms include diminished hand dexterity and subtle changes in balance and gait with leg stiffness, incoordination, and/or weakness. Patients may present with frequent falls. Initial sensory complaints are often predominant in the upper extremities.

Compromised bladder or bowel function is less common, but when present is associated with greater disease severity.

Occipital headache, neck and/or upper extremity pain from associated radiculopathy is common.

Physical Examination
Spastic paraplegia is a typical finding reflecting early involvement of the corticospinal tracts.

Pathological reflexes such as Hoffman sign, Babinski sign, hyperreflexia in lower extremity muscle stretch reflexes (MSR), and clonus are consistent with cord compression. A normal jaw MSR helps to distinguish CSM from intracranial pathology. The presence of concomitant lumbar stenosis may mask lower extremity hyperreflexia.

Upper motor neuron signs may be accompanied by lower motor neuron signs such as hyporeflexia and fasciculations in the upper extremities at the level of cord or root compression (e.g., shoulder girdle muscle wasting and fasciculations at C5-C6 or intrinsic hand muscle atrophy at C8-T1).

Sensory changes vary according to the location and extent of spinal cord dysfunction. Altered vibratory and proprioceptive changes are often present. Posterior column dysfunction may result in ataxia, positive Rhomberg's sign, and a wide-based gait.

Patients with CSM who develop a central cord syndrome after hyperextension injury typically manifest with disproportionately greater upper extremity than lower extremity weakness and relative sacral sensory sparing.

Limited neck range of motion reflects underlying spondylosis. Patients may exhibit L'hermittes phenomenon upon neck flexion, characterized by a brief shock-like sensation down the spine and extremities.

Assessment of Impairment and Function
Grip strength evaluation with a dynamometer, the 10-second step test, and the 10-second open-and-close-hand test are valid measures for assessment of impairment and are useful tools to measure natural history and treatment efficacy. Normal subjects can perform the latter two tests more than 15 and 20 times respectively.

Gait analysis including changes in walking speed has been shown to be a reliable method of monitoring response to treatment.

Scales for evaluation of CSM include the modified Japanese Orthopedic Association (mJOA) scale which assesses items related to motor and sensory function of upper and lower extremities and bladder function. The myelopathy disability index (MDI) is another instrument that includes items regarding activities of daily living (ADL) that are commonly affected by CSM.

Diagnostic Tests
Imaging
Imaging is the key to diagnosis. Antero-posterior, lateral, and oblique radiographs should be performed in those with suspected CSM.

Spondylotic changes such as disk space narrowing and osteophyte formation and listhesis are often present (although should be interpreted with the awareness that such changes are common with increasing age even in the absence of CSM). Any decrease in segmental and global lumbar lordosis should be noted.

The absolute sagittal diameter of the spinal canal should be measured from the posterior aspect of the mid-vertebral body to the spinolaminar line. The sagittal canal diameter to 13 mm or less at C3 to C7 is considered stenotic, but the absolute measurement is affected by the degree of magnification of the radiograph. The ratio of the sagittal canal diameter to mid-vertebral body diameter (Torg-Pavlov ratio) of 0.8 or less on a standard lateral radiograph is considered evidence of spinal canal stenosis (Table 13.1). Calculating this ratio eliminates the influence of magnification differences between radiographs,

Table 13.1
Torg-Pavlov Ratio

Measured on a Conventional Lateral Radiograph

Ratio of:

a. The sagittal diameter of the spinal canal (measured as the shortest distance from the midpoint of the posterior surface of the vertebral body to the spinolaminar line), and

b. Sagittal diameter of the vertebral body (measured between the midpoints of the anterior and posterior surfaces of the vertebral body)

Ratio of a/b <0.8 is considered to be significant for cervical spinal stenosis (normal ratio of a/b is ~1.0)

Using a ratio vs the absolute canal diameter eliminates influence of magnification differences between radiographs

Limitations:

Considered to be highly sensitive but of low predictive value

Does not take into account spondylotic changes that occur in the vicinity of the intervertebral disk, or the contribution of soft tissue to canal narrowing

Clinical relevance, by itself, to predict risk of myelopathy after trauma is uncertain

Should not be used as an indication in itself to perform prophylactic surgery

---

and offers a universally comparable numeric value. Although some correlation has been suggested, the role of the Torg-Pavlov ratio for predicting clinically relevant risk of occurrence of SCI after a traumatic event has not been conclusively established.

Lateral flexion and extension radiographs provide assessment of range of motion and instability.

Magnetic resonance imaging (MRI) is useful for evaluation of the soft tissues and neural elements. The effect of CSM on the size and shape of the spinal cord should be assessed. Relatively good correlation has been reported between clinical severity of CSM and the presence of a region of high signal intensity in T2-weighted MR images. CT myelography has a limited role but may provide additional information regarding the bony architecture and stenosing osseous structures.

Lumbar spinal imaging may be indicated in cases of suspected concomitant lumbar spinal stenosis.

Laboratory studies are primarily done to rule out other etiologies in the differential diagnosis of CSM.

Electrodiagnostic testing is helpful for evaluating root involvement and to exclude coexisting or other differentials such as amyotrophic lateral sclerosis or neuropathies.

Evoked potential testing may have a useful role in certain specific situations for diagnosis and prognosis, and in intra-operative monitoring during high risk spine surgery. Somatosensory evoked potentials (SSEP) can provide indication of posterior column function but don't provide information about motor tracts and are not sufficiently precise to localize the cord involvement. Motor evoked potential (MEP) elicited with transcranial magnetic stimulation evaluate motor tracts have been shown to correlate with clinical features and imaging. Normal MEPs predicted favorable prognosis in a study of patients with MRI features of asymptomatic CSM.

Differential Diagnosis
Although CSM is the most common cause of cervical myelopathy it is important to consider a broad differential diagnosis. This includes motor neuron disease, multiple sclerosis and other demyelinating conditions, other causes of spinal cord dysfunction (e.g., tumors, syringomyelia, infectious, inflammatory, and nutritional myelopathies), peripheral and entrapment neuropathies, intracranial pathology, and systemic causes of hyperreflexia.

It is important to remember that these conditions may coexist with CSM.

Management

The varied natural history of the disease makes evaluation of treatment options challenging. Definitive treatment guidelines for CSM are limited with several areas of controversy and lack of consensus.

Medical and Rehabilitative Management
Patients without major neurological deficits but with radiological evidence of cord compression may be treated conservatively and monitored. The role of surgical decompression in this setting remains controversial. A soft cervical collar may limit additional injury by acting as a restraint to extremes of movement and there are some reports of association of its use with neurological improvement although the evidence for this is limited. More rigid collars are often discarded if prescribed for long-term use. Discouragement from high risk and high impact activities is prudent. Nonsteroidal anti-inflammatory drugs (NSAIDS) are used for symptomatic pain management.

Rehabilitation interventions depend on the extent and type of neurological deficit. Mobility assessment, gait training, and fall risk management are important components in those with significant lower extremity neurological impairment. Patients with upper extremity weakness and impaired hand dexterity are candidates for ADL assessment and training and prescription of appropriate adaptive equipment. There is evidence to suggest that patients with spinal cord dysfunction due to CSM make significant functional gains with inpatient rehabilitation and can achieve functional outcomes similar to those with traumatic SCI.

Prompt management and secondary prevention of complications such as urinary incontinence, urinary tract infections, pressure ulcers, and venous thromboembolism is important in those with significant spinal cord dysfunction.

Surgical Management
In the setting of progressive neurological deficit with CSM, surgical decompression should be considered, although evidence-based consensus about the long-term effectiveness of surgical intervention and the specific surgical approach is still limited.

Both anterior and posterior surgical approaches have been used to treat CSM. The choice of technique depends upon factors including location of the primary compressive lesion, presence of spinal instability, spinal alignment, number of levels involved, and surgeon preference. Anterior approaches include anterior cervical discectomy and fusion or cervical corporectomy. The presence of cervical kyphosis usually requires an anterior approach. Patients who have widespread stenosis with multi-segmental cord compression, ligamentum flavum buckling, or technical/mechanical factors that interfere with an anterior approach, may be candidates for posterior decompression. Laminectomy alone carries the risk of developing postoperative kyphotic deformity which is lessened with other posterior approaches such as laminectomy with fusion, or laminoplasty. A high incidence of C5 motor root paralysis has been reported with laminoplasty. Disk arthroplasty in conjunction with decompression procedures has been hypothesized to decrease the incidence of adjacent level disease. While initial results have been promising longer follow-up is needed to justify the additional expense as well as to identify potential long-term complications.

Patient Education
Patients should be fully informed of the risk, benefits, and limitations of various surgical and nonsurgical treatment options so they can participate in making informed decisions about their care.

Practice Pearls

Routinely consider CSM in the differential diagnosis of unexplained subtle gait abnormalities or hyperreflexia in elderly patients.

Don't assume that CSM is the primary cause of neurological impairment just because there is radiological evidence of cervical spondylosis without evaluating for other conditions.

Remember that concomitant lumbar stenosis may cause diagnostic confusion by masking typical finding of CSM such as hyperreflexia.

KNOWLEDGE GAPS AND EMERGING CONCEPTS

Recent advances in novel neuroimaging techniques are likely to play a key future role in assessment and management of CSM. Spinal diffusion tensor imaging (DTI) analyzes movement of extracellular water within white matter fibers, provides ability to perform three-dimensional reconstruction of the spinal cord, and can help quantify severity of injury to individual white matter tracts. Magnetic resonance spectroscopy (MRS) offers metabolic information regarding cellular biochemistry and function of neural structures within the spinal cord. There is also emerging interest in using functional MRI of the brain to study cortical reorganization in response to CSM, which may provide an explanation of why some patients with radiological evidence of severe CSM are able to function with relatively minor neurological deficits.

Given the fact that some patients with CSM do not experience neurological improvement following surgery despite MRI evidence of alleviation of the spinal cord compression, there is growing interest in identifying cellular mechanisms affecting spinal cord function. There are efforts to develop appropriate chronic SCI animal models to study targeted therapies that directly address the biological injury on a molecular level.

There are controversies about the natural history of CSM as well as the role and long-term outcomes of conservative versus surgical treatment of patients with mild symptoms. Uniform consensus about the preferred surgical approaches is lacking. Randomized clinical studies are needed to resolve these issues.

SUGGESTED READING

Aebli N, Wicki AG, Rüegg TB, Petrou N, Eisenlohr H, Krebs J. The Torg-Pavlov ratio for the prediction of acute spinal cord injury after a minor trauma to the cervical spine. *Spine J.* 2013;13(6):605-612.

Edwards CC II, Riew KD, Anderson PA, Hilibrand AS, Vaccaro AF. Cervical myelopathy. Current diagnostic and treatment strategies. *Spine J.* 2003;3(1):68-81.

Ghogawala Z, Whitmore RG. Asymptomatic cervical canal stenosis: is there a risk of spinal cord injury? *Spine J.* 2013;13(6):613-614.

Karadimas SK, Erwin WM, Ely CG, Dettori JR, Fehlings MG. The pathophysiology and natural history of cervical spondylotic myelopathy. *Spine (Phila Pa 1976).* October 15, 2013;38(22)(suppl 1):S21-S36

Klineberg E. Cervical spondylotic myelopathy: a review of the evidence. *Orthop Clin North Am.* 2010;41(2):193-202.

Matz PG, Anderson PA, Holly LT, et al. Joint Section on Disorders of the Spine and Peripheral Nerves of the American Association of Neurological Surgeons and Congress of Neurological Surgeons. The natural history of cervical spondylotic myelopathy. *J Neurosurg Spine.* 2009;11(2):104-111.

McKinley WO, Tellis AA, Cifu DX, et al. Rehabilitation outcome of individuals with nontraumatic myelopathy resulting from spinal stenosis. *J Spinal Cord Med.* 1998;21(2):131-136.

Nikolaidis I, Fouyas IP, Sandercock PA, Statham PF. Surgery for cervical radiculopathy or myelopathy. *Cochrane Database Syst Rev.* 2010;(1):CD001466.

Sabharwal S. *Cervical Spondylotic Myelopathy.* PM&R Knowledge NOW/American Academy of Physical Medicine and Rehabilitation. http://now.aapmr.org/cns/sci-disorders/Pages/Cervical-Spondylotic-Myelopathy.aspx. Published November 3, 2012. Modified June 8, 2013.

CHAPTER 14

Nontraumatic Cauda Equina Syndrome

GENERAL PRINCIPLES

Cauda equina syndrome (CES) results from pathology involving multiple sacral and lumbar nerve roots within the lumbar spinal canal with resulting neurological deficit. Impairments may include bladder and bowel dysfunction, sensory impairment in the perineal saddle area, and variable lower extremity weakness and reflex changes.

Etiology

While CES can result from spinal trauma, there are several nontraumatic causes of CES. The most common among those is midline lumbar disk herniation. The most common site of disk herniation associated with CES is at the L4-5 level. Other causes include spinal stenosis, tumors, hematoma, abscess, or iatrogenic, for example due to direct injury to the cauda equina during surgery, compression from a postoperative hematoma, or spinal manipulation.

Epidemiology

While it is considered to be relatively rare, the reported incidence of CES varies considerably and is not well defined. It is estimated to occur in 1% to 6% of lumbar disk herniations that undergo surgical treatment.

Pathophysiology

The nerve roots that form the cauda equina may be particularly susceptible to injury from mechanical compression due to a relative lack of protective connective tissue covering. Unlike peripheral nerves that are covered by epineurium, perineurium, and endoneurium, nerve roots of the cauda equina only have endoneurium covering. In addition to the primary compressive injury, secondary injury mechanisms may including nerve root ischemia. Mechanical compression of the nerve roots may also impair nutrition of the nerve roots, cause venous stasis, and impede axonal flow. Some patients may be predisposed to cauda equina injury if they have a congenitally narrow spinal canal or have acquired spinal stenosis from a combination of degenerative changes of the disk and the segmental posterior joints and thickening of the ligamentum flavum.

Disease Course

The disease may present acutely with sudden onset or may have a much more gradual progression of neurological impairment over weeks or months.

CLINICAL CONSIDERATIONS

Assessment

History
Patients may present acutely with urinary retention, accompanied by sudden onset of low back pain with variable radiation to the legs, variable leg weakness, and perineal anesthesia (Table 14.1). Bowel disturbance may range from constipation to incontinence but is not always obvious in those with acute presentation due to loss of rectal sensation

Another subset of patients may have a much more insidious onset with slow progression of numbness, tingling, or urinary symptoms. They may notice perianal sensory impairment as an abnormal sensation while wiping themselves with toilet paper. Bladder dysfunction may not always be reported especially if patients don't have urinary incontinence, but large volumes may be noted on postvoid urine residuals on testing.

Impairment of sexual function may occur and genital sensory impairment may be reported with symptoms of reduced penile sensation or reduced sensation noted during sexual activity.

Some of these patients may have long-standing history of lumbar disk disease associated with low back pain. Those with preexisting lumbar spinal stenosis often have history of neurogenic claudication with pain that occurs while walking or prolonged standing, and improves with rest or flexion position.

Physical Examination
Assessment should include careful examination of the sacral and lumbar myotomes and dermatomes including testing of the perianal region for light touch and pin-prick sensation. Neurologic rectal examination includes determination of deep anal pressure and testing for voluntary contraction of the external anal sphincter around the examiner's finger. Anal wink and

Table 14.1

Comparison of Conus Medullaris and Cauda Equina Lesions[a]

Clinical Feature	Conus Medullaris	Cauda Equina
Pain	Less common	Frequent
Symmetry	More often symmetrical	Often asymmetrical
Sensory loss	Saddle distribution, may have dissociated loss of pain and temperature sensation	Radicular sensory loss, sensory loss is not dissociated
Muscle stretch reflexes	May be preserved	Often lost depending on the nerve roots involved
Anal and bulbocavernosus reflex	Often lost, but may be preserved in high conus lesions	Usually lost
Bowel and bladder reflexes	Usually absent, but may be preserved in high conus lesions	Usually absent
Prognosis for recovery	Less likely	More likely

[a]It is often difficult to clinically distinguish conus medullaris and cauda equina lesions due to overlapping features and usual concomitant involvement of lumbar roots with conus injuries. Isolated conus medullaris injuries are rare.

bulbocavernosus reflex should be examined to evaluate the sacral roots. Motor exam may reveal variable leg weakness and loss of reflexes.

Conus Medullaris vs. Cauda Equina Lesions

The neurological examination will vary with the location of damage and the relative involvement of the conus and cauda equina (Table 14.1). Conus medullaris lesions typically result in impaired sensation over the sacral dermatomes (saddle anesthesia), lax anal sphincter with loss of anal and bulbocavernosus reflexes, and sometimes weakness in the lower extremity muscles. Depending on the level of the lesion, this type of injury may manifest with a mixed picture of upper motor neuron and lower motor neuron signs. For example, with high lesions of the conus medullaris there may occasionally be preservation of the bulbocavernosus reflex and anal wink that are typically absent with lower lesions. Cauda equina involvement more often results in asymmetric atrophic, areflexic paralysis of the limbs, radicular sensory loss, and sphincter impairment. In some cases it may be difficult to clinically distinguish a conus medullaris injury from a cauda equina injury.

Diagnostic Tests

Magnetic resonance imaging is the imaging of choice because of its ability to visualize the soft tissues, including nerve roots, dural sac, ligamentous structures, intervertebral disks, and epidural or subdural hematomas.

Practice Pearls

Development of new symptoms of perianal sensory changes or bladder symptoms in patients with an increase in back pain or sciatica should be urgently investigated with appropriate diagnostic imaging and consultation as needed. There is sometimes a tendency to minimize new symptoms in those with long-standing back problems both on part of the patient and physician.

A high index of suspicion for a hematoma compressing the cauda equina is warranted in patients who are on anticoagulant therapy and develop bladder or sacral sensory impairments. Similarly, development of increasing back pain or persisting difficulty in voiding in the postoperative period after spine surgery requires a high index of suspicion and prompt evaluation.

Management

Prompt attention is typically warranted. Surgical decompression is indicated, often involving laminectomy and/or diskectomy, with nonsurgical management having a relatively limited role. Decompression should not be unduly delayed, and it is generally agreed that it should be performed within 24 to 48 hours. However, there is less consensus regarding even more urgent intervention, with some suggestion that waiting till the next morning when proper facilities are available may be preferable to performing an emergency procedure if the patient presents in the evening and optimal resources are not available without waiting overnight. Surgery can be technically demanding and care is needed to avoid causing further nerve root damage. Postoperatively, a comprehensive rehabilitation program may be indicated to address residual impairments and functional deficits in mobility and activities of daily living, and to address persisting problems with neurogenic bladder, bowel, and/or sexual dysfunction.

Prognosis: Incontinence at presentation is a poor prognostic feature. Those with incomplete CES without urinary retention have better prognosis for recovery than those with the full-blown syndrome. Recovery may continue for up to 1 year or longer after surgery.

KNOWLEDGE GAPS AND EMERGING CONCEPTS

Further evaluation of timing and urgency of surgical intervention is needed. Controversy currently exists in this regard. Some studies imply that outcome is independent of the timing of surgery. However, other studies have demonstrated that motor deficits are more likely to persist with delayed surgery. Outcome studies are needed to define which subgroups of CES may benefit from emergency surgery and which do not need such urgent intervention. The procedures performed for CES range from microdiskectomy to wide laminectomy, diskectomy, and open inspection of nerve roots but additional studies are needed to compare the effectiveness and outcomes of these various surgical procedures.

SUGGESTED READING

Fraser S, Roberts L, Murphy E. Cauda equina syndrome: a literature review of its definition and clinical presentation. *Arch Phys Med Rehabil.* 2009;90(11):1964-1968.

Hertzler DA II, DePowell JJ, Stevenson CB, Mangano FT. Tethered cord syndrome: a review of the literature from embryology to adult presentation. *Neurosurg Focus.* 2010;29(1):E1.

Lavy C, James A, Wilson-MacDonald J, Fairbank J. Cauda equina syndrome. *BMJ.* 2009;338:b936.

New PW. Cauda equina syndrome. Specialist rehabilitation. *BMJ.* 2009;338:b1725.

Spector LR, Madigan L, Rhyne A, Darden B II, Kim D. Cauda equina syndrome. *J Am Acad Orthop Surg.* 2008;16(8):471-479.

CHAPTER 15

Tumors of the Spine and Spinal Cord

GENERAL PRINCIPLES

Etiology and Epidemiology

Tumors involving the spine and spinal cord can be classified based on origin (primary or secondary) or based on location as extradural or intradural (i.e., outside or inside the thecal sac). Intradural tumors can be further divided into extramedullary or intramedullary (i.e., arising outside or within the spinal cord). Fifty-five percent to 60% of all spinal tumors are extradural, 35% to 40% are intradural-extramedullary, and 5% are intramedullary.

Extradural Tumors
Metastatic tumors account for over 98% of extradural spinal tumors, with primary vertebral tumors making up the remaining small fraction. About 1 in 20 patients with cancer develop spinal cord compression. Nearly all types of cancers can metastasize to the spine, but most common sources are lung, breast, prostate, kidney, lymphoma, and myeloma. The thoracic spine is the most common part of the vertebral column involved in metastatic disease, except in prostatic cancer where the lumbar spine is more often involved.

Intradural-Extramedullary Tumors
Extramedullary tumors are mostly benign. Meningiomas and neurofibromas/schwannomas account for the great majority. Meningiomas are often located posterior to the thoracic cord or near the foramen magnum, occur more often in females, and most often occur in the thoracic spine. Neurofibromas and schwannomas arise from Schwann cells of the nerve roots. Multiple neurofibromas suggest the likelihood of neurofibromatosis.

Intradural-Intramedullary Tumors
Intramedullary tumors are ependymomas, astrocytomas, or others (including hemangioblastoma and, occasionally, intramedullary metastases). Ependymomas are more common in adults; astrocytomas account for the majority of intramedullary tumors in children. Ependymomas arise from cells lining the

central canal; nearly all are benign; they are most commonly located in the cervical cord or in the vicinity of the cauda equina/filum terminale. Astrocytomas can vary in degree of invasiveness from low-grade to high-grade, and are most often cervical.

Disease Course

Extradural metastatic tumors have an acute or subacute onset. Intradural tumors grow slowly and have a gradual progression. Intramedullary tumors usually have an insidious disease course that develops over weeks or months.

CLINICAL CONSIDERATIONS

Assessment

History and Examination
The most common presenting symptom of spinal tumors is pain. Pain is often unremitting, worse in the supine position, and more noticeable at rest. Pain may be local or radicular.

Recent onset of persisting pain in the thoracic spine that awakens the patient at night and worsens with coughing or sneezing suggests that the possibility of vertebral metastasis should be considered. There is often a known history of the primary tumor, but in about 20% of cases spinal metastases are the initial presentation of cancer elsewhere. Local tenderness is usually present on palpation.

Neurological deficits can occur due to cord compression and/or local nerve root involvement. Distribution of deficits is based on the location of the lesion. Segmental pain and sensory loss can occur at the level of the tumor due to dorsal root irritation or compression. Segmental lower motor neuron loss may also be present at the level of the tumor, and upper motor neuron signs may be present below the level of the lesion. Sensory loss below the lesion level and sphincter involvement may also be present.

Intramedullary tumors often extend over multiple segments and may give a clinical picture similar to a syringomyelia (e.g., dissociated sensory loss, central cord syndrome).

The general physical examination may provide clues about the source of the tumor (e.g., primary site of metastatic cancer, café-au-lait spots suggestive of neurofibromatosis).

Diagnostic Tests
Magnetic resonance imaging (MRI) is the imaging of choice and provides excellent visualization of the tumor and the involved structures. It is also able to distinguish tumors from other masses, for example, abscess or hematoma.

Gadolinium-enhanced and noncontrasted MRI sequences are standard. Location and appearance can help characterize the type of spine or spinal cord tumor. Plain radiographs and bone scans have a limited role since they don't identify a substantial percent of tumors.

In case of a suspected metastatic lesion seen on MRI, the entire spine should be visualized since there are often additional silent metastases present. Testing to identify the primary source of tumor is needed if spinal metastasis is the first presentation of cancer, including possible tissue biopsy.

Management

Surgical Resection of Primary Spinal Tumors
Surgical removal is the treatment of choice for most extramedullary tumors (which are usually benign), and is curative in most cases. Intramedullary tumors are also removed surgically. Ependymomas are often well demarcated so amenable to complete removal. If astrocytoma removal is incomplete or there is histological evidence of malignancy, postoperative radiation is typically given.

Management of Metastatic Spinal Cord Compression
Metastatic spinal cord compression needs to be addressed urgently, typically with steroids (to reduce edema) and radiation. In addition, specific therapy is initiated once the tumor type is identified.

If not medically contraindicated, steroids are recommended for any patient with neurologic deficits who is suspected or confirmed to have metastatic extradural spinal cord compression. A uniform consensus on dose is lacking. A bolus of 8 to 10 mg dexamethasone (or equivalent) can be given, followed by 16 mg/d (usually in 2–4 divided doses for tolerance). Patients with complete paraplegia should be considered for higher bolus (up to 100 mg has been suggested) and high maintenance doses, but the risk of serious adverse reactions should be considered. Motor deficits that are established for over 12 hours and don't improve in 48 hours have a poor prognosis for recovery. Steroids are generally continued at a lower dose till radiotherapy is complete, and gradually tapered over several days. Patients with radiographic compression but no neurologic deficits generally do not require steroids.

Radiation therapy directed at the compressive tumor is also usually given, and should be started as early as possible. A typical regimen is 3000 cGY administered over 15 days. Surgical decompression with laminectomy is rarely done or needed with the use of radiation in this situation. However, with advances in surgical techniques, surgical interventions for controlling neurological deficit, pain, and instability, including minimally invasive surgery, have been advocated as a treatment option. It has been suggested that surgery followed by radiation may have better outcomes than radiation alone for patients in some situations; surgical morbidity needs to be factored in that decision.

Rehabilitation Management

Several reports have demonstrated that patients with functional loss from neoplastic spinal cord compression can make significant functional gains from inpatient rehabilitation. Rehabilitation treatment may focus on mobility, self-care, management of bladder and bowel dysfunction if present, and pain, mood, and/or fatigue management. Preservation of effects of rehabilitation has been reported postdischarge in patients who have survived, with demonstrated maintenance of function for self-care and mobility at several months after discharge.

KNOWLEDGE GAPS AND EMERGING CONCEPTS

Minimally invasive surgical techniques have been reported as a treatment option for spinal metastasis with good results. The role of stereotactic radiosurgery, to deliver a high dose of radiation to the target site while decreasing the amount delivered to the normal tissue, is being explored as a potential option for treatment of spinal metastasis.

SUGGESTED READING

Fattal C, Fabbro M, Gelis A, Bauchet L. Metastatic paraplegia and vital prognosis: perspectives and limitations for rehabilitation care. Part 1. *Arch Phys Med Rehabil.* 2011;92(1): 125-133. Doi: 10.1016/j.apmr.2010.09.017.

Fattal C, Fabbro M, Rouays-Mabit H, Verollet C, Bauchet L. Metastatic paraplegia and functional outcomes: perspectives and limitations for rehabilitation care. Part 2. *Arch Phys Med Rehabil.* 2011;92(1):134-145.

Huang ME, Sliwa JA. Inpatient rehabilitation of patients with cancer: efficacy and treatment considerations. *PM R.* 2011;3(8):746-757.

Loblaw DA, Mitera G, Ford M, Laperriere NJ. A 2011 updated systematic review and clinical practice guideline for the management of malignant extradural spinal cord compression. *Int J Radiat Oncol Biol Phys.* 2012;84(2):312-317. Doi: 10.1016/j.ijrobp.2012.01.014.

Mechtler LL, Nandigam K. Spinal cord tumors: new views and future directions. *Neurol Clin.* 2013;31(1):241-268. Doi: 10.1016/j.ncl.2012.09.011.

Raj VS, Lofton L. Rehabilitation and treatment of spinal cord tumors. *J Spinal Cord Med.* 2013;36(1):4-11. Doi: 10.1179/2045772312Y.0000000015.

Thakur NA, Daniels AH, Schiller J, et al. Benign tumors of the spine. *J Am Acad Orthop Surg.* 2012;20(11):715-724. Doi: 10.5435/JAAOS-20-11-715.

Wald JT. Imaging of spine neoplasm. *Radiol Clin North Am.* 2012;50(4):749-776. Doi: 10.1016/j. rcl.2012.04.002.

Waters JD, Peran EM, Ciacci J. Malignancies of the spinal cord. *Adv Exp Med Biol.* 2012; 760:101-113.

Zairi F, Marinho P, Bouras A, Allaoui M, Assaker R. Recent concepts in the management of thoracolumbar spine metastasis. *J Neurosurg Sci.* 2013;57(1):45-54.

CHAPTER 16

Vascular Myelopathy—Spinal Cord Infarction

Myelopathy due to a vascular cause can be secondary to:

- Spinal cord infarction, or
- Hemorrhage which could be
  - Within the spinal cord (hematomyelia)
  - In the epidural or subdural space, causing spinal cord compression

GENERAL CONSIDERATIONS

Etiology

Spinal cord ischemia can be caused either by systemic hypoperfusion or by focal interruption of blood supply. A definite etiology may not be identified in a significant proportion of cases.

Most common causes of spinal cord infarction are:

- Aortic surgery, instrumentation, or cross-clamping
- Dissecting aortic aneurysm
- Profound systemic hypotension

Other causes include:

- Cardiac embolism
- Atherosclerosis, atherothrombosis, and atheroembolism
- Vertebral artery dissection from cervical trauma or manipulation
- Vertebral or aortic angiography
- Arteritis (e.g., due to collagen vascular disease such as polyarteritis nodosa, systemic lupus erythematosus [SLE], or Sjögren syndrome, sarcoidosis, syphilis, tuberculosis, or cocaine use)
- Venous thrombophlebitis
- Hematological (due to procoagulant states, thrombocytosis, or sickle cell disease)

- Fibrocartilaginous embolism (from nucleus pulposus material following intervertebral disk rupture or trauma)
- As a complication of epidural injection
- Air embolism (from nitrogen bubbles in decompression sickness)

Epidemiology

Spinal cord infarction is a relatively rare cause of myelopathy. Age and gender distribution depends on the underlying etiology. Given the most frequent causes, it is most commonly seen in middle to older age.

Paraplegia is much more common than tetraplegia, with the mid-thoracic spinal cord being the most commonly involved region. With aortic aneurysm surgery, spinal cord infarction may occur in up to 5% to 10% of thoraco-abdominal aneurysm repairs, but is very rare in procedures below the infrarenal segment.

Pathophysiology

Important aspects of the blood supply of the spinal cord that affect the pathophysiology of spinal cord ischemia are summarized in Table 16.1.

Disease Course

Onset is typically acute with rapid progression. Initial flaccid paralysis may evolve to spastic paralysis with signs of upper motor neuron weakness or a mixed picture during the course of the disease. Those with complete paralysis have poor prognosis for neurological recovery. Some reports suggest that sphincter or sensory impairments are less likely to improve than motor weakness.

CLINICAL CONSIDERATIONS

Assessment

History and Physical Examination
Presentation is usually sudden. Radicular or trunk/back pain sometimes heralds the onset, and may be severe. Depending on the location of involvement, pain may be interscapular, referred to the shoulders or chest (mimicking cardiac pain), abdomen, anterior thighs, or buttocks.

Weakness and sensory loss are based on the level and distribution of ischemia. An anterior cord syndrome is typical with loss of pain and temperature and preserved touch, vibration, and position sense accompanying the paralysis, but other distribution of deficits may occur including those consistent with a complete transverse myelopathy, Brown-Sequard syndrome, central cord syndrome, or, rarely, a posterior cord syndrome. Typically, the paralysis is initially flaccid, accompanied by loss of muscle stretch reflexes and flaccid sphincters. It may evolve over days or weeks to spastic paralysis with hyperreflexia and

Table 16.1
Significant Clinical Implications of Spinal Cord Blood Supply

Blood Supply of the Spinal Cord	Clinical Significance
Single anterior spinal artery with discontinuous reinforcement by segmental arteries supplying the anterior two-thirds of the cord, versus two posterior spinal arteries with relatively robust segmental reinforcement throughout the length of the spinal cord supplying the posterior third	Spinal cord infarction often causes an anterior cord syndrome with paralysis and impaired pin-prick and temperature sensations, and relative sparing of the posterior columns and touch, position, and vibration sensations
Relatively avascular watershed area in the mid-thoracic region between the more robust anterior spinal artery rostrally and the artery of Adamkiewicz caudally	Mid-thoracic (T4–T8) level is the most common site of spinal cord infarction
Artery of Adamkiewicz, the major segmental artery supplying the lower spinal cord, most commonly arises between T10 and T12 on the left, but may arise anywhere between T5 and L2, and the extent of area supplied by it is variable	Because of variations in vascular supply, the effects of aortic injury, dissection, or cross-clamping at a particular level differ between individuals
Anterior horn cells are especially vulnerable to ischemia due to high metabolic demands	Preferential ischemic injury to anterior horn cells can cause a predominantly flaccid paralysis
Cross-sectional border zone in the spinal cord between the penetrating arteries from the anterior and posterior circulation can be relatively avascular	May be a contributing factor in the pathogenesis of central cord syndrome

upgoing plantar reflexes. Mixed or lower motor neuron paralysis may persist in those with significant anterior horn cell or cauda equina involvement.

Bladder, bowel, and sexual dysfunction are common. As with the paralysis, initial flaccid bladder with urinary retention and bowel paralysis with ileus, may evolve to features consistent with upper motor neuron involvement. While less common (based on the typical distribution of spinal cord involvement), more rostral levels of involvement with cervical or upper thoracic level of injury may be accompanied by additional symptoms and signs of autonomic dysfunction such as orthostatic hypotension, impaired thermoregulaton, and autonomic dysreflexia.

Diagnostic Tests
Magnetic resonance imaging (MRI) is the imaging of choice. However, it is sometimes normal in the first few hours. Subsequently, lesions are visible on T2 sequences that likely reflect edema, which can extend over several levels. There may be some enhancement after gadolinium infusion. In the more chronic stage, the infarcted region of the cord is often atrophic with an attenuated signal on MRI.

Additional diagnostic testing may be indicated to determine the etiology of infarction, if not otherwise obvious, including tests for immune mediated disorders, sarcoidosis, or infections (Chapter 12, Table 12.4).

Urodynamic testing is often indicated since the nature of bladder involvement is variable and is often hard to determine clinically. It may reveal detrusor areflexia, especially in the first few weeks, but later show evidence of detrusor hyperreflexia and detrusor-sphincter dysynergia (DSD).

Management

Treatment of identified underlying disease should be undertaken if/as feasible.

However, management in most cases is primarily limited to symptom management, and prevention and treatment of complications. As with other causes of myelopathy this includes appropriately addressing impairments in mobility and activities of daily living, bladder, bowel, and sexual dysfunction, prevention and management of complications such as pressure ulcers, pain, and spasticity, and addressing effects on psychosocial function and participation.

Issues related to a sense of blame or hostility of the patient and/or family towards the surgeon or treatment team that may arise in cases of iatrogenic, or perceived iatrogenic, injury need to be addressed appropriately, as do any issues of self-blame and regret in cases that occur after elective procedures.

KNOWLEDGE GAPS AND EMERGING CONCEPTS

Various techniques to prevent or minimize the occurrence of spinal cord ischemia during aortic surgery are being developed and implemented, but most need further evaluation and demonstration of effectiveness prior to widespread adoption.

Outcomes of spinal cord infarction have been systemically evaluated and reported to a much more limited extent than traumatic spinal cord injury, and further research in this area is warranted.

SUGGESTED READING

Kamin S, Gurstang S. Vascular disease of the spinal cord. *Top Spinal Cord Inj Rehabil.* 2008;14(2): 42-52.
Novy J, Carruzzo A, Maeder P, Bogousslavsky J. Spinal cord ischemia: clinical and imaging patterns, pathogenesis, and outcomes in 27 patients. *Arch Neurol.* 2006;63(8):1113-1120.
Salvador de la Barrera S, Barca-Buyo A, Montoto-Marqués A, Ferreiro-Velasco ME, Cidoncha-Dans M, Rodriguez-Sotillo A. Spinal cord infarction: prognosis and recovery in a series of 36 patients. *Spinal Cord.* 2001;39(10):520-525.

CHAPTER 17

Spinal Cord Hemorrhage and Spinal Arteriovenous Malformations

GENERAL PRINCIPLES

Hemorrhagic involvement of the spinal cord can be due to:

- Bleeding within the spinal cord (hematomyelia) or
- External compression from bleeding within the epidural or subdural space. Subarachnoid hemorrhage does not cause cord compression because blood is able to spread in the cerebrospinal fluid throughout the subarachnoid space.

Etiology

Causes of bleeding either within the spinal cord or in the epidural or subdural space include:

- Arteriovenous malformations (AVM)
- Anticoagulant therapy
- Bleeding disorders
- Bleeding into a vascular neoplasm of the spine or spinal cord
- Vasculitis
- As a rare complication of epidural or lumbar puncture or injection
- Trauma

Various classifications of AVM have been proposed. Morphologically, AVM can be:

- Arteriovenous fistulas, which represent a direct connection between arteries and veins without interposition of a pathological nidus, or
- True malformations with a vascular network that is interposed between the feeding arteries and draining veins

Table 17.1

Mechanisms by Which AVM Can Cause Myelopathy

Venous congestion and venous hypertension

Vascular steal

Compression due to mass effect

Hemorrhage inside the spinal cord (hematomyelia)

Epidural hemorrhage causing cord compression

AVM can also be classified by location, which could be dural, intradural, or intramedullary. Dural AV fistulas, also referred to as Type I AVM, are the commonest type. Intramedullary AVM with a true nidus within the spinal cord are also referred to as Type II.

Epidemiology

AVM can either be congenital or acquired. Age and gender distribution depends on the type but overall they are more common in middle-aged or older men. Type I AVM is the most common and is considered to be acquired in most cases. These are most often located in the lower thoracic cord or the conus.

Pathophysiology

AVM can affect the spinal cord in multiple ways including spinal cord compression, venous hypertension due to congestion, vascular steal, and hemorrhage (Table 17.1). Venous hypertension is thought to play a primary role in the pathophysiology of myelopathy associated with Type I AV fistulas. Hemorrhage within the cord can result from Type II AVM.

Disease Course

Patients often have a gradually progressive course, especially in those with Type I lesions. A stepwise course is considered classic, although is seen in only a minority of patients. This saltatory evolution is presumed to be due to fluctuating venous congestion within the cord. Acute onset of symptoms can occur when there is significant hemorrhage.

CLINICAL CONSIDERATIONS

Assessment

History and Physical Examination
Sensory impairment and/or weakness are common initial symptoms. Leg weakness and wasting with accompanying numbness and paresthesias in the

same distribution may be present. Some patients may have pain in the form of backache or sciatica. Claudication symptoms have also been reported. Gait impairment and urinary problems often develop.

A bruit may sometimes be heard over the spine at the site of the AVM. Occasionally, patients will have other cutaneous angiomas, or a nevus may be seen on the skin of the back overlying the site of the AVM.

Evolution is variable, ranging from abrupt and apoplectic to worsening over several months. With the progressive or stepwise course, symptoms may be present for years before a diagnosis is made. The severity and distribution of symptoms is also variable.

Diagnostic Tests
Magnetic resonance imaging (MRI) or computed tomography (CT) myelography may show the presence of enlarged serpiginous blood vessels, but may not be able to identify these in some cases. MRI may show myelomalacia, edema, or bleeding. Appearance and signal intensity of the bleed on MRI may help determine its duration, but the correlation can be variable.

Spinal angiography is used for definitive diagnosis and to identify the vascular anatomy for surgical planning. It can be technically challenging and may need to be performed at a specialized center.

Management

Management of acute epidural hematoma includes urgent surgical decompression and treatment for any identified underlying clotting disorder.

AVM associated with progressive neurological impairment or recurrent bleeding should be evaluated for potential therapeutic intervention. Endovascular techniques, embolization, and microsurgical correction of AVM are now increasingly possible. More extensive surgical resection or ligation may be needed in some cases and successful correction is not always feasible. Focal radiation therapy has also been used, but its effectiveness is not clear

Ongoing supportive treatment to address neurological impairment and function is needed for persisting deficits.

Practice Pearl

A vascular malformation is not always identified on MRI, so the possibility and further testing should be considered in the differential diagnosis of otherwise unexplained myelopathy with signs of cord congestion and edema on MRI even when no lesion is visible.

KNOWLEDGE GAPS AND EMERGING CONCEPTS

Ongoing advances in selective spinal angiography and microsurgery are making precise visualization and treatment of vascular lesions increasingly feasible. Further studies are needed to compare effectiveness and long-term outcomes of existing and evolving techniques.

SUGGESTED READING

Bostroem A, Thron A, Hans FJ, Krings T. Spinal vascular malformations—typical and atypical findings. *Zentralbl Neurochir.* 2007;68(4):205-213.

Caragine LP Jr, Halbach VV, Ng PP, Dowd CF. Vascular myelopathies-vascular malformations of the spinal cord: presentation and endovascular surgical management. *Semin Neurol.* 2002;22(2):123-132.

Rodesch G, Lasjaunias P. Spinal cord arteriovenous shunts: from imaging to management. *Eur J Radiol.* 2003;46(3):221-132.

Spetzler RF, Detwiler PW, Riina HA, Porter RW. Modified classification of spinal cord vascular lesions. *J Neurosurg.* 2002;96(2 suppl):145-156.

Zozulya YP, Slin'ko EI, Al-Qashqish II. Spinal arteriovenous malformations: new classification and surgical treatment. *Neurosurg Focus.* 2006;20(5):E7.

CHAPTER 18

Multiple Sclerosis

GENERAL PRINCIPLES

Multiple Sclerosis (MS) is a chronic disorder of the central nervous system (CNS), characterized by immune mediated inflammation, demyelination, glial scarring, and neuronal loss. It is typically disseminated in time and space, that is, lesions occur at different times and in different CNS locations.

Etiology

Both genetic and environmental factors are likely involved. Monozygotic twin studies and family aggregation studies provide evidence of genetic susceptibility. Epidemiological data and migration studies have suggested that exposure to an environmental agent within the first 15 years of life seems to trigger subsequent MS. Low levels of vitamin D and infectious agents, particularly the Epstein-Barr virus, are among the proposed environmental culprits.

Epidemiology

MS is a leading cause of neurological disability in young adults. Its prevalence has increased steadily over the past four to five decades in several regions of the world. It affects about 400,000 individuals in the United States and 2.5 million people worldwide.

It is rare in children but its onset increases steadily from adolescence to age 35, and then gradually decreases. Onset after age 65 is rare. Women are affected two to three times as often as men. White populations are at higher risk than blacks or Asians. MS is more common in countries with temperate climates and there is a higher rate of prevalence in northern United States and Canada compared to the south. The environmental association with higher altitudes and lower sunlight exposure provides support to the proposed role of lower vitamin D levels in pathogenesis.

Pathophysiology

New MS lesions are associated with perivascular infiltration of T cells and macrophages. B cells are also involved with evidence of myelin-specific antibodies on damaged myelin sheaths. There is breakdown of the blood-brain barrier (BBB), as demonstrated in magnetic resonance imaging (MRI) with use of gadolinium contrast, which may persist for 6 to 8 weeks.

Demyelinating plaques are the hallmark of the disease, with acute plaques being distinguished by the presence of inflammation. As lesions evolve, astrocytic proliferation or gliosis becomes predominant. A degree of repair with remyelination occurs but may be partial, with remyelinating axons showing thinner myelin sheaths than normal. Loss of myelin leads to disruption of the normal saltatory nerve conduction with reduced conduction velocity and conduction block. Conduction block may be incomplete, affecting high but not slow-frequency impulses.

Worsening of conduction block with raised body temperature and metabolic activity may explain clinical worsening with fever, high environmental temperature, or strenuous physical activity.

Astrocytic scarring may interfere with complete remyelination. Although axonal sparing is typical, MS is not solely a disease of the myelin. The importance of associated neuronal damage and gray matter involvement in contributing to permanent neurological disability, and to the development of spinal cord and brain tissue atrophy seen in some cases, is being increasingly recognized. Lack of proper myelin may adversely affect trophic nutritional support to the neuron, and the redistribution of sodium channels along the axons instead of the normal concentration at the nodes of Ranvier could increase susceptibility to free radical damage, leading to future neuronal damage.

Common sites of MS lesions include:

- Periventricular white matter of the cerebral hemispheres
- Spinal cord (especially the subpial regions)
- Brainstem
- Cerebellum
- Optic nerves

Disease Course

Onset of MS may be abrupt or insidious. The severity and course of the disease varies significantly amongst individuals. Four clinical forms of MS have been described based on disease course:

- *Relapsing-remitting MS (RRMS)*. This is the most common form, accounting for over 85% of all cases at onset of the disease. Patients have discrete attacks that evolve over hours, days, to weeks with recovery over the following weeks to months, remaining neurologically stable between relapses.
- *Secondary progressive MS (SPMS)*. SPMS begins as RRMS, but during the course of the disease patients begin to experience progressive deterioration unrelated to acute relapses. The risk of developing SPMS is

estimated to be around 2% each year for patients with RRMS, so eventually a majority of those patients evolve to SPMS.

▓ *Primary-progressive MS (PPMS)*. This accounts for about 10% to 15% of
all MS diagnoses. These patients have a steady neurological and functional worsening but don't experience discrete attacks. PPMS often
beings at an older age and with a more even sex distribution than other
forms of MS.

▓ *Progressive-relapsing MS (PRMS)*. It accounts for about 5% of cases and
is characterized by steady worsening from the onset, but with superim-
posed acute attacks as in those with SPMS.

In addition, a clinically isolated syndrome (CIS), has been described to refer
to patients who have one demyelinating event accompanied by MRI and cerebrospinal fluid (CSF) findings supportive of MS, although a single episode of
inflammation, whether unifocal or multifocal, cannot be classified as MS. Some
patients will have no further episodes or evidence of the disease, but the majority eventually develops future relapses and a diagnosis of MS. The estimated
risk of developing MS after 20 years is around 60%, increasing to 80% if the initial MRI showed abnormalities in addition to the expected clinically significant
lesion based on presentation.

Prognosis for Long-Term Disability
Adverse and favorable prognostic factors for long-term disability are summarized in Table 18.1.

The Kurtzke Expanded Disability Status Scale (EDSS) is used to measure the
disability status (Table 18.2). It focuses primarily on mobility and ranges
from 0 (no impairment) to 10 (death) with half-point increments in between.
While useful in quantifying MS-related disability, it has significant limitations (e.g., the scale is not linear, changes of one point between lower scores
do not equate to single point change at higher scores, and there is no measure
of cognition).

Table 18.1

Prognostic Factors for Long-Term Disability in MS	
Favorable Factors	**Adverse Factors**
Early age of onset	Late age of onset
Female sex	Male sex
Sensory dysfunction (paresthesia) at onset	Cerebellar dysfunction (ataxia) at onset, insidious motor onset
Relapsing-remitting clinical course	Progressive clinical course
Longer inter-attack interval; low initial relapse rate	Short interval between first two relapses
Fewer lesions on baseline MRI	High lesion load on MRI at presentation

Table 18.2
Kurtzke Expanded Disability Status Scale (EDSS)

0.0 = Normal neurologic exam (all grade 0 in functional status [FS])

1.0 = No disability, minimal signs in one FS (i.e., grade 1)

1.5 = No disability, minimal signs in more than one FS (more than one grade 1)

2.0 = Minimal disability in one FS (one FS grade 2, others 0 or 1)

2.5 = Minimal disability in two FS (two FS grade 2, others 0 or 1)

3.0 = Moderate disability in one FS (one FS grade 3, others 0 or 1) or mild disability in three or four FS (three/four FS grade 2, others 0 or 1) though fully ambulatory

3.5 = Fully ambulatory but with moderate disability in one FS (one grade 3) and one or two FS grade 2; or two FS grade 3; or five FS grade 2 (others 0 or 1)

4.0 = Ambulatory without aid or rest for ~500 m

4.5 = Ambulatory without aid or rest for ~300 m

5.0 = Ambulatory without aid or rest for ~200 m

5.5 = Ambulatory without aid or rest for ~100 m

6.0 = Unilateral assistance required to walk about 100 m with or without resting

6.5 = Constant bilateral assistance required to walk about 20 m without resting

7.0 = Unable to walk beyond about 5 m even with aid; essentially restricted to wheelchair; wheels self and transfers alone

7.5 = Unable to take more than a few steps; restricted to wheelchair; may need aid to transfer

8.0 = Essentially restricted to bed or chair or perambulated in wheelchair, but out of bed most of day; retains many self-care functions; generally has effective use of arms

8.5 = Essentially restricted to bed much of the day; has some effective use of arm(s); retains some self-care functions

9.0 = Helpless bed patient; can communicate and eat

9.5 = Totally helpless bed patient; unable to communicate or eat

10.0 = Death due to MS

MS Variants

Neuromyelitis optica (NMO) or Devic's disease is a necrotizing inflammatory disorder that primarily involves the optic nerves and spinal cord. It is now considered to be distinct from MS. It is a syndrome with diverse causes including systemic autoimmune disorders and acute viral infections, but is often idiopathic. It is often disabling over time with a high percent eventually developing blindness and permanent paralysis.

Acute disseminated encephalomyelitis (ADEM) and acute transverse myelitis: Isolated transverse myelitis can be an initial presentation of MS, but is often a postinfectious phenomenon. ADEM is an autoimmune disorder characterized by widespread perivenular inflammation and demyelination of the brain and spinal cord, most commonly as a result of antecedent viral infection. It has also been reported as a rare complication of vaccinations. It is more common in children than in adults and has a monophasic course. Permanent neurological sequelae are common, but some patients make remarkable recovery.

CLINICAL CONSIDERATIONS

History and Physical Examination (Table 18.3)

Presentation of MS may be acute or insidious, and is very diverse.

Common initial symptoms, in decreasing order, are: sensory loss, visual impairment, weakness, paresthesias, gait or balance problems, diplopia, or vertigo. A small percent present with paroxysmal attacks or bladder dysfunction.

Over the course of the disease over 80% of patients develop weakness, sensory disturbances, and ataxia, and bladder-related symptoms. Various other symptoms develop as the disease evolves (Table 18.3). Fatigue and worsening of symptoms with heat or exercise is common. Other ancillary symptoms include Lhermitte's symptom/sign (with an electric shock-like sensation radiating down the back on neck flexion), paroxysmal symptoms, and trigeminal neuralgia. Cognitive dysfunction and depression may occur.

Table 18.3
Clinical Manifestations of MS

Clinical Manifestation	Involved Structure/ Process	Features
Sensory		
Sensory loss, paresthesias	Sensory tracts	Most common initial manifestation of MS
Sensory level	Spinal cord	Often accompanying band-like sensation on torso
Pain	Varies	Pain is common during course of the disease, and can change locations over time. Can be nociceptive or neuropathic in origin
Lherrmitte's symptom	Cervical spinal cord	Electric shock-like sensation radiating down the back on neck flexion; can also occur with other disorders of the cervical spinal cord
Facial pain/ trigeminal neuralgia	Root entry zone of the trigeminal nerve	Brief, lancinating facial pain, often triggered by afferent input from face or teeth; most cases are not related to MS but early age of onset, bilateral involvement, and sensory loss on exam should raise suspicion
Motor		
Weakness	Corticospinal tracts	Limb weakness, loss of dexterity, z and gait impairment may occur

(continued)

Clinical Manifestation	Involved Structure/ Process	Features
Motor		
Spasticity	Corticospinal tracts	Especially involves the legs, with accompanying hyperreflexia and Babinski sign, associated with painful spasms, interference with function
Ataxia	Cerebellar tracts or dorsal column	Often have accompanying cerebellar signs
Tremor	Cerebellar tracts	Intention tremor worse at the end of a purposeful movement, often accompanying postural tremor of head and trunk
Facial weakness	Facial nerve/nucleus in the pons	Spared loss of ipsilateral taste sensation and lack of retroauricular pain differentiate it from Bell's palsy
Facial myokymia	Corticobulbar tracts or brainstem course of the facial nerve	Chronic flickering contractions of the orbicularis oculi and other facial muscles
Visual		
Deceased visual acuity and color perception	Optic neuritis (ON)	Generally monocular symptoms but occasionally bilateral, ranging from mild to complete visual loss of the eye; preceding or accompanying periorbital pain; scotoma in central field of vision; optic disk may be normal, swollen, or pale
Diplopia	Medial longitudinal fasciculus causing internuclear ophthalmoplegia (INO), or due to sixth, third, or fourth nerve paralysis	INO has impaired adduction of ipsilateral eye with nystagmus in the abducting eye; bilateral INO is especially suggestive of MS; blurring resolves when either eye is covered unlike with ON
Speech and swallowing		
Dysarthria	Cerebellar, brainstem, or corticobulbar tract	Speech impairment is common; can have cerebellar dysarthria with scanning speech, tongue weakness from lower brainstem involvement, or corticobulbar-related spastic dysarthria
Dysphagia	Brainstem	May develop later in the course of disease with choking on thin liquids

(continued)

Table 18.3
Clinical Manifestations of MS (*continued*)

Clinical Manifestation	Involved Structure/ Process	Features
Autonomic		
Bladder and bowel dysfunction	Autonomic tracts	Urinary frequency, urgency, nocturia, incontinence, or hesitancy may occur; constipation is the most frequent manifestation of MS-related bowel dysfunction, and may be worsened by medication side-effects or decreased fluid intake to counter urinary problems.
Sexual dysfunction	Autonomic tracts	Impaired erection and ejaculation in men, impaired vaginal lubrication in women; reduced libido, adductor spasms may interfere with sex
Systemic		
Cognitive dysfunction	Cerebral cortex	May manifest as problems with information processing, attention, problem solving, multitasking, abstract thinking, short-term memory, or word finding. More common in progressive forms, correlates with cerebral atrophy and "black holes" on MRI; depression and fatigue may also cause or worsen it; some patients develop "la belle indifference" or even striking euphoria
Depression	Multifactorial	Lifetime prevalence of around 50%; can be reactive, endogenous, or part of illness itself; symptoms may overlap and be confused with MS symptoms
Fatigue	Multifactorial	Common, may be a debilitating; manifestation of the disease itself, or caused or worsened by depression or sleep disturbance
Ancillary symptoms		
Heat sensitivity (Uhtoff's phenomenon)	Worsening of conduction block	Symptoms worsen with hot shower, exercise, or fever
Paroxysmal phenomena	Epiphatic (nonsynaptic) transmission and spontaneous discharges arising from edges of demyelinating plaques may contribute to the mechanism	Lasts from seconds to minutes, often in clusters; may include paroxysmal sensory disturbances of a body part, e.g., facial pain or limb dysesthesia, or paroxysmal tonic contractions

Examination findings depend on the location of the lesion, and key features are summarized in Table 18.3. In addition to a focused exam based on the presenting symptoms, a careful and comprehensive neurological assessment including cranial nerves, motor, reflexes, posture, balance, coordination, sensory examination, and mental status examination may identify other impairments and disseminated effects of the disease. A general assessment may identify secondary effects of the disease and, if indicated, a more comprehensive assessment for depression or cognitive function may be warranted.

Assessment of mobility and activities of daily living is needed to define the effect of the neurological impairments on function, identify needed interventions and establish a baseline for future progression or for monitoring efficacy of treatment. Detailed psychosocial assessment may identify barriers and facilitators for participation in life activities.

Diagnostic Tests

MRI has transformed the diagnosis and management of MS. However, while the central role of MRI in diagnosis has resulted in adjustments to criteria of diagnosis for MS, the fundamental principles for making the diagnosis have not changed, that is, neurological impairments compatible with MS, where alternatives have been excluded, and with evidence for dissemination of lesions in both time and space.

MRI abnormalities are seen in the vast majority of patients, though a large percent are asymptomatic. In people presenting spinal cord syndromes that could potentially be due to demyelination, MRI of both spine and brain is usually done. While MS lesions are associated with certain typical characteristics (Table 18.4), those are not specific to MS and several other conditions (e.g., vasculitis, small vessel disease) may produce similar looking lesions.

The central role of MRI is reflected in the updated McDonald criteria for diagnosing MS (Table 18.5). MRI can be used to demonstrate dissemination of the lesions in time and in space.

MRI criteria acceptable for showing dissemination in space include three of the following four criteria on brain and spinal cord imaging:

1. One gadolinium-enhancing lesion or nine T2-hyperintense lesions if there is no gadolinium-enhancing lesion
2. At least one infratentorial lesion
3. At least one juxtacortical lesion
4. At least three periventricular lesions
   Note: A spinal cord lesion can be considered equivalent to a brain infratentorial lesion; and enhancing spinal cord lesion is considered equivalent to an enhancing brain lesion; and individual spinal cord lesions can contribute together with individual brain lesions to reach the required number of T2 lesions.

Table 18.4

Characteristics of MS Lesions on MRI

Multifocal white matter lesions

Increased signal intensity on T2-weighted image

Often ovoid or round; homogeneous or may possess a rim of altered signal intensity

New (or reactivated chronic) lesions show gadolinium enhancement, which is a reflection of leakage due to inflammation and breakdown of the blood-brain barrier

Periventricular, white matter, brain stem, corpus callosum, cerebellum, or spinal cord locations are typical

Lesions are often perpendicular to the ventricular surface reflecting perivenous demyelination ("Dawson's fingers") seen on sagittal image

MRI criteria for showing dissemination of lesions in time are fulfilled by one of the following two ways:

1. Detection of gadolinium enhancement at least 3 months after the onset of the initial clinical event, if not at the site corresponding to the initial clinical event, or
2. Detection of a new T2 lesion if it appears at any time compared with a reference scan done at least 30 days after the onset of the initial clinical event.

MRI also has a role in assessing disease burden and has prognostic value. Evidence of brain atrophy may be seen in those with long-standing MS.

Evoked potentials, including visual evoked potentials, brainstem auditory evoked potentials, and somatosensory evoked potentials, can be useful for demonstrating dissemination of lesions in space even if impairment of those pathways is not clinically evident. However, MRI of the brain and spinal cord has limited the utility of evoked potentials to a large extent.

CSF electrophorsesis to detect oligoclonocal immunological bands can also assist in diagnosis, although it is not always needed or indicated. The presence of oligoclonal bands in the CSF and not in the serum (indicating intrathecal production of IgG), together with typical MRI changes and the appropriate clinical context strongly support the diagnosis of MS. IgG/albumin ratio is raised in the CSF and the IgG index, which compares IgG/albumin ratio in the CSF and blood, is abnormal in the majority of patients with MS, but is not exclusive to this condition.

The differential diagnosis for MS is extensive including infectious, autoimmune, vascular, neoplastic, and genetic disorders as well as other demyelinating disorders of the CNS, including NMO (Devic's disease) and ADEM. In addition to brain and spinal cord MRI, tests to exclude other causes of the neurological impairment commonly include antinuclear antibodies, Lyme titers, venereal disease research laboratory test (VDRL) or rapid plasma regain (RPR),

Table 18.5

The McDonald Criteria for Making a Diagnosis of MS (Based on Demonstration of Dissemination in Space and Time)

Clinical Presentation	Additional Data Needed for MS Diagnosis
Two or more attacks; objective clinical evidence of two or more lesions or objective clinical evidence of one lesion with reasonable historical evidence of a prior attack	None
Two or more attacks; objective clinical evidence of one lesion	Dissemination in space, demonstrated by: - One T2 lesion on MRI in at least two out of four MS-typical regions of the CNS (periventricular, juxtacortical, infratentorial, or spinal cord) OR - Await a further clinical attack implicating a different CNS site
One attack; objective clinical evidence of two or more lesions	Dissemination in time, demonstrated by: - Simultaneous presence of asymptomatic gadolinium-enhancing and nonenhancing lesions at any time OR - A new T2 and/or gadolinium-enhancing lesion(s) on follow-up MRI, irrespective of its timing with reference to a baseline scan OR - Await a second clinical attack
One attack; objective clinical evidence of one lesion (clinically isolated syndrome)	Dissemination in space and time, demonstrated by: For dissemination in space: - One T2 lesion in at least two out of four MS-typical regions of the CNS (periventricular, juxtacortical, infratentorial, or spinal cord) OR - Await a second clinical attack implicating a different CNS site AND For dissemination in time: - Simultaneous presence of asymptomatic gadolinium-enhancing and nonenhancing lesions at any time OR - A new T2 and/or gadolinium-enhancing lesion(s) on follow-up MRI, irrespective of its timing with reference to a baseline scan OR - Await a second clinical attack

(continued)

Table 18.5

The McDonald Criteria for Making a Diagnosis of MS (Based on Demonstration of Dissemination in Space and Time) (*continued*)

Clinical Presentation	Additional Data Needed for MS Diagnosis
Insidious neurologic progression suggestive of MS (PPMS)	One yr of disease progression (retrospectively or prospectively determined) PLUS Two out of the three following criteria: - Evidence for dissemination in space in the brain based on one T2+ lesions in the MS-characteristic periventricular, juxtacortical, or infratentorial regions - Evidence for dissemination in space in the spinal cord based on two T2+ lesions in the cord - Positive CSF (isoelectric focusing evidence of oligoclonal bands and/or elevated IgG index)

vitamin B12 levels, and thyroid stimulating hormone. Additional studies may be indicated based on clinical context. Also see Chapter 12 and Table 12.4 for diagnoses and tests that are often considered in the differential diagnosis of acute myelopathy.

Management

Management of MS can be grouped into three main categories: treatment of acute relapses; treatment with immunomodulatory disease-modifying drugs aimed at ameliorating the underlying disease course, and symptomatic management.

Treatment of Acute Relapses

- Standard treatment for acute relapses is with intravenous steroids using 500 to 1000 mg/d for 3 to 5 days, with or without follow-up taper with oral prednisone over 1 to 2 weeks
- Therapy reduces severity and duration of attacks, but it is not clear if it has any long-term benefit
- Acute relapses should be differentiated from pseudo-exacerbations (e.g., those precipitated by heat, infection, or excess activity) for which glucocorticoids are not useful
- Therapy to counter side effects of short-term glucocorticoids may include: low-salt, potassium rich diet, prophylaxis for gastritis or peptic ulcer disease, and management of any worsening of emotional lability (e.g., with lithium carbonate), anxiety, or sleep disturbance
- Alternatives therapeutic options to intravenous steroids for acute relapses include: oral steroids (but these have higher gastrointestinal and psychiatric side effect profile), adrenocorticotropic hormone (ACTH) injection (infrequently used now), plasmapheresis

(removal, separation, and replacement of plasma to bloodstream for those unresponsive to steroid treatment), and intravenous immunoglobulin (IVIg)

■ Addition of short-term physical and occupational therapy interventions is often helpful

Disease Modifying Therapies (Table 18.6)
The three forms of beta-interferon and glatiramer acetate all have been shown to be modestly effective at reducing relapse rate (by approximately 30%), are administered by injection, and have a relatively mild side effect profile. One of these drugs is often initiated as the first line treatment for RRMS, and choice amongst those may be based on route of administration and side effect profile (Table 18.6). Interferon beta-1a or 1b suppress T-helper cell response and glatiramer acetate alters T-cell activation.

Natalizumab, a monoclonal antibody that blocks T-cell migration across the BBB, is more effective in reducing relapses (at about 70%) than first-line agents. However, it has significant side effects including the rare but potentially fatal development of progressive multifocal leukoencephalopathy (PML).

Mitoxantrone, an immunosuppressive agent that inhibits cell replication, is the only agent currently available that may be effective in PRMS and SPMS in addition to RRMS, but has serious dose-limiting cardiotoxicity. Stronger treatments, therefore, carry a more significant side effect profile, so it is important that the treatment be matched to the patient.

Fingolimod, a sphigosine-1 receptor agonist, represented a milestone following its approval as an oral drug for MS in 2010, offering patients a much more convenient administration route. However, association with cardiovascular complications has led to a more cautious approach in its initial prescribing.

Dimethyl fumarate and teriflunomide are two additional orally administered agents that have been approved in 2013 for the treatment of RRMS. Dimethyl fumarate is available as an enteric-coated preparation. It is thought to act by enhancing cellular response to oxidative stress through activation of a nuclear factor-like 2 (Nrf2) pathway. Side effects include flushing, gastrointestinal events, and lymphopenia.

Teriflunomide is an orally administered pyrimidine synthesis inhibitor; its mechanism of action in MS may involve a decrease in the number of activated lymphocytes in the CNS. It may cause liver function test abnormalities and has a boxed warning for hepatotoxicity. Additional side effects include decreased white cell count and a potential for teratogenicity (based on animal data).

Symptomatic Treatment (Table 18.7)
Because MS can cause a variety of neurological impairments, functional deficits, and secondary complications, symptomatic management plays a prominent

Table 18.6
Disease Modifying Drugs for Multiple Sclerosis

Drug (Brand Name)	Administration Route/ Frequency	Mechanism of Action[a]	Side Effects
IFN-β-1a (Avonex)	IM injection weekly	Suppress T cell response, inhibit T-cell migration across BBB	Flu-like symptoms, injection site reactions, neutralizing antibodies can reduce efficacy
IFN-β-1a (Rebif)	SQ injection weekly		
IFN-β-1b (Betaseron)	SQ injection three times a week		
Glatiramer acetate (Copaxone)	SQ injection daily	Alter T-cell activation, reduce inflammatory cytokine production	Site reactions, postinjection reaction
Mitoxantrone (Novantrone)	IV injection every 3 months	Immunosuppressive agent that inhibits cell replication	Dose-limiting cardio-toxicity, infections, leukopenia
Natalizumab (Tysabri)	IV injection monthly	Monoclonal antibody against an adhesion molecule on lymphocytes, blocks T-cell migration across BBB	Rare but potentially fatal PML
Fingolimod (Gilenya)	PO once daily	Traps lymphocytes in the periphery which prevents them from reaching the brain	First-degree heart block and bradycardia, LFT or WBC count abnormalities (often mild)
Dimethyl fumarate (Tecfidera)	PO twice a day	Enhances cellular response to oxidative stress	Flushing, gastrointestinal events, and lymphopenia
Teriflunomide (Aubagio)	PO once daily	Pyrimidine synthesis inhibitor; action in MS may involve a decrease in the number of activated lymphocytes in the CNS	LFT and WBC count abnormalities, has a boxed warning for hepatotoxicity, potential for teratogenicity (based on animal data)

Abbreviations: BBB, blood-brain barrier; CNS, central nervous system; IFN-β, interferon β; IM, intramuscular; IV, intravenous; LFT, liver function tests; PML, progressive multifocal leukoencephalopathy; PO, oral; SQ, subcutaneous; WBC, white blood cells.
[a] The mechanism of action of several of the listed drugs is only partially understood at present.

Table 18.7

Symptomatic Management of the Major Manifestations of MS

Manifestation	Management

Fatigue	- Energy conservation techniques
	- Identify and treat secondary causes (sleep disorder, nocturia, depression), heat sensitivity (see below)
	- Medications for primary MS fatigue:
	  • Amantadine 100 mg twice daily
	  • Modafinil 100–400 mg every morning
	  • Methylphenidate 5–20 mg twice daily

Heat sensitivity	- Heat avoidance - Air conditioning, cooling vests
Spasticity	- Stretching, positioning, exercise, modalities - Identify and treat exacerbating factors (e.g., infection) - Medications: Baclofen, tizanidine, diazepam, dantrolene, cyclobenzaprine; baclofen intrathecal pump; local chemodenervation - See Chapter 38A for details

Pain	- Identify and treat mechanical or nociceptive causes
	- Neuropathic pain can be severe and difficult to treat
	- Medications for neuropathic pain
	  • Anticonvulsants (e.g., carbamazepine, phenytoin, gabapentin, pregablin)
	  • Antidepressants (e.g., amitriptyline)
	  • Antiarrhythmics (e.g., mexiletine)
	- Cognitive behavioral therapy
	- See Chapter 38C for details

Paroxysmal symptoms (e.g., trigeminal neuralgia)	- Often responsive to anticonvulsant medications (carbamazepine, gabapentin, pregablin) in modest doses - Milder cases of trigeminal neuralgia may respond to local anesthetic ointment
Bladder dysfunction	- Guided by urodynamic testing - Antimuscarinic agents for detrusor hyperreflexia - Alpha blockers, intermittent catheterization for DSD - Prompt identification and management of urinary infections - See Chapter 34A for details
Bowel dysfunction/ constipation	- Adequate fluid and fiber intake - Review medications for constipating side effects - Bowel medications, bowel management as needed - See Chapter 36A for details
Sexual dysfunction	- Address secondary factors such as pain, positioning, fatigue, spasticity - PDE-5 inhibitors (sildenafil, tadalafil, vardenafil) for erectile dysfunction - See Chapter 35 for details

(continued)

Table 18.7

Symptomatic Management of the Major Manifestations of MS (*continued*)

Manifestation	Management
Gait impairment, weakness	- Potassium channel blocker 4-amino pyridine (4-AP) has been demonstrated to improve some aspects of ambulation, and is available as an FDA-approved agent, dalfampridine given at 20 mg/d - Assistive devices and task-specific therapy as needed
Tremor/ataxia	- Can be poorly responsive to treatment - Medications include clonazepam, isoniazid, mysoline, propranolol, though efficacy is limited - Weighted wrist cuffs, arm rests, weighted walkers may help - Deep-brain stimulation and thalamotomy have been tried with limited success
Impaired function and ADL	- Identify and address specific contributing impairments - Physical and occupational therapy, task-specific therapeutic exercise, assistive devices as indicated
Dysphagia and dysarthria	- Swallowing evaluation including videoflouroscopy as indicated - Dietary modification, postural techniques as appropriate - Speech therapy
Visual problems	- Eye patch for persistent diplopia - Eye prisms for severe nystagmus
Depression	- Antidepressant medication (SSRI, tricyclic antidepressants) - Behavioral interventions, counseling
Cognitive impairment	- Detailed testing to identify specific deficits - Compensatory strategies (lists, pacing, electronic aids) - May try the cholinesterase inhibitor donepazil 10 mg/d though not approved for use in MS - Identify and address secondary factors (fatigue, disturbed sleep, depression)
Lifestyle management	- Healthy diet, correct any nutritional deficiencies - Regular exercise per tolerance, swimming and water aerobics are often well tolerated, avoiding hot water temperature above 30°C for heat sensitivity - General health promotion and disease prevention, influenza vaccination shown to be safe and effective but should be delayed for 4–6 weeks after acute relapse - Support social and vocational participation

Abbreviations: ADL, activities of daily living; DSD, detrusor sphincter dyssynergia; PDE-5, phosphodiesterase-5 inhibitors; SSRI, selective serotonin reuptake inhibitors.

role in the overall care of people with MS. Table 18.7 provides a summary of symptomatic management of the major manifestations of MS. Several of these, for example, management of spasticity, pain, and bladder, bowel, and sexual dysfunction, are covered in greater detail in separate chapters dedicated to those problems in other sections of this book.

KNOWLEDGE GAPS AND EMERGING CONCEPTS

Available tools to measure the impact of MS and MS related disability have several limitations and better outcome measures are needed to assess the efficacy of treatments.

Most currently available disease-modifying therapies have been compared to placebo often using different criteria to measure effectiveness, and direct comparative studies between different agents are limited.

As mentioned previously, new oral agents for MS have been approved recently. Several investigative therapies are at various stages of development and undergoing clinical trials. These include combination therapies, additional monoclonal antibodies targeting lymphocyte receptors, use of myelin basic protein (MBP) to induce antigen-specific tolerance and the prospect of developing a vaccine for MS, and bone marrow transplant.

SUGGESTED READING

Barten LJ, Allington DR, Procacci KA, Rivey MP. New approaches in the management of multiple sclerosis. *Drug Des Devel Ther.* 2010;4:343-466.

Ben-Zacharia AB. Therapeutics for multiple sclerosis symptoms. *Mt Sinai J Med.* 2011;78(2): 176-191.

Crayton HJ, Rossman HS. Managing the symptoms of multiple sclerosis: a multimodal approach. *Clin Ther.* 2006;28(4):445-460.

Crayton HJ, Heyman RA, Rossman HS. A multimodal approach to managing the symptoms of multiple sclerosis. *Neurology.* 2004;63(11 suppl 5):S12-S18.

Derwenskus J. Current disease-modifying treatment of multiple sclerosis. *Mt Sinai J Med.* 2011;78(2):161-175.

Freeman JA. Improving mobility and functional independence in persons with multiple sclerosis. *J Neurol.* 2001;248(4):255-259.

Hartung HP, Montalban X, Sorensen PS, Vermersch P, Olsson T. Principles of a new treatment algorithm in multiple sclerosis. *Expert Rev Neurother.* 2011;11(3):351-362.

Khan F, Turner-Stokes L, Ng L, Kilpatrick T. Multidisciplinary rehabilitation for adults with multiple sclerosis. *Cochrane Database Syst Rev.* 2007 Apr18;(2):CD006036.

Matsuda PN, Shumway-Cook A, Bamer AM, Johnson SL, Amtmann D, Kraft GH. Falls in multiple sclerosis. *PM R.* 2011;3(7):624-632.

Noseworthy JH, Lucchinetti C, Rodriguez M, Weinshenker BG. Multiple sclerosis. *N Engl J Med.* 2000;343(13):938-952.

Samkoff LM, Goodman AD. Symptomatic management in multiple sclerosis. *Neurol Clin.* 2011;29(2):449-463.

Souza A, Kelleher A, Cooper R, Cooper RA, Iezzoni LI, Collins DM. Multiple sclerosis and mobility-related assistive technology: systematic review of literature. *JRRD.* 2010;47(3):213-224.

CHAPTER 19

Spinal Arachnoiditis

GENERAL PRINCIPLES

Arachnoiditis is an inflammatory process of the spinal meninges that results in increased fibrous tissue within the subarachnoid space.

Etiology

Arachnoiditis may occur as a consequence of spinal surgery, intrathecal administration of certain agents such as some contrast media used for myelography, infectious meningitis, or subarachnoid hemorrhage.

Epidemiology

Arachnoiditis encountered in current practice is most frequently limited to involvement of either the cauda equina or to single nerve roots.

Pathophysiology

While the arachnoid itself is avascular, the reactive inflammatory response to irritation or injury can occur in the surrounding vascular pia and dura. This leads to adhesions and chronic thickening of the arachnoid with obliteration of the subarachnoid space. The adjoining nerve roots and spinal cord may be compromised by compression and vascular occlusion from the fibrous connective tissue.

Disease Course

Presentation may be delayed for weeks, months, or even a year after exposure to the precipitating cause. Rarely, arachnoiditis may be complicated by development of a syrinx, presumably related to altered cerebrospinal fluid flow.

CLINICAL CONSIDERATIONS

Assessment

History and Physical Examination
History of the underlying preceding event may provide a clue to the diagnosis, although presentation may be delayed.

The condition may remain asymptomatic despite radiological evidence of pathology.

Distribution of symptoms and signs depends on the location of the arachnoiditis and the affected structures. Sensory root involvement often causes pain, sometimes in a radicular distribution, as well as depressed muscle stretch reflexes. Low back pain with radiation to the legs is a common presentation. Involvement of the cauda equina can present with muscle atrophy, lower motor neuron leg weakness, and bladder and bowel dysfunction. Spinal cord compression may result in spastic paraplegia, sometimes months or years following radicular symptoms.

Diagnostic Tests
Diagnostic imaging includes myelogram, computed tomography myelogram, or magnetic resonance imaging (MRI), which shows clumping of the nerve roots and obliterated subarachnoid space and thecal sac.

Management

The condition is typically resistant to curative treatment. Steroids have not been shown to be effective. Surgery has been reported to help occasionally when the condition is confined to a relatively localized area, but that is uncommon.

Symptomatic treatment is needed for pain and other chronic symptoms.

KNOWLEDGE GAPS AND EMERGING CONCEPTS

It has been suggested that there are individual genetic characteristics that may increase susceptibility to develop arachnoiditis, but these have not been well defined and further research is needed.

SUGGESTED READING

Vloeberghs M, Herregodts P, Stadnik T, Goossens A, D'Haens J. Spinal arachnoiditis mimicking a spinal cord tumor: a case report and review of the literature. *Surg Neurol.* 1992;37(3):211-215.
Wright MH, Denney LC. A comprehensive review of spinal arachnoiditis. *Orthop Nurs.* 2003;22(3):215-219.

CHAPTER 20

Infections of the Spine and Spinal Cord

GENERAL PRINCIPLES

Infections involving the spine and spinal cord can be categorized based on location, and include infections of the vertebral column, spinal canal, or spinal cord.

Infections of the Vertebral Column

These include vertebral osteomyelitis (pyogenic, mycobacterial, or fungal) and disk space infection. Features of pyogenic osteomyelitis are summarized in Table 20.1.

Tuberculosis of the spine is common in developing countries. Although infrequent in the United States, its prevalence is higher amongst immigrant, immune compromised or homeless individuals. Clinical presentation can be similar to that for pyogenic infections (Table 20.1), though onset is often more sub-acute or chronic. Vertebral destruction and paravertebral abscess formation is seen on imaging but, unlike pyogenic infections, vertebral end-plates and inter-vertebral disks are often preserved. Treatment involves several months of multi-drug chemotherapy for tuberculosis after obtaining tissue biopsy and culture.

Infections in the Spinal Canal

These primarily include epidural abscess, which is summarized in Table 20.2. Subdural abscess is much less common than epidural.

Infections of the Spinal Cord

Infectious involvement of the spinal cord can be bacterial, viral, fungal, or parasitic. Bacterial infections of the spinal cord itself in the form of intramedullary abscess are very rare. The spinal cord can be involved in neurosyphilis. Tabes dorsalis due to untreated syphilis involves the posterior columns. Several viruses can affect the spinal cord. Human immunodeficiency virus (HIV) is associated with a vacuolar myelopathy that predominantly affects the posterior and lateral columns and occurs in late stages of the disease (Table 20.3). Other viral infections can occur in people with HIV or other

Table 20.1

Pyogenic Vertebral Osteomyelitis/Discitis	
Etiology	- Hematogenous spread is most common, may occasionally be affected by contiguous spread or direct inoculation (e.g., penetrating trauma, surgical contamination) - *Staphylococcus aureus* is most common agent - *Pseudomonas* may be seen in drug abusers, *Salmonella* may occur with sickle cell anemia
Epidemiology	- More common in immune compromised, diabetics, elderly, intravenous drug abusers - Lumbar spine is most frequently involved, followed by thoracic
Clinical presentation	- Commonly present with low back pain - Fever, chills, night sweats may provide clue to presence of infection - Localized tenderness over involved vertebra - Rapidity of progression depend on virulence of underlying organism - Risk factors and source of infection may be detected (e.g., peripheral lines for vascular access, urinary infection)
Imaging	- Plain films show decreased disk space height, erosion of vertebral end plates (an important indication of pyogenic infection), but may be normal in first few days - MRI with gadolinium is imaging of choice for early detection; bone marrow edema is an early finding (hypointense signal on T1-weighted image, hyperintense on T2-weighted) - Radionuclide scans (technetium, gallium) have high sensitivity but low specificity; can be used for monitoring treatment
Other tests	- ESR, CRP usually high; can be used to monitor response to treatment
Management	- Tissue biopsy and culture should be obtained prior to antibiotics if at all feasible - Pyogenic osteomyelitis usually need 4–6 weeks of intravenous antibiotics often followed by oral antibiotics for several weeks; surgical decompression and fusion may be needed for instability, deformity

Abbreviations: CRP, C-reactive protein; ESR, Erythrocyte sedimentation rate; MRI, magnetic resonance imaging.

Table 20.2

Epidural Abscess

Etiology	- *Staphylococcus aureus* is most common agent - Other organisms include gram negative bacteria, anaerobes, fungal, mycobacterial - May occur due to hematogenous spread from infections of the skin, soft tissue, or other organs - Can also occur as a direct extension of vertebral osteomyelitis/discitis
Epidemiology	- Risk factors include immune compromise (diabetes, malignancy, alcoholism), intravenous drug abuse, infections at distant sites
Clinical presentation	- Clinical triad of midline back pain, fever, and progressive limb weakness is typical - Once signs of myelopathy appear, they may progress rapidly; bladder dysfunction may develop
Imaging	- MRI scan identifies the abscess and its extent, and distinguishes it from other conditions
Other tests	- Increased white cell count, blood culture may be positive - ESR, CRP usually high; can be used to monitor response to treatment
Management	- Usually a combination of decompressive surgery and long course of antibiotics - Surgery prevents development or progression of paralysis but established deficits of several days duration may not improve. - Broad spectrum antibiotics can be started after culture is obtained and modified based on results of culture; often need to be continued for 4–6 weeks

Abbreviations: CRP, C-reactive protein; ESR, Erythrocyte sedimentation rate; MRI, magnetic resonance imaging.

Table 20.3

HIV-Associated Myelopathy

Primary HIV myelopathy is a vacuolar myelopathy that occurs in late stages of the disease. Incidence has decreased since the introduction of highly active antiretroviral therapy

It predominantly involves the posterior (and sometimes lateral) columns, and often presents with sensory ataxia and spastic weakness

Pathogenesis is unknown. Possibility of inability to utilize Vitamin B12 has been suggested with similarity in the distribution of pathological findings in the spinal cord to those seen with Vitamin B12 deficiency

Other causes of myelopathy in HIV positive individuals include opportunistic or coinfections. Infections can be bacterial (pyogenic, tuberculosis, syphilis), viral (e.g., cytomegalovirus, herpes simplex, varicella zoster), fungal (e.g., cryptococcosis), or parasitic (e.g., toxoplasmosis)

Treatment of primary HIV myelopathy is mainly supportive. Prognosis is poor

Abbreviation: HIV, human immunodeficiency virus.

immunocompromised individuals, for example, cytomegalovirus, herpes simplex, or varicella zoster. Parasitic infections of the spinal cord such as toxoplasmosis can occur in HIV positive individuals. Other parasitic infections include cysticercosis and schistosomiasis, which are rare in the United States, but common worldwide.

SUGGESTED READING

Garg RK, Somvanshi DS. Spinal tuberculosis: a review. *J Spinal Cord Med*. 2011;34(5): 440-454.

Go JL, Rothman S, Prosper A, Silbergleit R, Lerner A. Spine infections. *Neuroimaging Clin N Am*. 2012;22(4):755-772.

Gray F, Gherardi R, Trotot P, Fenelon G, Poirier J. Spinal cord lesions in the acquired immune deficiency syndrome (AIDS). *Neurosurg Rev*. 1990;13(3):189-194.

Ho EL. Infectious etiologies of myelopathy. *Semin Neurol*. 2012;32(2):154-160.

Richie MB, Pruitt AA. Spinal cord infections. *Neurol Clin*. 2013;31(1):19-53.

CHAPTER 21

Nutritional, Toxic, and Environmental Myelopathies

GENERAL PRINCIPLES

Nutritional Myelopathies

The most significant nutritional myelopathy is subacute combined degeneration (SACD) from vitamin B12 deficiency (Table 21.1). Copper deficiency is a rare cause of myelopathy that has been recognized in the last decade and may present similarly to SACD. Case reports have been associated with upper gastrointestinal bariatric surgery, malabsorption, and zinc overload all of which interfere with copper absorption.

Toxic Myelopathies

As indicated in Chapter 12, Table 12.1, there are several toxic and environmental elements that can cause myelopathy. Although very uncommon in the United States, worldwide, predominantly in parts of Asia, Africa, and the Caribbean, lathyrism is an important cause of toxic myelopathy. It is caused by ingesting a certain variety of legume, the *Lathyrus* grain, in high concentration. These grains have a neurotoxin that causes spastic paralysis.

Physical/Environmental Causes of Myelopathy (Electrical, Decompression, Radiation)

Electrical Trauma and Lightning Strikes
These are rare causes of spinal cord injury (SCI), though precise incidence is not known. SCI can result from direct injury by the electric current or occur indirectly due to fall from a height after sustaining electric injury. Key features are summarized in Table 21.2.

Decompression Sickness
Myelopathy can be a manifestation of decompression sickness in scuba divers who rapidly return to surface from depth after under-water diving. Its features are summarized in Table 21.3.

Table 21.1

Key Features of Subacute Combined Degeneration (SACD) Due to Vitamin B12 Deficiency

Etiology	- Due to Vitamin B12 (cobalamin) deficiency - Most common cause is pernicious anemia, due to intrinsic factor antibodies that prevent absorption of B12 from the terminal ileum - Other causes include malabsorption, gastric resection, terminal ileum disease, and dietary deficiency. Nitrous oxide anesthesia or inhalation has been reported to cause it through inactivation of B12 metabolism
Epidemiology	- Prevalence varies depending on population studied - Higher prevalence of deficiency in elderly individuals or coexistent alcohol abuse
Pathophysiology	- B12 is involved in enzymatic reactions for myelin and neurotransmitter synthesis, but the significance of this role in pathogenesis of SACD is unclear - Up-regulation of neurotoxic cytokines and down-regulation of neurotrophic factors may be involved in pathogenesis
Pathology	- Degenerative changes are seen in peripheral and central nervous system (myelin breakdown and vacuolation, early involvement of posterior columns, later spreading to the corticospinal tracts)
Associated conditions	- Other effects of B12 deficiency include megaloblastic anemia, peripheral neuropathy, and dementia
Clinical presentation	- Early sensory symptoms in the legs with loss of vibratory and position sense - There may be combined features of UMN and LMN involvement in the legs (loss of ankle reflexes with hyperreflexia at the knees, muscle atrophy with spasticity and positive Babinski sign) - Sensory ataxia and/or spastic paraplegia may predominate - Sphincter involvement is uncommon
Diagnostic tests	- Low Vitamin B12 level - Reduced sensory nerve conduction on electrophysiological testing - MRI findings predominantly affecting the posterior columns
Management	- Vitamin B12 replacement (oral supplementation 1,000 μg daily or intramuscular injection)

Abbreviations: LMN, lower motor neuron; MRI, magnetic resonance imaging; UMN, upper motor neuron.

III. Nontraumatic Myelopathies

Table 21.2

Spinal Cord Injury Due to Electrical Trauma or Lightning Strike

Etiology and pathophysiology	- Electrical or lightning injury is a rare cause of myelopathy - Exposure of cord parenchyma to electric current causes tissue damage due to heating, altered cell membrane permeability, or denaturation of cellular protein - Mechanical injury due to fall from a height after sustaining an electrical injury is an additional indirect mechanism of SCI
Associated conditions	- The electrical shock or lightning strike can also cause • Skin burns • Brain injury due to cardio-pulmonary arrest and hypoxia • Peripheral nerve injury from electrical current or from compartment syndrome • Muscle injury that can cause weakness, myoglobinuria, renal damage, or compartment syndrome • Vascular injury including venous wall injury with risk of venous thrombosis • Autonomic dysfunction with cardiac arrhythmias, bradycardia, or cardiac arrest
Clinical presentation	- Presentation can be varied • Acute and transient flaccid paralysis that resolves in 24 hrs • Immediate paralysis with persistent deficits • Delayed onset of myelopathy with sensory and motor symptoms appearing after days or weeks, that usually persist • Myelopathy due to fall after sustaining electric injury presents as a traumatic injury - Presenting features of associated conditions
Diagnostic tests	- Imaging may show evidence of fall-related vertebral trauma and cord injury
Management	- Management may be complicated by associated conditions mentioned above - Late deterioration or progression of neurological deficits may occur in some

Table 21.3

Myelopathy Associated With Decompression Sickness

Etiology and pathophysiology	- Occurs in scuba divers who rapidly return to surface from depth after under-water diving. There are also case reports associated with loss of aircraft cabin pressure

(continued)

	- Upon rapid ascent and decompression, nitrogen gas previously forced under pressure in the blood, bubbles back out into blood stream and tissues - Exact pathogenesis is not understood but is thought to involve venous congestion
Associated conditions	- Associated problems can be varied depending on location of air bubbles - Large joint involvement causes aching pain ("bends") - Brain involvement may cause confusion or behavior changes, headache, visual problems - Skin involvement manifests as itching or burning sensation, or rash - Shortness of breath or cough may occur with pulmonary involvement - Inner ear involvement can cause dizziness, vertigo, nausea, and vomiting
Clinical presentation	- Usually immediate onset but may be delayed for several hours (or may occasionally develop during subsequent air flight with ascent to altitude) - Low back pain and/or pain in girdle-like distribution - Paralysis, paresthesias, and sphincter involvement may occur due to myelopathy - Symptoms of associated conditions mentioned above
Diagnostic tests	- MRI may show white matter and dorsal column involvement but findings are varied and may be nonspecific
Management	- Prompt identification and treatment is important and improves prognosis for recovery - Management primarily involves rapid recompression in a specialized chamber - Hyperbaric oxygen therapy is also beneficial

Abbreviation: MRI, magnetic resonance imaging.

Radiation Myelopathies

Radiation myelopathy is a rare form of myelopathy that result from radiation exposure of the spinal cord during radiotherapy of primary or metastatic tumors of the spinal cord or of malignancies in adjacent areas. Spinal cord involvement by tumor needs to be ruled out prior to making the diagnosis. Myelopathy due to radiation can be early (usually transient) or delayed (permanent); features of these two types of radiation myelopathy are compared in Table 21.4.

Table 21.4

Radiation Myelopathy: Early and Delayed Forms

Feature	Early	Delayed
Onset	6 weeks to 6 months after radiation	More than 6 months after radiation, rarely earlier; average 1–2 yrs after, may occur up to 4 yrs later
Course/prognosis	Transient with full recovery	Usually permanent neurological deficits
Prevalence	Infrequent, but more common than delayed	Rare
Dose relationship	No clear dose relationship	Dose dependent; usually with radiation doses above 5,000 cGY
Presentation	Limb paresthesias, electric shock-like sensation radiating down the back on neck flexion (Lhermitte's sign); may be intermittent; resolve over few months	Gradual onset of spastic paralysis and impaired sensation below the level of irradiation; sphincter disturbance may occur
Pathology	Thought to involve transient demyelination of white matter tracts, especially the posterior columns	White matter involvement (demyelination, cellular infiltrate), vascular involvement (thrombosis and areas of infarction)
Treatment	Usually none needed	Primarily supportive; no established primary treatment but reports have included steroids, anticoagulants, hyperbaric oxygen, and, recently, use of angiogenesis inhibitors

SUGGESTED READING

Jaiser SR, Winston GP. Copper deficiency myelopathy. *J Neurol*. 2010;257(6):869-881.
Kumar N. Metabolic and toxic myelopathies. *Semin Neurol*. 2012;32(2):123-136.
Lammertse DP. Neurorehabilitation of spinal cord injuries following lightning and electrical trauma. *NeuroRehabilitation*. 2005;20(1):9-14.

Scalabrino G. Subacute combined degeneration one century later. The neurotrophic action of cobalamin (vitamin B12) revisited. *J Neuropathol Exp Neurol*. 2001;60(2):109-120.

Schwendimann RN. Metabolic, nutritional, and toxic myelopathies. *Neurol Clin*. 2013;31(1): 207-218.

Vollmann R, Lamperti M, Magyar M, Simbrunner J. Magnetic resonance imaging of the spine in a patient with decompression sickness. *Clin Neuroradiol*. 2011;21(4):231-233.

CHAPTER 22

Spina Bifida/ Myelomeningocele

GENERAL PRINCIPLES

Spina bifida or spinal dysraphisms refers to congenital conditions with neural tube defects that result from a failure of closure of the posterior arch of the spine. These can be broadly categorized as open (defect in the overlying skin with exposure of neural tissue) or closed (neural tissue is covered by skin).

The most significant of these is myelomeningocele (MMC), which makes up more than 90% of open spinal dysraphisms and is associated with neurological defects.

Etiology

Both genetic and environmental factors are thought to be involved. Risk is increased in those with a positive family history. While most children with MMC are born to families without a previous affected child, risk of recurrence increases to 2–5% with one affected child and to 10–15% with two affected siblings. If one parent has spina bifida, there is a 4% risk of having a child with the same condition. Several environmental factors have been implicated in etiology of MMC including folic acid deficiency, exposure to certain medications during early pregnancy (especially carbamazepine and valproate), occupational exposure to certain solvents, and maternal diabetes.

Epidemiology

Incidence of MMC seems to be decreasing worldwide and in the United States (U.S.). Possible reasons may include increased intake of folate supplementation in women of childbearing age, mandatory fortification of grain products, and more widespread screening leading to higher rates of elective termination. Estimated rates of MMC in the U.S. are just under 2/1000 births though there is some geographical variation.

Pathophysiology

MMC and other neural tube defects occur because of failure of closure of the neural tube in the third and fourth weeks of gestation.

152

Prevention and Prenatal Counseling

All women of childbearing age are recommended to consume folic acid supplements (0.4 mg daily). Those who have had a previous affected pregnancy should consume higher amounts from 1 month prior to conception through the end of the first trimester of pregnancy.

Prenatal screening involves testing of maternal serum α-fetoprotein between the 16th and 18th weeks of gestation. High level ultrasound can confirm the diagnosis in most instances. In the small percent where good images can't be obtained to make a definitive diagnosis, amniocentesis to test amniotic fluid α-fetoprotein levels can be done. After diagnosis is established, genetic counseling and discussion of management options should be done.

CLINICAL CONSIDERATIONS

Assessment and Management

MMC has direct or indirect effect on multiple body systems. Key features in assessment and management of the most important consequences and complications of MMC are summarized in Table 22.1.

Table 22.1

Multisystem Consequences and Complications of Myelomeningocele (MMC)

Body System/Problem	Considerations
Neurological	
Primary neural defect	- Lumbosacral level is most common (~70%) - Early closure of back defect (within 72 hrs of delivery) is indicated to prevent infection
Associated or secondary neurological problems	- Includes hydrocephalus, hydromyelia, Chiari malformation, tethered cord (see Table 22.2)
Physical/functional	- Mobility depends on neurological level - Those with thoracic MMC are nonambulatory, high or mid lumbar may have limited ambulation as children but lose that with age, low lumbar and sacral are community ambulators, though may have decreased endurance
Musculoskeletal	
Scoliosis	- Can be congenital (due to vertebral abnormalities) and/or paralytic (most likely with thoracic MMC) - Syringomyelia or tethered cord may also be factors
Contracture/dislocation	- Unopposed hip flexion and adduction can cause hip dislocations, especially in thoracic to L4 level (especially common in those with L3 level) - Foot deformities (most commonly equinus or equinovarus) are common

(continued)

Table 22.1

Multisystem Consequences and Complications of Myelomeningocele (MMC) (*continued*)

Body System/Problem	Considerations
	- Often need surgical correction with heel cord lengthening and/or tendon transfer
Fractures	- Osteoporosis and pathological fractures may occur
Bladder/genitourinary	- Neurogenic bladder with poor compliance and contractility is common - Sphincter incompetence with incontinence is common; some may have detrusor-sphincter dyssynergia - Reflux and hydronephrosis may occur - Early and ongoing attention is needed to minimize upper tract complications (see Chapter 34A)
Bowel function	- Neurogenic bowel is common - Principles of bowel management apply (see Chapter 36A); antegrade continence enema (ACE) is a surgical option
Skin	- Pressure ulcers are an important cause of morbidity (see Chapter 37)
Latex allergy	- High prevalence in children with MMC - Related to repeated exposure to latex-containing products, medical supplies - Immunoglobulin E-mediated reaction - Reaction can occur intra-operatively due to mucosal exposure during surgical handling and be life-threatening if not promptly recognized and treated - Should be cared for in a latex-free environment, wear medical alert, and carry auto-injectable epinephrine
Endocrine/metabolic	- Short stature and disturbed growth are common; possible role of growth hormone - Obesity is common and is multifactorial - Precocious puberty may occur (possibly due to increased pressure on hypothalamus causing premature activation) - Female fertility is normal; males have high infertility rates
Cognitive/behavioral	- On average have a lower IQ score than peers - Behavioral problems are common
Psychosocial	- Caregiver burden/expense can be significant - Learning difficulties, medical issues can impact education - Transition to adulthood may be associated with system of care challenges - Vocational, relationship, independent living issues often arise

Associated Neurological Conditions

Neurological deficits depend on the site of the defect, and include motor, sensory, bowel, and bladder dysfunction. Deficits related to the primary MMC are static from birth and don't evolve further. However, several associated conditions commonly occur that can cause additional neurological deficits. Associated neurological problems include hydrocephalus, coexisting Chiari malformation (type II, also see Chapter 23), hydromyelia, and tethered cord. Most patients require shunt placement to manage the associated hydrocephalus, but shunt malfunction is common. Clinical presentation and management of each of these neurological conditions is summarized in Table 22.2.

Ambulation and Mobility
Functional goals and mobility outcomes depend on the level of the MMC.

Table 22.2

Neurological Conditions Associated With Myelomeningocele		
Condition	**Key Points**	**Clinical Presentation**
Hydrocephalus	- Develops in over 90% of cases - Most require placement of a ventriculoperitoneal shunt - Shunt malfunction is common and presents with similar findings as for hydrocephalus	- Headache, irritability, lethargy, vomiting - Increasing head circumference in infants, bulging anterior fontanel - Strabismus may be associated - May present with subtle cognitive changes
Chiari malformation (Type II)	- Present in over 90% of cases - One of the main causes of death during infancy in MMC - Caudal displacement and deformation of cerebellar tonsils, vermis, fourth ventricle and medulla through the foramen magnum - Symptoms may respond to shunting of hydrocephalus; some require posterior fossa decompression	- Symptoms reflect lower brainstem dysfunction - Dysphagia, nasal regurgitation, choking - Hoarseness or stridor - Cyanosis - Apnea, breath-holding, sleep apnea - Nystagmus - Upper extremity weakness - Opisthotonus, torticollis
Hydromyelia/ syringomyelia	- Confirmed by MRI	- May be asymptomatic - Progressive scoliosis - New motor deficits - Change in spasticity
Tethered cord syndrome	- Associated with arachnoiditis and fibrosis after MMC repair which tether the cord to low lumbar or sacral region - Commonly seen on MRI; surgical treatment only if symptoms develop - May increase during period of rapid growth in adolescence	- Worsening leg weakness and/or gait - Progressive scoliosis - Pain in back or legs - Leg muscle atrophy - Loss of tendon reflexes - Change in bowel or bladder function - New contracture (e.g., pes cavus)

Thoracic level MMC requires wheelchair mobility. Dynamic or static standers can be used between 1 and 2 years of age. Reciprocating gait orthoses can be tried in young children but usually have to be discontinued in childhood. Scoliosis is very common at this level and requires consideration of a thoracolumbar spinal orthosis (TLSO) and/or surgical correction.

Upper lumbar level MMC is commonly associated with hip dislocation due to unopposed hip flexors and adductors. Ankle foot orthoses or knee-ankle-foot orthoses are used along with assistive gait aids such as walker or crutches. Most of these children need to transition to wheelchair as they grow older.

Children with lower lumbar level MMC (L4-5) can walk with crutches and braces, but several eventually transition to wheelchair.

Those with sacral level MMC usually walk without braces or gait aids. Foot deformities may occur due to intrinsic foot muscle weakness and may negatively impact walking endurance.

Other Systemic Effects
These include osteoporosis with risk of pathological fractures, lower limb contractures, pressure ulcers, neurogenic bowel, bladder, and sexual dysfunction, and endocrine problems including short stature and precocious puberty (Table 22.1). Obesity is common, with significant medical and functional implications. Latex allergy is common. Cognitive and behavioral problems often coexist, and can adversely affect education and schooling.

Transition to Adulthood
Around 80% of individuals with MMC now survive into adulthood. Transition from long-standing and often comprehensive pediatric care to less cohesive adult health care can be associated with challenges related to access and coordination.

Continued problems in adulthood include late neurological changes, overuse musculoskeletal injuries, pathological fractures, and ongoing urological complications. Attention to relationships, sexual and reproductive health is important starting in adolescence. Women with MMC who are sexually active should take folic acid at a higher dose (4 mg daily) than otherwise recommended. Issues related to employment and independent living commonly need to be addressed. Regular preventive health care and management of unrelated medical problems should be integrated as part of ongoing primary care.

KNOWLEDGE GAPS AND EMERGING CONCEPTS

A prospective randomized controlled trial demonstrated that fetal surgery with in-utero repair of the MMC before 26 weeks gestation may preserve neurological function, reverse the hindbrain herniation of the Chiari II malformation, and reduce the need for postnatal placement of a ventriculoperitoneal shunt. However, there were significant associated risks including premature birth.

Further research should expand understanding of the pathophysiology of MMC, evaluate long-term impact of in-utero intervention, and refine timing and technique of fetal MMC surgery.

SUGGESTED READING

Adzick NS. Fetal surgery for spina bifida: past, present, future. *Semin Pediatr Surg.* 2013;22(1):10-17.

Dicianno BE, Kurowski BG, Yang JM, et al. Rehabilitation and medical management of the adult with spina bifida. *Am J Phys Med Rehabil.* 2008;87(12):1027-1050.

Liptak GS, Dosa NP. Myelomeningocele. *Pediatr Rev.* 2010;31(11):443-450.

Liptak GS, El Samra A. Optimizing health care for children with spina bifida. *Dev Disabil Res Rev.* 2010;16(1):66-75.

Sandler AD. Children with spina bifida: key clinical issues. *Pediatr Clin North Am.* 2010;57(4):879-892.

CHAPTER 23

Chiari Malformation and Developmental Syringomyelia

GENERAL PRINCIPLES

Chiari malformations are developmental abnormalities of the hindbrain that are characterized by caudal displacement of part of the cerebellum and, in some instances, the lower brainstem, through the foramen magnum into the cervical spinal canal. These are classified by the parts of the hindbrain that protrude into the spinal canal and the associated anatomic abnormalities. Type I involves herniation of the cerebellar tonsils below the foramen magnum, and is the common form. Type II involves displacement and deformation of both the cerebellum and medulla (Table 23.1).

Etiology/Epidemiology

Spinal cord involvement varies with the type of Chiari malformation (Table 23.1).

- Syringomyelia, that is, cavity formation within the spinal cord, is present in over 30% of Type I Chiari malformation cases, and the majority of cases of developmental syringomyelia are associated with Type I Chiari malformation.
- Type II Chiari malformation, on the other hand, is usually associated with myelomeningocele (Chapter 22).

Some patients may have associated hydrocephalus, although this is much less common with type I than with type II malformation.

Pathophysiology

The precise mechanisms underlying the development of syringomyelia are not known, though obstruction of cerebrospinal fluid (CSF) flow and related abnormalities in CSF pressure are likely contributing factors. The syrinx is often in the mid-cervical region but may extend caudally or rostrally.

Table 23.1

Chiari Malformation		
Type	Abnormality	Spinal Cord Involvement
Type I	Herniation of the cerebellar tonsils below the foramen magnum	Syringomyelia in over 30%
Type II	Displacement and deformation of cerebellar tonsils, vermis, and medulla through the foramen magnum	Myelomeningocele is commonly present, often have a tethered cord, filum terminale lipoma may be present

Disease Course

Type I Chiari malformation may remain asymptomatic. Insidious symptoms may develop in adolescence or adulthood, often presenting in the 20s or 30s. The clinical course is variable and unpredictable.

Type II malformations often present in infancy or early childhood, and are discussed further in Chapter 22 along with myelomeningocele.

CLINICAL CONSIDERATIONS

Assessment

History and Physical Examination
In type I Chiari malformation, neck pain or occipital headache is a common initial symptom, and may be exacerbated by activity, stooping, or with Valsalva maneuver, for example, with sneezing or coughing. This may occur with Chiari malformation even without the presence of a syrinx, in which case it is probably attributable to compression or stretching of cervical roots.

An aching or burning pain that is often asymmetrical and involving the neck, shoulder, and arm, often at the border of sensory impairment is common in those with syringomyelia.

The classic presentation of syringomyelia is a dissociated sensory loss of pain and temperature sensation with preserved touch and vibration in a cape distribution over the neck, shoulders, and arms (Table 23.2). Most cases begin asymmetrically and may present with injuries or burns to the hand because of impaired sensation. Muscle weakness and wasting with loss of reflexes in the upper extremities may occur with extension of the syrinx into gray matter.

Table 23.2

Neurological Manifestations of Syringomyelia

Deficit	Spinal Cord Structures Involved
Dissociated pain and temperature sensory loss in a "cape distribution"; hand injuries or burns	Decussating spinothalamic tract fibers
Hand, arm, or shoulder wasting and weakness; loss of upper extremities reflexes	Anterior horn cells in the cervical spinal cord
Horner's syndrome	Descending sympathetic pathways or cells in the intermediolateral column at T1 and T2
Spastic paralysis of the legs	Corticospinal tract
Bowel and bladder dysfunction	Descending sympathetic fibers
Vocal cord or palatal paralysis with dysarthria, dysphagia, aspiration; nystagmus, dizziness, tongue atrophy and weakness	Brainstem and cranial nerve nuclei involved in case of rostral extension

Claw hand deformity of the hands may occur as a result. With progressive enlargement of the syrinx and compression of the spinal tracts, spastic paralysis of the legs, bowel and bladder dysfunction, and a Horner's syndrome may occur. Extension of the syrinx into the brainstem (syringobulbia) with cranial nerve involvement can cause dysarthria, aspiration due to dysphagia, nystagmus, dizziness, or tongue atrophy.

It may be difficult to separate symptoms and signs caused by the Chiari malformation itself (e.g., nystagmus, ataxia, dizziness, head, and neck pain) from those caused by the syrinx when the two disorders coexist.

Children with syringomyelia often develop progressive scoliosis, though that is uncommon with adult-onset presentation because of skeletal maturity.

In some cases there may be associated craniovertebral abnormalities, for example, Klippel-Feil abnormality with fusion of the C2 and C3 vertebra and a short neck and low hairline on examination.

Diagnostic Tests
Diagnosis of Chiari malformation is confirmed with magnetic resonance imaging (MRI) which shows the cerebellar displacement. The entire spinal cord should be imaged to identify and define the extent of associated syringomyelia. The signal from the syrinx is usually similar to signal from the CSF, unless it is loculated and contains protienaceous or blood breakdown material. Brain MRI will detect associated hydrocephalus, if present.

Practice Pearl

It is important to rule out underlying abnormalities such as Chiari malformation or syringomyelia in patients who present with "idiopathic" scoliosis.

Management

Surgical decompression of the posterior fossa for the Chiari tonsillar herniation with suboccipital craniectomy, with or without duraplasty and cervical laminectomy, is indicated for symptomatic patients.

Shunting of the syrinx may improve or stabilize the neurological deficit in some patients, although results are often unpredictable and the additional benefit provided by this procedure is not clear. If hydrocephalus is present, that should be addressed with shunt placement before attempting to correct the syrinx.

KNOWLEDGE GAPS AND EMERGING CONCEPTS

The role and indications of direct decompression or drainage of the syrinx is not well established and needs to be further defined.

SUGGESTED READING

deSouza RM, Zador Z, Frim DM. Chiari malformation type I: related conditions. *Neurol Res.* 2011;33(3):278-284.

Roy AK, Slimack NP, Ganju A. Idiopathic syringomyelia: retrospective case series, comprehensive review, and update on management. *Neurosurg Focus.* 2011;31(6):E15.

Sekula RF Jr, Arnone GD, Crocker C, Aziz KM, Alperin N. The pathogenesis of Chiari I malformation and syringomyelia. *Neurol Res.* 2011;33(3):232-239.

CHAPTER 24

Hereditary Spastic Paraplegia

GENERAL PRINCIPLES

Hereditary spastic paraplegia (HSP) includes a group of clinically and genetically diverse inherited neurodegenerative disorders that cause lower limb spasticity and weakness.

It can be classified as uncomplicated or complicated. Uncomplicated HSP is the most common and is characterized purely by spastic paraplegia, whereas complicated HSP is associated with a wide variety of associated conditions, such as deafness, amyotrophy in the upper limbs, ichthyosis, optic neuropathy, dementia, and mental retardation.

Etiology

The genetics of HSP are complex and heterogeneous. Several spastic paraplegia gene (SPG) loci have been mapped, and multiple genes have been identified to date. The mode of inheritance for HSP can be autosomal dominant, recessive, or X-linked. Autosomal dominant HSP is the most prevalent form and accounts for the majority of cases. Most cases of uncomplicated (pure) HSP are inherited in an autosomal dominant fashion. The most common HSP-related genes that account for over 50% of the cases are SPAST (also known as SPG4) and SPG3A. In contrast, autosomal recessive inheritance is more common for the complicated forms.

Epidemiology

The prevalence of HSP is estimated to be at 3 to 10 cases per 100,000. The clinical onset of the disease can begin anywhere from early childhood to 70 years of age or older.

Pathophysiology

The common pathologic feature in HSP is retrograde degeneration of the distal portion of the longest nerve fibers in the corticospinal tracts and posterior columns. It is believed that HSP is associated with a disruption of axonal transport and membrane trafficking, which is critical to axonal health and function. The long axons of the corticospinal tracts and posterior columns are particularly reliant on such processes. In some cases, mitochondrial dysfunction may also be associated with HSP.

Disease Course

This is a slowly progressive neurodegenerative disease process, which gradually results in spasticity and weakness in bilateral lower extremities. Although there is clinical variability in HSP onset and progression, abrupt onset or rapid symptom progression are not characteristic and should suggest a different diagnosis. When HSP manifests in the first two years of life, it is often nonprogressive for a couple of decades followed by slow worsening thereafter. Later onset of symptoms in early childhood or in adults is characterized by slow, gradual progression. Lifespan is often normal in many cases of uncomplicated HSP.

It is important to recognize that there is often variation in the severity and progression within and between HSP families. Caution is warranted in estimating the degree of eventual disability as a result of this variation. In general, subjects from families with well-documented uncomplicated HSP are not likely to develop complicated HSP. This is helpful in predicting outcomes, because uncomplicated HSP makes upper extremity functional impairment, speech or swallowing problems, or a significantly reduced lifespan much less likely.

CLINICAL CONSIDERATIONS

Assessment

History
Typically, patients have a history of normal gestation, delivery, and early childhood with the subsequent development of increased tone in the legs and gait disturbance.

Onset of HSP is subtle, with development of leg stiffness. The insidious development of these symptoms can arise anywhere from early childhood to mid-to-late adulthood. Lower extremity spasticity is often reported to be worse in cold weather, following exertion, and at the end of the day.

The development of neurogenic bladder is a common late manifestation of the disease process, and typically presents as urinary urgency. Cognitive impairment may occur, especially with some forms of complicated HSP.

A thorough family history is essential for patients with HSP. The presence of typical clinical features in other family members strongly supports the diagnosis, but the absence of family history does not exclude the diagnosis. Family history may be absent because of gene mutation, late age of symptom onset, mild symptoms that are attributed to other causes, or autosomal recessive or X-linked inheritance, in which carriers are often asymptomatic.

Physical Examination
Examination of the lower extremities in patients with HSP typically reveals spasticity and weakness that is mostly symmetric. The extent of weakness is variable and may be mild, especially with early-onset disease, even in the presence of severe spasticity. Spasticity is especially prominent in the hamstrings, adductor, and gastroc-soleus muscles, and weakness is often most obvious in the hamstrings, iliopsoas, and tibialis anterior muscles. This is often accompanied by brisk reflexes, extensor planter responses, decreased vibratory sensation in the toes, and pes cavus.

Decreased vibratory sensation may be present in the toes, but severe dorsal column impairment is not typical of uncomplicated HSP. Although hyperreflexia in the upper extremities may be present, significant spasticity or weakness in the arms should lead to questioning of the diagnosis, as should the presence of bulbar muscle weakness, the presence of a sensory level, or markedly asymmetric involvement.

Gait abnormalities depend on the extent, and distribution of leg weakness and spasticity, and may include reduced stride length, toe walking, circumduction, dragging of toes, scissoring, hyperlordosis, or hyperextension at the knees.

For the complicated subtype of HSP, multiple abnormalities may coexist with spastic paraplegia, including but not limited to: mental retardation, ataxia, extrapyramidal signs, hypoplasia of corpus callosum, hydrocephalus, seizures, amyotrophy, and deafness. Eye exam may reveal optic neuropathy, cataracts, retinal degeneration, and/or ophthalmoplegia. Ichthyosis or hyperbilirubinemia may occur in some patients.

Diagnostic Tests
Genetic testing has an important diagnostic role. The mapping and cloning of HSP genes has led to increasing availability of specific molecular genetic tests, although gene testing is commercially available for only a subset of genes. A genetic diagnosis can now be made in over 50% of cases of autosomal dominant HSP by screening the two most common HSP-related genes, SPAST (SPG4) and SPG3A. Additional genetic testing may be available on a research basis.

The primary role of additional laboratory testing is to exclude alternative diagnoses. Investigations may include tests for vitamin B12, copper, ceruloplasmin, very long chain fatty acids, white cell enzymes, plasma amino acids, serum lipoprotein analysis, serology for syphilis, and human immunodeficiency virus.

Magnetic resonance imaging (MRI) of the brain and spinal cord can exclude other disorders, such as multiple sclerosis, leukodystrophies, and structural abnormalities. MRI of the brain may reveal possible hypoplasia of the corpus callosum in some patients with complicated HSP. MRI of the spine may reveal thinning of the spinal cord, especially in the thoracic region.

Electromyography and nerve conduction studies are usually normal in uncomplicated HSP, but some forms of complicated HSP may be associated with peripheral neuropathy and evidence of lower motor involvement.

Management

There is no available treatment to slow or reverse the disease process.

Management of HSP is done with the goal of maintaining the greatest degree of functional independence for each patient.

Contracture prevention and spasticity management are important for many of these individuals and can include stretching, splinting, antispasticity medications (e.g., baclofen, tizanidine, or dantrolene sodium), and intrathecal baclofen pump placement.

Physical therapy and occupational therapy should be initiated to assess functional mobility and activities of daily living. A regularly followed exercise regimen should incorporate daily or twice daily stretching and daily exercises to promote improved endurance and activity tolerance and to prevent deconditioning. Ankle-foot orthoses can be helpful to reduce toe dragging. Canes, walkers, or wheelchairs may eventually be required, though some individuals with HSP never require assistive devices for ambulation.

Education on prevention of pressure ulcer formation and appropriate neurogenic bowel and bladder management should also be initiated. Medications, such as oxybutynin, are helpful in managing urinary urgency.

Patient and Family Education
The availability of gene testing can improve genetic counseling in HSP. The limitations in the ability to predict prognosis and variability in disease onset and progression between and within families should be kept in mind when providing counseling to patients and families with HSP. Support groups and other forums that facilitate interaction with others who have the same disorder may be helpful.

Practice Pearl

A significant proportion of undiagnosed spastic paraplegia is genetic in origin. Consider the possibility of HSP in adults with gradual onset of spastic paraplegia, where a cause cannot be determined, even in the absence of an obvious family history. A detailed family investigation is important in such cases, keeping in mind that some affected individuals may have very mild or subtle symptoms.

KNOWLEDGE GAPS AND EMERGING CONCEPTS

Novel insights into the processes that maintain axons and advances in the cellular mechanisms involving axonal transport and membrane trafficking, and the potential for pharmacologic manipulation of these pathways, should help identify potential therapeutic solutions for HSP and other neurodegenerative disorders with axonal pathology in the future.

The increasing number of genes being identified in association with HSP has led to the growing recognition about the heterogeneous nature of this disorder. With advances in gene sequencing technology, more genes for HSP and related disorders are very likely to be uncovered in the near future.

SUGGESTED READING

Blackstone C. Cellular pathways of hereditary spastic paraplegia. *Annu Rev Neurosci.* 2012;35:25-47. Doi: 10.1146/annurev-neuro-062111-150400.

Depienne C, Stevanin G, Brice A, Durr A. Hereditary spastic paraplegias: an update. *Curr Opin Neurol.* 2007;20(6):674-680.

Sabharwal S, Brown MS. *Hereditary Spastic Paraplegia.* PM&R Knowledge NOW/American Academy of Physical Medicine and Rehabilitation. http://now.aapmr.org/cns/sci-disorders/Pages/Hereditary-Spastic-Paraplegia.aspx. Published September 20, 2013.

Salinas S, Proukakis C, Crosby A, Warner TT. Hereditary spastic paraplegia: clinical features and pathogenetic mechanisms. *Lancet Neurol.* 2008;7(12):1127-1138.

Schüle R, Schöls L. Genetics of hereditary spastic paraplegias. *Semin Neurol.* 2011;31(5): 484-493.

CHAPTER 25

Amyotrophic Lateral Sclerosis/ Adult Motor Neuron Disease

GENERAL PRINCIPLES

Motor neuron diseases are a heterogeneous group of diseases involving the irreversible loss of motor neurons. Amyotrophic lateral sclerosis (ALS) is the most common form of progressive motor neuron disease in adults, and the terms are sometimes used synonymously. ALS affects both the lower motor neurons in the spinal cord and brainstem, and the upper motor neurons in the motor cortex. ALS is the primary focus of this chapter. Phenotypic variants of ALS are listed in Table 25.1.

Etiology

There is growing evidence suggesting that ALS should be considered a spectrum of disorders rather than a single entity. ALS is traditionally classified into two categories that are clinically very similar: familial and sporadic, with sporadic accounting for over 90% of cases.

Familial ALS accounts for about 5% to 10% of cases and most of these are autosomal dominant in inheritance. It involves mutations in a heterogeneous group of genes. At least 16 gene mutations have been identified. Mutation involving the enzyme superoxide dismutase 1 (SOD1) was the first mutation to be identified, accounting for about 20% of familial ALS cases.

Patients who do not have affected relatives are considered to have the sporadic form of ALS; however some may be misclassified due to incomplete penetrance. Sporadic ALS is considered to be a complex entity, in which genetic and environmental factors combine to increase the risk of developing the condition. While there have been suggestions of weak and inconsistent associations with various chemicals, pesticides, and electromagnetic radiations, no definite environmental factors have been identified.

Table 25.1

ALS and Related Phenotypes

Entity	Features	Median Survival
ALS	Both upper and lower motor neuron signs. Most common form of adult-onset motor neuron disease	3–4 yrs (although 5%–10% may survive for ≥10 yrs)
Primary lateral sclerosis	Upper motor neuron signs only. Up to 75% of patients develop ALS within 3–4 yrs	20 yrs or more for those who do not progress to ALS
Progressive muscular atrophy	Lower motor neuron signs only. Variable evolution to ALS	Typically 5 yrs, but a subset survive for over 20 yrs
Progressive bulbar palsy	Bulbar involvement with swallowing and speech impairments. Aspiration pneumonia is the usual cause of death	2–3 yrs

Abbreviation: ALS, amyotrophic lateral sclerosis.

Epidemiology

Risk of developing ALS peaks between ages 50 and 75. Men are more often affected than women, with a male to female ratio of about 1.5:1.0. The annual incidence of ALS among adults is estimated to be between 2.5 and 3.0 per 100,000.

A study released by the Institute of Medicine in 2006, based on review of the literature, concluded that there is limited and suggestive evidence of an association between military service and later development of ALS, although no association with location of service or history of combat exposure was noted. ALS has been declared a presumptively-compensable illness for all Veterans with 90 days of continuously active service in the military.

Pathophysiology

The precise mechanisms underlying neurodegeneration in ALS have not been well-defined but are suggested to involve a combination of glutamate excitotoxicity, generation of free radicals, mutant SOD1 enzymes, along with abnormalities in mitochondrial function and axonal transport processes associated with accumulation of neurofilament intracellular aggregates. Whether these aggregates or inclusions exert direct toxic effects, e.g., by sequestering factors that are essential for cellular function, is not established.

Disease Course

Although the presentation and progression varies considerably, ALS typically has a relentlessly progressive disease course with a median time of survival between 24 to 48 months. Over 60% patients die within 3 years of presentation. Of the remaining, 10% survive for over 8 years.

Prognostic Factors

Adverse and favorable prognostic factors for rate of progression and life expectancy are summarized in Table 25.2. Younger age of presentation has better prognosis. Disease starting in the limbs has better prognosis than bulbar or respiratory onset. Women more often present with bulbar onset than men, and have a somewhat worse overall prognosis. Among those with limb-onset disease, lower limb onset seems to have better prognosis than upper limb. Reduced vital capacity (VC) to less than 50% of normal, impaired executive and cognitive function, and significant weight loss at time of presentation are also negative prognostic factors.

CLINICAL CONSIDERATIONS

Assessment

History

ALS typically presents in an insidious, progressive manner. Symptoms at onset are usually asymmetrical. As times passes and more muscles are involved, the condition becomes more symmetrical.

Initial symptoms may be nonspecific and include muscle cramping, twitching, fatigue, and ill-defined weakness. Lower limb involvement may present with gait impairment such as tripping or dragging one leg. Upper limb involvement may present with problems in fine motor movement such as doing buttons with distal involvement or with difficulty lifting arms for activities such as

Table 25.2

Prognostic Factors in ALS	
Favorable Factors	**Adverse Factors**
Age <50 yrs	Age >65 yrs
Male sex	Female sex
Lower limb onset	Bulbar or respiratory onset
Long interval from first symptom to diagnosis	Short interval from first symptom to diagnosis
Variants such as pure upper motor conditions (primary lateral sclerosis)	Rapidly declining function, forced vital capacity <50%, impaired executive function, weight loss at presentation

Abbreviation: ALS, amyotrophic lateral sclerosis.

hair brushing due to proximal weakness. Twenty-five percent have a bulbar onset and may present with drooling (sialorrhea), dysarthria, and/or difficulty chewing, or nasal regurgitation due to dysphagia.

Respiratory symptoms may develop as the disease progresses or, occasionally, patients may present with those. Symptoms of respiratory insufficiency may include dyspnea, orthopnea, poor sleep and sleep fragmentation, nightmares, early morning headaches, worsened daytime somnolence, and attention/concentration problems.

Sphincter disturbances are usually absent, at least initially. Minor sensory symptoms may be present in some but should not be prominent. While fasciculations are painless, painful cramps (in limb, abdominal, and/or paraspinal muscles) may develop as the disease progresses.

Up to 50% patients with ALS may experience pseudobulbar affect or emotional lability with uncontrollable laughter or crying. Cognitive and/or behavioral impairment may be present in some cases. Up to 15% of patients may have associated features of frontotemporal dementia characterized by personality changes, irritability, and persisting impairment of executive function such as impaired judgment and impulsivity.

Detailed family history may identify potential familial disease with reduced penetrance.

Physical Examination
The typical feature of ALS on examination is the presence of widespread pure motor signs of both upper and lower motor neuron dysfunction, which are not attributable to other causes. Lower motor neuron signs may occur in the same limb as upper motor neuron signs. Weak and wasted muscles with retained or increased reflexes should raise suspicion of ALS.

Lower motor signs include weakness, fasciculations, atrophy, and hyporeflexia. Fasciculations and atrophy may be noted in the tongue as well as limbs. Facial and bulbar muscle weakness may be noted on cranial nerve exam. Ocular movements are typically preserved. Head drop may occur due to neck muscle weakness. Upper motor signs include hyperreflexia, clonus, spasticity, and pathological reflexes such as Babinski sign, Hoffmann sign, snout and palmomental reflexes, and jaw jerk.

Diagnostic Tests
Laboratory Tests
There is no established biomarker of the disease, and lab tests are done primarily to exclude other conditions. Tests typically include complete blood count, chemistry panel, erythrocyte sedimentation rate, serum and urine electrophoresis, thyroid function tests, parathyroid levels, serum calcium, and phosphate. Depending on the clinical presentation, other tests may include

Vitamin B12 level, Lyme serology, human immunodeficiency virus (HIV) serology, serology for immune mediated disease, anti-ganglioside antibodies, and muscle enzymes. Heavy metal screen may be done in those with a potential history of exposure. Lumbar puncture for cerebrospinal fluid analysis and/or muscle or nerve biopsy may be indicated in select cases.

Neuroimaging

Magnetic resonance imaging (MRI) of the cervical spine should be done to rule out cervical myelopathy, other causes of cord compression, or syringomyelia as the cause for the neurological impairment. Cranial MRI, to look for brainstem involvement by other pathology, is also done, especially in those who present with bulbar involvement.

Electrodiagnostic Testing

Electromyography (EMG) is a key ancillary test in patients with suspected motor neuron disease. Fasciculations, fibrillations, and positive sharp waves on EMG indicate ongoing motor neuron loss, and large polyphasic motor units are indicative of reinnervation. Significant abnormalities in nerve conduction studies may suggest alternative diagnoses.

Genetic Testing

Genetic counseling is required prior to any genetic testing. Screening of patients with known familial ALS to look for mutations of known genes may offer some benefit, although its precise role is still evolving. The role of screening of asymptomatic first degree relatives of familial ALS is not well defined at this time, and needs to be limited to a strictly voluntary basis.

Diagnostic Criteria for ALS

The diagnosis of ALS requires simultaneous upper and lower motor neuron involvement with progressive weakness, and exclusion of alternative diagnoses. A committee of the World Federation of Neurology established diagnostic guidelines for ALS. The original El Escoril clinical criteria for ALS have been modified to incorporate electrodiagnostic testing, which has improved diagnostic sensitivity without increasing false-positives. Based on the criteria, the diagnosis of ALS is ranked as "definite," "probable," and "possible" (Table 25.3).

Differential Diagnosis

Careful consideration and exclusion of alternate diagnoses is essential before establishing the diagnosis of ALS, given the prognostic implications and potential treatability of several conditions. The absence of disease progression in patients diagnosed with ALS, or evolution of atypical features (e.g. significant sensory, sphincter, visual, autonomic, or basal ganglia dysfunction), should trigger review of diagnosis and suspicion of alternate conditions.

ALS-Related Phenotypes

Related phenotypes of ALS include primary lateral sclerosis, progressive muscular atrophy, and progressive bulbar palsy (Table 25.1).

Table 25.3

Criteria for Diagnosis of ALS

The patient must have: clinical signs and symptoms of disease; progression of signs and symptoms over time; and no electromyographic or neuroimaging evidence of another disease process.

Definite ALS	Probable ALS	Possible ALS
Clinical or electrophys-iological evidence, demonstrated by the presence of upper and lower motor neuron signs in the bulbar region and at least two spinal regions, or the presence of upper and lower motor neuron signs in three spinal regions[a]	Clinical or electrophys-iological evidence, demonstrated by upper and lower motor neuron signs in at least two spinal regions, with some upper motor neuron signs necessarily rostral to the lower motor neuron signs	Clinical or electrophysio-logical signs of upper and lower motor neuron dysfunction in only one region, or upper motor neuron signs alone in two or more regions, or lower motor neuron signs rostral to upper motor neuron signs

Abbreviation: ALS, amyotrophic lateral sclerosis.

[a]Four anatomic regions are defined as: (1) bulbar, (2) cervical (includes upper limb), (3) thoracic (includes abdominal muscles), and (4) Lumbar (includes lower limb).

Post-Polio Syndrome

Post-polio syndrome (PPS) is a condition developing many years following paralytic polio in which the muscle strength and clinical function are slowly deteriorating, usually without the dramatic loss of muscle strength as seen in ALS. The diagnosis of PPS requires the following criteria:

1. Prior paralytic poliomyelitis with evidence of motor neuron loss, as confirmed by history of the acute paralytic illness, signs of residual weakness, atrophy of muscles on neurological examination, and signs of denervation on EMG
2. A period of partial or complete functional recovery after acute paralytic poliomyelitis, followed by an interval (usually 15 years or more) of stable neurologic function
3. Gradual or sudden onset of progressive and persistent muscle weakness or abnormal muscle fatigability (decreased endurance), with or without generalized fatigue, muscle atrophy, or muscle and joint pain
4. Symptoms persist for at least a year
5. Exclusion of other neurologic, medical, and orthopedic problems as causes of symptoms

Other Conditions

Cervical spondylotic myelopathy (Chapter 13) and multifocal motor neuropathy are two of the conditions most commonly mistaken for ALS.

The list of differential diagnosis of ALS includes hereditary conditions (e.g., spinobulbar muscular atrophy, hereditary spastic paraplegia, fascioscapulohumeral muscular dystrophy), metabolic and toxic conditions (e.g., hyperthyroidism, hyperparathyroidism, heavy metal intoxication, lathyrism), immune-mediated conditions (including multifocal motor neuropathy with conduction block, chronic inflammatory demyelinating polyneuropathy, myasthenia gravis, polymyositis, multiple sclerosis, paraneoplastic disorders), structural disorders (e.g., cervical spondylotic myelopathy, syringomyelia or syringobulbia, postradiation myelopathy or plexopathy, tumor, or cerebrovascular disease), and other neurodegenerative conditions.

Fasciculation without progressive weakness is a common and usually benign phenomenon.

Management

Breaking the News
While the content, diagnostic information and prognostic implications differ for ALS, many of the principles applicable to breaking news about other serious conditions also apply here (Chapter 48). These include not being rushed, providing the diagnosis in person rather than on phone, asking whether patients wish their family member to be with them for the discussion, finding out what the patient already knows or suspects, providing information in small chunks, stopping between each chunk to evaluate response and proceeding accordingly. One should avoid withholding the diagnosis, providing insufficient information, delivering information callously, or taking away or not providing hope. It is important to summarize the discussion, and provide a plan and contact information for follow-up. Referral to an ALS support group may be helpful.

Providing a timely diagnosis is important for resolving uncertainty, allowing patients to better plan the remaining part of their life, avoiding unnecessary additional diagnostic testing, and having the opportunity to initiate neuroprotective treatment when fewer cells are irreversibly compromised.

Multidisciplinary ALS Teams
Multidisciplinary clinics have been shown to improve quality of life and function of patients with ALS in some studies. The core multidisciplinary team often includes a physician specializing in neuromuscular disease, nurse, physical therapist, occupational therapist, speech and language pathologists, nutritionist, social worker, and respiratory therapist. Consulting specialties often include pulmonology, gastroenterology, psychology, and spiritual counseling. Good ongoing communication and coordination within the team, and with the patient's primary care provider, is essential.

Neuroprotective Treatment/Riluzole
While there are ongoing clinical trials of several potentially promising agents, the only evidence-based neuroprotective medication at present is riluzole. Its mechanism of action in ALS is unknown, although it does reduce glutamate-induced excitotoxicity. Analysis of published literature has suggested that riluzole increases the probability of surviving one year by 10% to 15% and, on average, adds about 3 months to patient survival. It is generally well-tolerated; fatigue, gastrointestinal side effects, and elevated liver enzymes occur occasionally. Realistic expectations for treatment effects and potential side effects need to be discussed with the patient and caregivers. Treatment with riluzole 50 mg twice daily should be initiated as early as possible after the diagnosis once a decision to treat is made after considering expected therapeutic benefits and potential side effects.

Symptomatic Treatment (Table 25.4)
Symptomatic management forms the mainstay of ALS treatment with the goal to treat troublesome symptoms, alleviate suffering, and improve quality of life. Sialorrhoea (drooling or excessive salivation) due to bulbar involvement is common and may be socially disabling. It is treated with anticholinergic medications, and in resistant cases, with botulinum toxin injection or irradiation of the salivary glands. With bulbar weakness, attention to swallowing and nutrition is necessary. Percutaneous endoscopic gastrostomy is a standard procedure for enteral nutrition. It requires mild sedation, which poses risk in those with advanced respiratory impairment, so should be performed before VC falls below 50%. Percutaneous radiologic gastrostomy is an alternative that does not require sedation. Various low tech and high tech alternatives to augmentative and alternative communication can be used to improve communication when severe dysarthria develops. As limb weakness progresses, various mobility aids and assistive devices can be provided, depending on the extent of impairment.

Spasticity and painful muscle cramps may require treatment. Sleep impairment, fatigue, depression, and anxiety can arise from a number of factors, and should be adequately treated along with identification and management of causative factors. Cognitive and/or executive function impairment may occur in a significant proportion so vigilance to identify and manage these is important.

Table 25.4 provides a summary of symptomatic management of the major manifestations of ALS.

Respiratory Management
Monitoring Respiratory Function
Respiratory failure, with or without pneumonia, is the most common cause of death in ALS.

(text continued on page 178)

Table 25.4

Symptomatic Management in ALS

Manifestation	Management
Inspiratory weakness/hypoventilation	- Monitor pulmonary function, FVC - Consider NIPPV for FVC <50% - Discussion and informed decision about tracheostomy and mechanical ventilation, incorporated in advance directives - Avoid unnecessary oxygen administration - Manage anxiety and discomfort of severe dyspnea with benzodiazepines and/or opiates
Impaired cough and secretion management	- Mechanical insufflation-exsufflation with cough assist device • E.g., 4 treatments a day and as needed, 5 coughing cycles per sequence followed by 30 s of rest; 5 sequences for each treatment. Initial pressures of +15 cm H_2O insufflation and –15 cm H_2O exsufflation gradually increased to a goal of +40 and –40 cm H_2O - Breath-stacking and manually-assisted cough techniques - Mechanical suction device - Treated tenacious secretions with adequate hydration, mucolytic agents such as acetylcysteine (200–400 mg three times daily), and/or a nebulizer

Sialorrhea (drooling)	- Anticholinergic medication
	  • Amitriptyline 10 mg three times a day
	  • Atropine drops, sublingually 3–4 times a day
	  • Glycopyrrolate 1–2 mg three times a day
	  • Transdermal scopolamine patch, every 3 days
	- Botulinum toxin injection into parotid and/or submandibular gland, as a second line agent
	- Irradiation of salivary glands in refractory cases

(continued)

Table 25.4

Symptomatic Management in ALS (continued)

Manifestation	Management
Swallowing and nutrition	- Monitor bulbar impairment and nutritional status - Refer to speech pathologist and dietician - Swallowing evaluation, and if needed, videofluoroscopy - Thick liquids, modified food consistency - Swallowing techniques (supra-glottic swallow, postural change, chin-tuck maneuver) - Calorie-dense meals, protein supplements - Early consideration of feeding tube. The timing of PEG or PRG should be individualized. Nasogastric tube feeding may be used in the short-term
Dysarthria/impaired communication	- Techniques to improve speech intelligibility (slow rate, over-articulation) with early impairment - Use of gestures, head-nodding, word lists, and communication boards to augment communication - Electronic augmentative and alternative communication devices (voice synthesizers, head or eye gaze controlled communication devices)
Impaired mobility, gait	- Assistive devices and mobility aids based on extent of impairment (e.g., cane, AFO for foot drop, rolling walker, power wheelchair) - Transfer devices, lifts, hospital bed
Impaired function and ADL	- Assistive devices for dressing, grooming, feeding, toileting - Home modifications - Caregiving assistance
Fatigue	- Identify and treat secondary causes (hypoventilation, sleep disturbance, depression) - Medications for debilitating fatigue: • Modafinil 100–400 mg every morning
Painful muscle cramps	- Massage and stretching - Hydrotherapy in heated pool

(continued)

Manifestation	Management

	- Medications
	  • Levetiracetam may be tried
	  • Quinine sulphate 200 mg twice daily may help but is no longer recommended by FDA

Spasticity	- Stretching and positioning - Antispasticity medications (baclofen, tizanidine, diazepam, dantrolene) although ALS-specific literature is sparse. See Chapter 38A for details. - Baclofen pump may be considered in select patients

Insomnia	- Hypnotic agents, e.g., eszopiclone or zolpidem
	- Identify and treat contributing factors
	  • Depression and anxiety (see below)
	  • Hypoventilation—consider NIPPV
	  • Gagging on secretions—treat excess mucus and sialorrhea, elevate head end of bed
	  • Inability to turn due to weakness—hospital bed, repositioning by caregiver

Depression and anxiety	- Antidepressant medication (SSRI, tricyclic antidepressants) See Chapter 41 - Benzodiazepines for anxiety - Behavioral interventions, support and counseling
Impaired cognitive and executive function	- Screening for cognitive impairment - Detailed neuropsychological testing in those with positive screen or suggestive symptoms - Caregivers and health care provider should be aware and trained to adapt interactions accordingly - Consider impact on new learning, informed consent, and decision-making capacity - Identify and address secondary factors (fatigue, disturbed sleep, depression)
Pseudobulbar emotional lability	- Explanation about causation being an effect of ALS rather than an additional mood or psychological disorder - If troublesome, can try SSRI or amitriptyline

(continued)

Table 25.4

Symptomatic Management in ALS (continued)

Manifestation	Management
Caregiver burden	- Support groups, emotional and spiritual support - Respite care and caregiving assistance
End of life care	- Discussion about end-of-life decisions and advance medical directives early in the disease course - Reassurance about availability of comfort measures to minimize pain and suffering - Opioids and benzodiazepines for dyspnea and/or pain - Timely referral/coordination with palliative care teams - Options for hospice care, including home hospice - Bereavement counseling and support for caregivers

Abbreviations: ADL, activities of daily living; AFO, ankle-foot orthosis; ALS, amyotrophic lateral sclerosis; FDA, Food and Drug Administration; FVC, forced vital capacity; NIPPV, noninvasive positive pressure ventilation; PEG, percutaneous endoscopic gastrostomy; PRG, percutaneous radiologic gastrostomy; SSRI, selective serotonin uptake inhibitors.

Early symptoms of respiratory dysfunction should be actively sought at each clinic visit. Pulmonary function should be tested every few months to measure respiratory muscle strength. Testing most commonly includes VC; additional tests may include maximum inspiratory mouth pressure, maximum expiratory mouth pressure, sniff nasal inspiratory pressure, and nocturnal pulse oximetry. Cough effectiveness can be assessed by measuring peak cough flow.

Noninvasive Positive Pressure Ventilation

Noninvasive positive pressure ventilation (NIPPV) has several demonstrated benefits in ALS (Table 25.5). If tolerated, NIPPV may prolong survival (particularly in patients who are able to use it for more than 5 hours per day, and those without severe bulbar dysfunction), improve symptoms of hypoventilation (such as fragmented sleep, morning headache, daytime somnolence, and cognitive function), and improve quality of life without increasing caregiver burden or stress.

The decision to prescribe NIPPV should be based on a combination of evidence of respiratory muscle weakness and respiratory symptoms, although consensus about explicit criteria is lacking. NIPPV should be considered in ALS patients with symptoms of respiratory insufficiency and forced vital capacity (FVC) less than 50%; some evidence supports consideration of NIPPV at FVC

Table 25.5

Potential Benefits of NIPPV in ALS

Prolonged survival

Improved symptoms of hypoventilation (disturbed sleep, morning headache, daytime somnolence)

Improved cognitive function

Improved quality of life without added caregiver burden or stress

Abbreviations: ALS, amyotrophic lateral sclerosis; NIPPV, noninvasive positive pressure ventilation.

less than 50% even in the absence of respiratory symptoms or with higher FVC in the presence of symptomatic respiratory weakness.

NIPPV is typically delivered with bi-level positive airway pressure devices. Various nasal or oronasal mask interfaces can be used. Treatment is usually initiated at night to alleviate symptoms of nocturnal hypoventilation. Patients who rely on NIPPV need to have an alternative power source available. ALS patients and caregivers need training about trouble-shooting and emergency contact information for equipment malfunction.

Oxygen therapy is not needed and should be avoided in most instances of respiratory insufficiency in patients with ALS. It can worsen carbon dioxide retention and oral dryness.

Secretion Management and Cough Assistance

In addition to inspiratory weakness, which is assisted by NIPPV, patients with ALS also have expiratory muscle weakness with impaired cough. Cough-assistance devices that provide mechanical insufflation-exsufflation (MI-E) can be of benefit in patients with reduced peak cough expiratory flow (2–3 L/s or less). Goal MI-E pressures are +40 cm H_2O for insufflation and -40 cm H_2O for exsufflation, given that +35/-35 cm H_2O are the minimum pressures needed to clear airway secretions.

Breath stacking and manually assisted cough techniques can also be used to improve peak cough flow. With breath stacking, multiple inspiratory volumes occur without expiration. Thus inspiratory volumes summate or stack to result in a larger lung volume to be used for a spontaneous or manual-assisted cough. Breath stacking requires the patient be able to voluntarily close the glottis between inspiratory efforts to prevent loss of inspired volume. This may be difficult for the ALS patient. Alternatively, expiration can be occluded with a one-way valve that only allows airflow with inspiration. Given that inspiratory muscles are likely to be weak when breath stacking is considered to augment peak cough flow, the inspired volumes can be manually provided with a resuscitation bag.

Techniques to reduce the risk of aspiration should be introduced, including suction machines, alteration in food texture, and advice regarding swallowing. Tenacious secretions should be treated by ensuring adequate hydration, the use of mucolytic agents such as acetylcysteine (200–400 mg three times daily), or the use of a saline nebulizer with β-receptor antagonists.

Mechanical Ventilation
Less than 10% of patients choose tracheostomy and long-term invasive mechanical ventilation. The patient and family should be fully informed of the burdens and benefits before making a decision, and the conversation should happen prior to severe respiratory compromise rather than in an emergency, and incorporated into advance directives. The inadvertent initiation of tracheostomy and mechanical ventilation in an emergency situation in a patient without advance directives poses difficult ethical and clinical challenges since most patients are not able to wean off the ventilator once initiated. Although tracheostomy with mechanical ventilation will avoid death from respiratory failure, median ALS patient survival after its initiation is around 1 to 3 years, with respiratory infection being the most common cause of death. Caregivers of ALS patients with tracheostomy and mechanical ventilation report poor quality of life and may require significant psychosocial support. The right of the patient with ALS to refuse or withdraw any treatment, including mechanical ventilation, should be respected. If ventilation is withdrawn, adequate opiate and benzodiazepine dosage should be used to relieve dyspnea and anxiety.

Other Respiratory Interventions
Anecdotal success has been reported with high frequency chest wall oscillation for secretion management, but it has not been tested systematically. A possible role of diaphragmatic pacing stimulators has been suggested, but additional study is needed to establish its role in routine clinical practice.

Caregiver Burden and Support
ALS is associated with significant caregiver burden, which increases with disease progression and loss of independence. It can lead to problems with burnout, stress, depression, social isolation, and guilt in caregivers, and health problems resulting from ignoring their own care needs. There may also be considerable financial burden. Support groups may be helpful. Access to respite care and caregiving assistance should be facilitated as feasible. Maintaining communication between patients and caregivers is important. Attention to the caregiver's own physical, psychological, and spiritual needs is important.

End of Life Care
End of life care planning should be addressed early in the course of disease, including discussion about advance medical directives (living will, health care proxy, durable power of attorney), which should be readdressed every few months. Patients and caregivers are often anxious about distress from choking,

dyspnea, or pain at end of life and should be reassured about availability of effective comfort measures to make end of life peaceful and comfortable. Opioids (e.g., parenteral morphine) and benzodiazepines can be administered for dyspnea and/or pain, and titration of doses against clinical symptoms usually does not cause life-threatening respiratory depression. Neuroleptics such as chlorpromazine can be used for terminal restlessness and confusion. Timely referral and coordination with palliative care teams, options for hospice care, including home hospice, should be provided. Bereavement counseling and support should be available for caregivers.

KNOWLEDGE GAPS AND EMERGING CONCEPTS

One of the recent mutations identified in ALS involves an abnormal repeated expansion of a sequence of nucleotides in a cytoplasmic protein (C9ORF72) that has been found in 40% of families with ALS, but also in about 7% of patients with supposed sporadic ALS suggesting that apparent sporadic ALS can be inherited. It further reinforces the concept that ALS pathogenesis involves several different pathways. It has also been shown that this same mutation can give rise to ALS phenotype in some family members and a frontotemporal dementia phenotype in others, providing even stronger evidence that these conditions are likely the manifestations of a clinico-pathological spectrum.

There has been tremendous progress in understanding of the mechanism underlying ALS, but many questions remain including the factors that contribute to increasing the vulnerability of motor neurons in sporadic ALS. Large population-based cohort studies are needed to try to conclusively establish environmental risk factors for ALS. Efforts to identify biomarkers of ALS, to aid diagnosis and monitoring, are ongoing.

Greater understanding of mechanisms underlying the development of ALS creates potential therapeutic opportunities. Trials involving human neural stem cell transplantation into the spinal cord of patients with ALS have been initiated.

SUGGESTED READING

Blackhall LJ. Amyotrophic lateral sclerosis and palliative care: where we are, and the road ahead. *Muscle Nerve*. 2012;45(3):311-318.

Costa J, Swash M, de Carvalho M. Awaji criteria for the diagnosis of amyotrophic lateral sclerosis:a systematic review. *Arch Neurol*. 2012;69(11):1410-1416.

de Almeida JP, Silvestre R, Pinto AC, de Carvalho M. Exercise and amyotrophic lateral sclerosis. *Neurol Sci*. 2012;33(1):9-15.

EFNS Task Force on Diagnosis and Management of Amyotrophic Lateral Sclerosis; Andersen PM, Abrahams S, et al. EFNS guidelines on the clinical management of amyotrophic lateral sclerosis (MALS)—revised report of an EFNS task force. *Eur J Neurol*. 2012;19(3): 360-375.

Gruis KL, Lechtzin N. Respiratory therapies for amyotrophic lateral sclerosis: a primer. *Muscle Nerve.* 2012;46(3):313-331.

Hardiman O, van den Berg LH, Kiernan MC. Clinical diagnosis and management of amyotrophic lateral sclerosis. *Nat Rev Neurol.* 2011;7(11):639-649.

Ludolph AC, Brettschneider J, Weishaupt JH. Amyotrophic lateral sclerosis. *Curr Opin Neurol.* 2012;25(5):530-535.

Phukan J, Hardiman O. The management of amyotrophic lateral sclerosis. *J Neurol.* 2009; 256(2):176-186.

Robberecht W, Philips T. The changing scene of amyotrophic lateral sclerosis. *Nat Rev Neurosci.* 2013;14(4):248-264.

Turner MR, Hardiman O, Benatar M, et al. Controversies and priorities in amyotrophic lateral sclerosis. *Lancet Neurol.* 2013;12(3):310-322.

Williams TL. Motor neurone disease: diagnostic pitfalls. *Clin Med.* 2013;13(1):97-100.

IV. Physical Function and Rehabilitation

CHAPTER 26

Functional Outcomes Following SCI

GENERAL PRINCIPLES

Outcome Measures

In discussing measures of functional outcomes, it is useful to consider the International Classification of Functioning (ICF) as a conceptual framework. The ICF, developed by the World Health Organization, includes three broad domains: body functions and structure, activity, and participation (each of which can be influenced by environmental and personal factors). While the primary focus of this chapter is on functional activities, it is important to recognize that the three domains of the ICF interact with and influence each other.

As applied to spinal cord injury (SCI), examples of the most pertinent measures for the three domains of the ICF are listed below. Measures of activity limitations and overall functional independence in SCI (which are the ones most pertinent to this chapter) are reviewed in further detail in Table 26.1.

- *Body functions and structure*: International Standards for Neurological Classification of SCI (ISNCSCI). See Chapter 10 for details about the ISNCSCI.
- *Activities*: Functional Independence Measure (FIM), Spinal Cord Independence Measure (SCIM), Modified Barthel Index (MBI), and Quadriplegia Index of Function (QIF) (Table 26.1). In addition to these measures of overall functioning, there are measures of specific activities that are covered elsewhere in this book, for example, measures specific for walking (Chapter 30) or for specific aspects of upper extremity function (Chapter 28).
- *Participation*: Craig Handicap Assessment and Reporting Technique (CHART). This is discussed further in Chapter 42.

Factors Affecting Functional Outcomes

Neurological function, specifically motor function, is the primary determinant of overall functional outcomes after SCI.

Additional factors, such as age, comorbid conditions, pain, spasticity, body habitus, and psychosocial and environmental factors, also affect function, and can play a major role in determining functional outcomes.

Motor Recovery

Since neurological/motor function is the primary determinant of overall function after SCI, knowledge of motor recovery outcomes is particularly relevant to prediction of functional outcomes.

Neurological impairment is characterized by the ISNCSCI (Chapter 10). The ISNCSCI exam performed after 72 hours can be used to estimate prognosis

Table 26.1

Measures of Activity Limitation and Overall Functional Independence in SCI

Measure	Items Assessed	Scoring	Comments/ Considerations
Functional Independence Measure (FIM)	18 items (13 motor and 5 cognitive); Subscales under these 2 domains include: Self-care, Sphincter control, Transfers, Locomotion, Communication, Social cognition	Each item is scored from 1–7; Score of 1–5 implies helper is needed 1 = total assist 2 = max assist 3 = mod assist 4 = min assist 5 = supervision 6 = modified independence (device) 7 = complete independence Total FIM score range from 18–126 Provides subscores for the 2 domains: motor and cognitive	Most widely used disability measure Excellent inter-rater reliability Telephone and pediatric versions available Measures burden of care Does not measure ease of independent activity (effort, cosmesis) Not SCI-specific, e.g., respiration not measured Cognitive subscore less meaningful in SCI Substantial floor and ceiling effects May fail to detect meaningful functional change *(continued)*

Measure	Items Assessed	Scoring	Comments/ Considerations
Spinal Cord Independence Measure (SCIM-III)	19 items, divided into 3 subscales of function (Self-care, Respiratory and sphincter management, and Mobility)	Scoring range varies for individual items; item scores are weighted relative to the overall activity Total score ranges from 0–100	Specifically designed for people with SCI More precise and sensitive to changes than FIM Excellent inter-rater reliability Has been modified, SCIM-III is the third version Not as widely used as FIM, although its use is increasing
Modified Barthel Index (MBI)	10 items related to self-care, continence, and mobility	Total score ranges from 0–100	Measures burden of care Not SCI-specific and rarely used in SCI practice Measures basic activities of living, more complex skills are not assessed
Quadriplegia Index of Function (QIF)	Contains two parts: first part assesses 9 categories of function with multiple items under each category, second part is a questionnaire that assesses understanding of personal care via multiple choice questions	Each item is scored from 0–4 in order of increasing independence and added to give category scores for each category, category scores are then weighted based on assigned weights to each category Total score ranges from 0–100	Developed for individuals with tetraplegia Does not assess walking, so less applicable to ambulatory patients A shorter version is available Not in widespread clinical use at present

regarding neurological recovery. Reliability of earlier exam, for example in the first 24 hours, is decreased due to factors such as sedation, pain, intoxication, hemodynamic instability, and anxiety that can influence exam findings.

It should be recognized that, while several useful generalizations can be made in estimating prognosis for motor recovery, there are few absolutes in this regard. Estimates that apply to a particular category of patients with SCI will not be true for every individual patient within that category.

Overall Timing of Motor Recovery
The majority of recovery of motor function after SCI occurs in the first 6 months, most rapidly in the first 2 months after SCI. Recovery is faster in those with incomplete injury. In people with incomplete SCI, neurological improvement at a slower pace can continue up to 2 years and beyond.

Conversion of Complete to Incomplete SCI
While ~10% to 20% of patients with American Spinal Injury Association (ASIA) Impairment Scale (AIS) A, that is, complete injury, noted on the initial exam (conducted between 72 hours and 1-month post injury in different studies) convert to incomplete injury by one year, a much smaller percentage (3%–6%) recover functional strength in the legs. For reasons that are not completely clear, some recent studies have reported slightly higher rates of conversion from complete to incomplete. Differences between various studies may reflect timing of the initial exam (e.g., initial exam at 1-month is likely to have lower one-year conversion rate than a 72-hour or 1-week initial exam), and the accuracy of the initial exam. To document recovery, neurological function should be monitored periodically till it reaches a plateau.

Zone of Injury Recovery
Recovery of motor function in the zone of injury has been studied in complete tetraplegia. Because there are no key muscles in the thoracic region, and lumbar level lesions usually represent cauda equina injuries, it is not possible to clinically study zone-of-injury motor recovery in paraplegia.

While less than 10% of individuals with complete tetraplegia get any motor recovery in the legs, most patients with complete tetraplegia do gain motor function in the upper extremity within two to three motor segments below the initial neurological level, and gain one motor level (i.e., the next rostral key muscle recovers to grade 3 or better) after injury.

▩ Muscles with some motor power below an antigravity muscle (i.e., grade 1 or 2 strength) have a better prognosis than muscles with no motor power. Studies have found that if the next rostral key upper extremity muscle has some initial strength (grade 1 or 2), 90% will reach antigravity strength by 1 year. If the next rostral muscle has zero initial strength, 45% will gain antigravity strength by 1 year and 64% will gain antigravity strength by 2 years.
▩ The rate of zone of injury recovery decreases as more time passes without evidence of return of strength in the rostral muscles. For example, in individuals with motor complete tetraplegia, 97% of upper extremity key muscles with a muscle grade 1 or 2 at 1 month recovered to at least grade 3 by 1 year. Only 10% of upper extremity

muscles with no motor power at 1 month reached grade 3 strength by 1 year.

▨ There are some differences depending on the initial motor level of injury, with conversion rates being slightly higher overall for C6 to C7 (85%), followed by C5 to C6 (75%), and then C4 to C5 (70%).

This information on expected neurological recovery, and the likelihood of gaining one motor level in complete tetraplegia, can help in setting long-term goals during the acute period.

Ambulation Potential
Community ambulators have been defined by ability to walk greater than or equal to 150 feet, in addition to being able to transfer from sit to stand, and don and doff orthotics independently. Several criteria have been used to predict ambulation potential.

Based on Initial ASIA Impairment Scale

▨ Of patients with AIS A (complete) SCI, on initial exam, only ~3% will get enough strength to ambulate in one year after injury.
▨ Sensory incomplete, motor complete (AIS B) individuals comprise ~10% of all new injuries. Overall, ~50% of those who are initially classified as AIS B will become ambulatory.
  ◉ Those AIS B individuals with preserved sacral pin sensation, have a better prognosis for lower extremity recovery approaching that of motor incomplete individuals, whereas for those without pin sensation, prognosis for recovery of ambulation ranges from 10% to 33%.
▨ For individuals with motor incomplete AIS C injuries, ~75% will become community ambulators. Age and the amount of preserved spinal cord function below the lesion influence recovery of ambulation. The greater the amount of function preserved, the better the prognosis for recovery of ambulation. Prognosis is poorer in those above 50 to 60 years of age.
▨ Prognosis for walking is excellent (~95%) for those initially classified as AIS D.

Based on Lower Extremity Motor Score
Lower Extremity Motor Score (LEMS) is the sum of the motor score of five key muscles in each extremity graded from 0 to 5, totaling a maximum of 50 for the lower limbs (Chapter 10).

While few patients with complete tetraplegia or complete paraplegia get significant improvement in LEMS over time, those with incomplete tetraplegia or incomplete paraplegia gain an average of ~12 points in LEMS between 1-month to 1-year postinjury (with relatively little additional improvement between the first and second year).

Table 26.2

Predicting Community Ambulation Based on 30-day Lower Extremity Motor Score (LEMS)[a]		
SCI Category	30-Day LEMS Score	Community Ambulators in 1 yr
Complete paraplegia	0	<1%
	1–9	45%
	>10	Not applicable
Incomplete paraplegia	0	33%
	1–9	70%
	>10	100%
Incomplete tetraplegia	0	0%
	1–9	21%
	10–19	63%
	>20	100%

[a]Based on Waters RL, Adkins R, Yakura J, Sie I. Donal Munro Lecture: Functional and neurologic recovery following acute SCI. *J Spinal Cord Med*. 1998;21(3):195-199 (and related studies by that group).

▓ The 30-day LEMS has been used to predict likelihood of community ambulation at 1 year. Table 26.2 provides specific percentages for different neurological categories. Patients with incomplete tetraplegia require greater lower extremity strength to ambulate than those with paraplegia because of decreased weight-bearing ability in the upper extremities.

Based on Other Clinical Exam Criteria

Hussey and Stauffer defined the following requirements for community ambulation in the 1970s:

▓ Bilateral hip flexion strength greater than or equal to 3/5; At least one side knee extension greater than or equal to 3/5, no more than one Knee-Ankle-Foot Orthosis (KAFO) and one Ankle-Foot orthosis (AFO) is needed (otherwise energy requirements would be too high for community ambulation); and intact proprioception at least at the hip and knees.

A clinical prediction rule for ambulation after traumatic SCI was published by the European Multicenter Study of Human SCI (EM-SCI) Study Group in 2011.

▓ Their prediction rule, which is based on a combination of age (<65 vs. ≥65 years) and four neurological tests—motor scores of the quadriceps femoris (L3), gastrocsoleus (S1) muscles, and light touch sensation of dermatomes L3 and S1—showed excellent discrimination in distinguishing independent walkers from dependent walkers and nonwalkers.

CLINICAL CONSIDERATIONS

Information about potential for motor recovery can be used to set functional goals and to plan for equipment needs, keeping in mind that individual factors and coexisting conditions may affect achievable goals.

Functional Outcomes After SCI

The Consortium for Spinal Cord Medicine has published guidelines on *Outcomes Following Traumatic Spinal Cord Injury*. Tables 26.3 to 26.5 summarize predicted functional outcomes, and related equipment needs for each level of motor complete SCI injury (functional outcomes following motor incomplete SCI will vary based on the extent of motor preservation).

It should be recognized that these outcomes reflect the level of independence that can be reached under optimal circumstances, without consideration of other personal and environmental factors that may apply to individual patients. An interdisciplinary approach, consideration of unique barriers and facilitators, and including the patient as an active participant in establishing goals are important elements in establishing an individualized rehabilitation program.

Individuals with SCI may experience changes in functional abilities over time for a variety of reasons. These include changes in neurological status, medical status and comorbidities, environment and living situation, psychosocial status, personal preferences and choices, or advancing age. Periodic assessment of functional abilities and the impact of these factors is important on an ongoing basis to optimize functional gains and/or to minimize potential functional losses.

KNOWLEDGE GAPS AND EMERGING CONCEPTS

Treatment effectiveness research is needed to better understand which program strategies efficiently produce the best outcomes. Research quantifying the expected impact of personal injury and environmental characteristics on the outcomes achieved is needed for greater accuracy in predicting outcomes and severity and for adjusting comparisons among programs.

Advanced imaging techniques such as diffusion tensor imaging, functional magnetic resonance imaging (fMRI), and magnetic resonance spectroscopy are being explored for potential applications to predict neurological and functional recovery. Similarly, advanced neurophysiological testing may have potential to supplement clinical testing to predict recovery of function.

Table 26.3

Pattern of Weakness and Functional Outcomes After Cervical Spinal Cord Injury[a]

Domain	C1–C4	C5	C6	C7–C8
Pattern of upper extremity weakness	Total paralysis of extremities	Absent elbow extension, pronation, all wrist and hand movements	Absent wrist flexion, elbow extension, and hand movement	Limited grasp release and hand dexterity due to intrinsic muscle weakness
Respiratory	Ventilator dependent (some C3, many C4 may be able to wean off ventilator)	Low endurance and vital capacity, may require assistance to clear secretions	Low endurance and vital capacity, may require assistance to clear secretions	Low endurance and vital capacity, may require assistance to clear secretions
Bowel management	Total assist	Total assist	Some to total assist	Some to total assist
Bladder management	Total assist	Total assist	Some to total assist with equipment, may be independent with leg bag emptying	Independent to some assist
Bed mobility	Total assist	Some assist	Some assist	Independent to some assist
Bed and wheelchair transfers	Total assist	Total assist	Level transfer: some assist to independent; uneven transfer: some to total assist	Level transfer: independent; uneven transfer: independent to some assist
Pressure relief/ positioning	Total assist, maybe independent with equipment	Independent with equipment	Independent with equipment and/or adapted techniques	Independent

Wheelchair propulsion	Manual: total assist, Power: Independent with equipment	Power: independent, Manual: independent to some assist indoor noncarpet surface, some to total assist outdoors	Power: independent with standard arm drive on all surfaces, Manual: independent indoors, some assist outdoors	Manual: independent on all indoor surfaces and level outdoor terrain, may need some assist or power for uneven terrain or long distances
Eating	Total assist	Total assist for setup, then independent eating with equipment	Independent with or without equipment, except total assist for cutting	Independent
Dressing	Total assist	Some assist upper extremities, total assist for lower extremities	Independent upper extremities, some to total assist lower extremities	Independent upper extremities, independent to some assist lower extremities
Homemaking	Total assist	Total assist	Some assist with light meal prep, total assist for other homemaking	Independent for light meal prep and homemaking, some assist with heavy household tasks
Driving	Total assist, attendant operated van (w/lift, tie downs)	Independent with highly specialized modified van	Independent driving a modified van from wheelchair	Car with hand controls or adapted van from captain's seat

aThese outcomes pertain to expected function after motor complete SCI; functional outcomes following motor incomplete SCI vary based on the extent of motor preservation.

Table 26.4

Typical Equipment Needs After Cervical Spinal Cord Injury

Equipment Category	C1–C4	C5	C6	C7–C8
Respiratory	Ventilator (if not ventilator free) and suction equipment			
Bed	Electric hospital bed, pressure relief mattress	Electric hospital bed, pressure relief mattress	Electric hospital bed or full to king standard bed, pressure relief mattress or overlay	Electric hospital bed or full to king standard bed, pressure relief mattress or overlay
Transfers	Power or mechanical lift, transfer board	Power or mechanical lift, transfer board	Mechanical lift, transfer board	Transfer board may be needed
Wheelchair	Power wheelchair with tilt and/ or recline (with postural support and head control devices as needed), vent tray, pressure relief cushion	Power wheelchair with tilt and/or recline with arm drive control, manual lightweight chair with hand rim modifications, pressure relief cushion	Lightweight manual wheelchair with hand rim modifications, may require power recline or standard upright power wheelchair, pressure relief cushion	Lightweight manual wheelchair with hand rim modifications, pressure relief cushion
Bathing, toileting	Reclining padded shower-commode chair (if roll-in shower available), shampoo tray, handheld shower	Padded shower-commode chair or padded transfer tub bench with commode cut-out, handheld shower	Padded transfer tub bench with commode cut-out or padded shower-commode chair, handheld shower	Padded transfer tub bench with commode cut-out or padded shower-commode chair, handheld shower

Eating, dressing, grooming	Total assist; specialized equipment, such as a balanced forearm orthosis, may allow for limited feeding ability in those with C4 SCI and minimal (<3/5) strength in deltoid and biceps	Long opponens splint (with pocket for inserting utensils), long-handled mirror, adaptive devices as needed	Short opponens splint, universal cuff, long-handled mirror, adapted devices as needed	Adapted devices as needed, long-handled mirror
Communication	Mouthstick, high-tech computer access, environmental control unit	Adaptive devices as needed (e.g., for page turning, writing, button pushing, computer access)	Adaptive devices as needed (e.g., tenodesis splint, writing splint)	Adaptive devices as needed
Transportation	Attendant operated van (w/lift, tie downs)	Highly specialized modified van with lift	Modified van w/lift, tie-downs, hand controls	Modified vehicle

Table 26.5

Expected Functional Outcomes for Motor Complete Thoracic, Lumbar, and Sacral Spinal Cord Injury

Domain	Expected Functional Outcome	Equipment
Bowel	Independent	Padded toilet seat
Bladder	Independent	
Bed mobility	Independent	Full to king size standard bed
Bed and wheelchair transfers	Independent	
Pressure relief	Independent	Wheelchair pressure relief cushion
Wheelchair propulsion	Independent indoor and outdoor	Manual lightweight wheelchair
Standing, ambulation	Standing: independent Ambulation: T1-T9: typically not functional T10-S5: functional, some assist to independent (T10-L2: household ambulation; L3-S5: community ambulation)	Standing frame Knee-ankle-foot orthosis or ankle-foot orthosis Forearm crutches or cane as indicated
Eating, grooming, dressing, bathing	Independent	Padded tub bench Hand-held shower
Communication	Independent	
Transportation	Independent in car, including loading and unloading wheelchair	Hand controls
Homemaking	Independent complex cooking and light housekeeping, some assist with heavy housekeeping	

Modified from Consortium for Spinal Cord Medicine. Outcomes Following Traumatic Spinal Cord Injury. Clinical Practice Guidelines for Health Care Professionals. Washington, DC, Paralyzed Veterans of America, 1999.

SUGGESTED READING

Alexander MS, Anderson KD, Biering-Sorensen F, et al. Outcome measures in spinal cord injury: recent assessments and recommendations for future directions. *Spinal Cord.* 2009;47(8):582-591.

Consortium for Spinal Cord Medicine. *Outcomes Following Traumatic Spinal Cord Injury. Clinical Practice Guidelines for Health Care Professionals.* Washington, DC: Paralyzed Veterans of America; 1999.

Horn SD, Smout RJ, DeJong G, et al. Association of various comorbidity measures with spinal cord injury rehabilitation outcomes. *Arch Phys Med Rehabil.* 2013;94(4 suppl):S75-S86.

Hussey RW, Stauffer ES. Spinal cord injury: requirements for ambulation. *Arch Phys Med Rehabil.* December 1973;54(12):544-547.

Kramer JL, Lammertse DP, Schubert M, Curt A, Steeves JD. Relationship between motor recovery and independence after sensorimotor-complete cervical spinal cord injury. *Neurorehabil Neural Repair.* 2012;26(9):1064-1071.

Marino RJ, Burns S, Graves DE, Leiby BE, Kirshblum S, Lammertse DP. Upper- and lower-extremity motor recovery after traumatic cervical spinal cord injury: an update from the national spinal cord injury database. *Arch Phys Med Rehabil.* 2011;92(3):369-375.

van Middendorp JJ, Hosman AJ, Donders AR, et al. A clinical prediction rule for ambulation outcomes after traumatic spinal cord injury: a longitudinal cohort study. *Lancet.* March 19, 2011;377(9770):1004-1010.

Waters RL, Adkins R, Yakura J, Sie I. Donal Munro Lecture: Functional and neurologic recovery following acute SCI. *J Spinal Cord Med.* 1998;21(3):195-199.

CHAPTER 27

Physical Rehabilitation Activities and Therapeutic Interventions in SCI

GENERAL PRINCIPLES

Early Acute Phase

Physical rehabilitation therapeutic interventions in the acute stage of spinal cord injury (SCI) focus on preventing secondary complications (Chapter 8). Activities include range of motion (ROM), positioning, passive and active assistive exercise, and therapeutic interventions for respiratory management and airway clearance. Transition to the upright position and early mobility is initiated in the absence of contraindications.

Rehabilitation Phase

In the rehabilitation phase, in addition to the above activities, therapy focuses on improving mobility and activities of daily living (ADL). Activities include bed mobility and mat exercises, transfer training, training in pressure relief techniques, wheelchair mobility, and, when applicable, gait training. Task-specific training in these areas is often accompanied by exercises to increase strength, flexibility, and endurance.

CLINICAL CONSIDERATIONS

Joint Protection and Positioning

Attention to joint protection is necessary not only to minimize discomfort but for long-term preservation of function.

During Physical Examination (or Other Encounters That Involve Physically Moving the Patient)
It is essential to protect joint integrity in the paralyzed limb and pay due attention to patient comfort and injury avoidance, not only during rehabilitation therapies but in all encounters that involve physically moving or positioning

Table 27.1

Moving and Positioning Patients With Paralysis in Bed During Physical Examination

- Avoid pulling on the paralyzed arm when turning or repositioning during the exam

- Try to maintain the paralyzed arm in a supported position at all times—during a turn, when lying supine (e.g., by placing it on the chest or on a pillow), or when side-lying

- Turning the paralyzed patient in bed (e.g., to examine the back) can be facilitated by crossing ankles in the direction of the turn or by bending the knee over the other leg prior to turning

- Maintain spinal precautions if applicable (e.g., when spinal instability is a concern)

- At the end of the exam make sure patients are left in a comfortable position, e.g., by adjusting the pillow or bedclothes as needed, since mobility impairments will not allow patients to readjust position themselves

- Make sure that any equipment or device that was moved during examination (e.g., call-light, bed side-rails, or wheelchair) is replaced in the proper original position at the end of the exam, and not left out of reach of the patient

---

of patients with SCI. For example, care should be taken to avoid pulling on the arm to turn the patient during physical examination (Table 27.1).

During Range of Motion
Particular attention is needed for joints below the neurological level of injury (NLI). While preservation of ROM is critical, care must also be taken not to overstretch soft tissues that provide the joint with structural stability (Table 27.2).

Positioning
For adequate stabilization and long-term health of the limb joints, proper positioning of the joint is necessary. Postures that stress the joint (e.g., hyperextension of the shoulder) should be minimized. When lying in bed, direct pressure on the shoulder should be avoided (e.g., by positioning slightly away from side-lying in the supine position), and the upper limb supported adequately, for example, with a pillow. In the supine position, the upper limb of patients with tetraplegia should be placed in abduction and external rotation on a periodic basis to avoid contractures. Prone positioning is a good option to provide stretching of the hip and knee flexors if tolerated and not precluded by the presence of medical devices.

During Activities
Activities such as transfers, weight-shifts, and wheelchair propulsion that are typically done throughout the day, day after day, are especially likely to result in overuse injuries including shoulder pain and carpal tunnel syndrome. Therefore, practice of correct technique to protect joints during these activities and minimize injuries is especially important (Table 27.3). Modifications of these activities (e.g., switching from a manual to power wheelchair, or addition of a transfer-assist device) may need to be considered if

Table 27.2

Special Precautions With Range of Motion Exercises in SCI

- When cervical spine instability is a concern, i.e., in the acute or postoperative phase, shoulder flexion or abduction beyond 90° may need to be avoided

- When thoracolumbar spine instability is a concern, hip flexion beyond 90° may need to be limited and straight leg raising restricted to a range that avoids pelvic tilting

- Extreme or forceful range of motion (ROM) should be avoided because of risk of soft tissue trauma, e.g., around the shoulder. It is especially important to support limbs during ROM when muscles are flaccid, as in the initial areflexive phase after injury

- Overstretching of finger flexors should be avoided in patients who may use a tenodesis grasp, i.e., in patients with C5, C6, or C7 motor level of injury, since that could lead to loss of a functional grasp

- Overstretching of back muscles should be avoided in patients with impaired trunk control since mild tightness of the back helps with balance in long and short sitting positions

Abbreviation: SCI, spinal cord injury.

problems arise. Extreme positions of the wrist, especially maximum extension, should be avoided as much as possible, for example, during weight-shifts or transfers. A combination of techniques should be used for these activities instead of repeated use of one technique. Potentially injurious or extreme positions of the shoulder should be avoided, such as maximum shoulder extension combined with internal rotation and abduction. Repetitive overhead activity that requires hand positioning above the shoulder can increase impingement and shoulder discomfort and should be minimized as feasible through use of equipment or environmental modification. Techniques to protect joints during wheelchair propulsion are summarized in Table 27.3 and also discussed in Chapter 29.

Range of Motion

Daily ROM exercise should be initiated as soon as the patient is medically stable, in order to prevent contractures and maintain function. Passive ROM is provided in areas of little or no strength, and active or active-assisted ROM in regions with some preserved strength. Self ROM exercises of the lower extremities may be taught to those with intact triceps and some hand function either without assistance or with assistance of leg-lift straps or loops.

Hip flexion and ankle plantar flexion contractures are prone to develop in the lower limbs with significant functional consequences, for example, interference with wheelchair seating. Patients with high tetraplegia tend to develop shoulder and scapular tightness, and those with C5 and C6 tetraplegia are especially prone to develop flexion and supination contractures due to unopposed action of elbow flexors.

Table 27.3

Techniques to Protect the Upper Extremities During Activities

Independent Transfers

-Teach patients to perform level transfer when possible
-Avoid placing either hand on a flat surface when a handgrip is possible during transfers. Avoid extremes of wrist extension
-For individuals who use tenodesis, transfers should be performed with fingers flexed and wrist extended to avoid overstretching the long finger flexors
-Avoid positions of impingement (e.g., internal rotation, flexion, and abduction of the shoulder) when possible (e.g., when transferring out of a tub; use a tub-bench instead)
-Vary the technique used and the arm that leads during transfer
-Consider the use of a transfer-assist device, such as a sliding board (which allows transfer to be broken down into smaller movements) especially in those with upper extremity

Weight Shifts

-Weight shifts for pressure relief should utilize a combination of techniques such as forward-leaning and side-to-side shifts, rather than relying primarily on repeated depression-style maneuvers

Overhead Activities

-Repetitive overhead activity that requires hand positioning above the shoulder can increase impingement and shoulder discomfort, and should be minimized as feasible through use of equipment or environmental modification
-Provide seat elevation or possibly a standing position to people with SCI who use power wheelchairs and have arm function

Manual Wheelchair Propulsion

-Also see Chapter 29
-Use a strong, fully customizable wheelchair made of the lightest possible material
-Adjust the rear axle of the wheelchair as far forward as feasible without compromising stability
-Use the correct seat height to minimize upper extremity forces during propulsion (i.e., when hand is placed at the top center position on the pushrim, the angle between upper arm and forearm should be between 100°–120°)
-Use long, smooth strokes in a semicircular pattern to limit high impact on the pushrim

Vocational, Avocational, and Home-Making Activities

-A thorough assessment of the patient's environment (including home, work, and/ or school) should be made. The environment should be altered and/or equipment provided to minimize overhead activities, reduce forces in the extremities, and reduce the frequency with which activities are performed.

Abbreviation: SCI, spinal cord injury.

In people with SCI, special precautions and considerations may apply to ROM, which are summarized in Table 27.2

Mat Activities and Bed Mobility

Progressive mat activities are initiated to work on balance and postural stability and as a foundation for training in sitting, reaching, and transfers.

These activities also provide strength and endurance benefits. The type of activities and postures practiced and the amount of assistance needed will vary with the available motor function and the level of SCI. Examples of basic positions practiced on the mat include prone on elbows, supine on elbows, long sitting (with legs extended out), and short sitting (similar to sitting in a chair). Transitions between positions and rolling are practiced. As appropriate, external challenges to balance and more challenging positions are added. These same skills are carried over to bed mobility. While the use of equipment for assisting with mobility can be useful, overreliance on equipment should be avoided and training should include strategies to maximize independence as appropriate in situations when that equipment is not available.

Transfers

Proper body position, including placement of the leading and trailing hands, leg and foot position, and proper setup are important prerequisites for mechanically efficient transfers. Wheelchair should be locked before transfer and placed in a proper position (at a 30°–45° angle to the other transferring surface, with footrest and armrest placed out of the way).

Depending on available motor function and strength, types of transfer training includes transfers between bed and wheelchair, toilet transfers, car transfers, and uneven transfers, for example, from floor to chair. Spasticity, contractures, and musculoskeletal pain can affect choice and feasibility of transfer techniques. In the absence of other comorbidities, most people with C7 NLI and below should be able to perform independent transfers, at least on level surfaces. Some patients with C6 NLI may be able to transfer independently with a sliding board, and others with C6 and those with C5 NLI need assistance with transfers with or without a sliding board. Those with motor complete injury at or above C4 are dependent for transfers and typically need a caregiver-operated mechanical lift (see Chapter 26 and Tables 26.3 and 26.4).

Transfer safety should be emphasized including avoidance of shear and skin protection, and fall prevention. One of the commonest circumstances for wheelchair-related fall occurrence in people with SCI is during transfers. As previously mentioned and summarized in Table 27.3 joint protection techniques should be incorporated into transfers.

Pressure Relief and Weight Shifts

Techniques for pressure relief and weight shift also depend on NLI and functional capability. Techniques of weight shift include anterior, lateral, pushup, and tilt-back. For patients with motor complete tetraplegia at C4 and above, weight shift is performed by an assistant or a powered system to tilt or recline the wheelchair. Anterior and lateral weight shift options can be accomplished by patients with NLI at C5 and below (although those with tetraplegia will need to learn techniques to recover from the forward position [e.g., by throwing one arm back to hook the back of the chair]). Pushup is feasible as an option in those with C7 and below since they have intact triceps but this puts additional stress on the shoulders and wrists. As mentioned previously, a combination of techniques is preferable to repeated use of a single technique to minimize overuse injury. Weight shifts need to be performed regularly (e.g., for 1–2 minutes every 15–30 minutes) while seated.

Additional Rehabilitation Training

Wheelchair skills training and prescription is discussed in Chapter 29. Gait training and ambulation are discussed in Chapter 30, including a discussion of approaches involving restorative therapies versus compensatory strategies to enhance function. ADL are further discussed in Chapter 28. Also see Chapters 43 and 45 for drivers training, adaptive sports, exercise, and recreation.

KNOWLEDGE GAPS AND EMERGING CONCEPTS

Effectiveness research is needed to better understand and optimize benefits of therapeutic interventions and strategies for physical rehabilitation. Timing of interventions and any additional benefit of periodic "tune-up" or review of task specific training in the postrehabilitation phase are also areas of needed research.

SUGGESTED READING

Hunt KJ, Fang J, Saengsuwan J, Grob M, Laubacher M. On the efficiency of FES cycling: a framework and systematic review. *Technol Health Care*. 2012;20(5):395-422.

Jones ML, Harness E, Denison P, Tefertiller C, Evans N, Larson CA. Activity-based therapies in spinal cord injury: clinical focus and empirical evidence in three independent programs. *Top Spinal Cord Inj Rehabil*. 2012;18(1):34-42.

Kirshblum S. New rehabilitation interventions in spinal cord injury. *J Spinal Cord Med*. 2004;27(4):342-350.

Morawietz C, Moffat F. Effects of locomotor training after incomplete spinal cord injury: a systematic review. *Arch Phys Med Rehabil*. 2013;94:2297-2308.

Paralyzed Veterans of America Consortium for Spinal Cord Medicine. Preservation of upper limb function following spinal cord injury: a clinical practice guideline for health-care professionals. *J Spinal Cord Med*. 2005;28(5):434-470.

Sabharwal S, Sebastian JL, Lanouette M. An educational intervention to teach medical students about examining disabled patients—Research Letter. *JAMA* 2000;284(9): 1080-1081.

CHAPTER 28

Upper Extremity Function in Tetraplegia

GENERAL PRINCIPLES

Loss of upper extremity function can severely limit functional ability and independence. Surveys have demonstrated that individuals with tetraplegia rank hand and arm function as their highest rated priorities for recovery, even more than walking or sexual function. Small gains in upper extremity function can significantly enhance quality of life in these individuals. Adequately addressing upper extremity function in tetraplegia is therefore of crucial importance.

Upper extremity function in tetraplegia is primarily affected by the extent of motor impairment based on the level and completeness of injury. Additional contributors to functional impairment include secondary complications such as contractures, spasticity, pain, and overuse injury.

Maximizing upper extremity function after tetraplegia therefore includes preserving function by preventing and treating secondary complications (such as contracture or overuse injury), compensating for impaired function through use of assistive devices and appropriate upper extremity orthoses, and resorting function through surgery, electrical stimulation, or other therapeutic interventions.

CLINICAL CONSIDERATIONS

Assessment

Measures of Neurological and Global Function
Neurological assessment in accordance with the International Standards for the Neurological Classification of Spinal Cord Injury (INSCSCI) (Chapter 10), global measures of functional assessment that incorporate upper-extremity related activities of daily living (ADLs) such as the Functional Independence Measure and/or the Spinal Cord Independence Measure III (Chapter 26), and

examination of upper extremity tone and range of motion (ROM) are integral parts of assessing upper extremity function. Instruments such as a grip
dynamometer and filament testing for two-point discrimination can be used
to further quantify motor or sensory impairments. Additional factors such as
static and dynamic sitting balance, which significantly influence upper extremity function, should be assessed.

Focused Assessment of Hand and Upper Limb Function
A functional assessment of use of the arm and hand evaluates the individual's
ability to use residual sensorimotor function to perform tasks. The ability to
perform gross motor tasks such as transfers and wheelchair propulsion is
evaluated. The ability to reach is a critical part of upper extremity assessment
since it allows the individual to use their hands or assistive devices to perform
various ADL. In those with hand function, the ability to perform fine motor
tasks using one hand as well as bi-manual tasks should be assessed. Different
grasping patterns may be evaluated including lateral or key pinch, tip pinch,
three-jaw chuck, and power grip.

The International Spinal Cord Injury Upper Extremity Basic Data Set
(currently in draft version, available for comments, at time of this writing)
groups hand function based on ability to reach and grasp (part of the Graded
Redefined Assessment of Strength, Sensibility, and Prehension [GRASSP] test).
Upper limb and shoulder function is categorized by determination of the
individual's ability to position hands on a desk, reach the mouth and head,
and overcome gravity. Hand grasp function is categorized into one of the following: 1. No hand function; 2. Passive tenodesis hand; 3. Active tenodesis
hand; 4. Active extrinsic-tenodesis hand (i.e., voluntary control of wrist and
some extrinsic hand muscles allowing for grasping but reduced dexterity); or
5. Active extrinsic-intrinsic hand (voluntary control of extrinsic and intrinsic
hand muscles and the ability to perform different grasp forms but potential
limitations of muscle strength and dexterity).

Several other direct or indirect measures of hand function in people with tetraplegia are available including the Capabilities of Upper Extremity instrument
and the Grasp and Release Test.

International Classification of Surgery of the Hand in Tetraplegia
The International Classification of Surgery of the Hand in Tetraplegia (ICSHT)
(Table 28.1) was developed specifically for surgical planning in the upper
extremity and to identify potentially available donor muscles for tendon transfers. While there is a correlation between the ICSHT group and SCI classification based on the INSCSCI, it is important to note that the ICSHT includes
evaluation of all upper extremity muscles below the shoulder (as opposed to
only five key muscles considered in the INSCSCI). Therefore, a single level
of injury (LOI) based on the INSCSCI can include multiple possible ICSHT

groups (Table 28.1). Moreover, to be considered functional in ICSHT, muscles have to be at least grade 4 in strength (vs. grade 3 strength used in classification based on the INSCSCI). This is because donor muscles often lose one grade of strength after transfer. Given the fairly ordered pattern segmental innervation of muscles of the upper extremity, each higher INSCSCI group adds an available muscle or muscles to the lower groups, although there can occasionally be exceptions to that.

The sensory portion of the ICSHT involves testing two-point discrimination on the thumb and index finger. Sensation is considered intact if two-point discrimination is less than or equal to 10 mm (classified as Cutaneous or Cu).

Table 28.1

International Classification of Surgery of the Hand in Tetraplegia (ICSHT)

Group	Muscles ≥ Grade 4 Strength	Function	Level of Injury (INSCSCI)
0	No muscles below elbow suitable for transfer		C5
1	Brachioradialis	Flexion of elbow	C5
2	Extensor carpi radialis longus	Weak wrist extension with radial deviation	C6
3	Extensor carpi radialis brevis	Wrist extension	C6
4	Pronator teres	Forearm pronation	C6, C7
5	Flexor carpi radialis	Wrist flexion	C7
6	Extensor digitorum communis and finger extensors	Extrinsic finger extension at metacarpophalangeal joint	C7
7	Extensor pollicis longus and thumb extensors	Extrinsic thumb interphalangeal joint extension	C7, C8
8	Digital flexors	Extrinsic finger flexion	C8
9	All muscles except intrinsics		C8
X	Exceptions		

Sensory (testing for two-point discrimination):
Cu (Cutaneous), if two-point discrimination in the thumb and index finger ≤ 10 mm
O (Ocular feedback only), if two-point discrimination in the thumb/index finger >10 mm or absent

Abbreviation: INSCSCI, International Standards for Neurological Classification of Spinal Cord Injury.

When two-point discrimination is greater than 10 mm, persons are considered to only have ocular input for hand function (classified as Ocular or O).

Management

Preservation of Upper Extremity Function by Preventing Secondary Complications
Proper positioning, ROM, and joint protection techniques are critical to preserve upper extremity function in people with tetraplegia and to prevent complications such as contractures, pain, and upper extremity overuse injury.

These aspects, and related precautions and preventive measures, are covered in further detail in Chapter 27 and Tables 27.1 to 27.3. Specific areas of attention may be warranted based on the LOI. Patients with C5 and some with C6 LOI are especially prone to get elbow flexion and/or forearm supination contractures because of muscle imbalance created by paralysis of opposing muscles, which can severely limit upper extremity function. Overstretching of finger flexors should be avoided in patients with C6 or C7 LOI who use a tenodesis grasp, since that could lead to loss of a functional grasp. Those with C8 LOI are prone to developing a claw hand (intrinsic minus) deformity that limits optimal hand opening and grasp.

Assistive Devices to Compensate for Loss of Upper Extremity Function
Table 28.2 lists examples of commonly used, relatively simple, assistive devices for various ADLs that compensate for upper extremity impairment and paralysis and can significantly increase functional independence.

More complex devices include electronic aids to independent living (E-ADLs), previously called environmental control units. The unit is controlled with a switch that is activated by a voluntary movement (e.g., voice activation, joystick, tongue control, or sip and puff). E-ADLs are available at different levels of complexity and cost and may be used to control multiple aspects of the environment such as lights, doors, intercom, bed, televisions/entertainment systems, telephones, and computer. Especially with these more complex devices, it is important to fit the device to the individual after consideration of their physical impairment, cognition, functional needs, goals, and preferences.

Advances in technology available to the general population through computers, tablets, and smart phones, and available software and adaptions to enhance access (including voice activation, head pointer, or eye-gaze systems) to these devices have opened up increasing avenues of communication and interaction.

Upper Extremity Orthoses
Upper extremity orthoses can be provided to maintain or enhance function, stabilize joints, relieve pain, and/or prevent deformity. These can be commercially

Table 28.2

Assistive Devices to Compensate for Impaired Hand and Upper Limb Function

Activity of Daily Living	Examples of Assistive Devices
Feeding	Plate guard
	Built-up or custom-handled utensils
	Angled spoon or fork
	Nonslip mat
	Nonspill cups
	Rocker knife
	Splints with slot for utensils
Dressing	Reacher
	Leg lift strap
	Dressing stick
	Button aids
	Velcro closures
	Velcro or elastic shoelaces
	Loops/zipper puller
	Sock aids
Grooming/bathing/toileting	Toothpaste squeezer
	Razor adaptor
	Electric shaver/toothbrush
	Wash mitt
	Liquid soap
	Long-handled mirror
	Catheter holder
	Adapted leg bag emptier
	Rectal stimulator device/Suppository inserter
Home-making	Button pushers
	Reachers
	Door knob gripper
	Adapted utensils for cutting, reaching, mixing

(continued)

Activity of Daily Living	Examples of Assistive Devices
Communication	Speaker phone
	Mouthstick
	Writing splint
	Typing peg
	Voice recognition software
	Adapted computer, smart phone, and tablet access

available off-the-shelf products or custom made. Orthoses can be static or dynamic (e.g., the wrist-driven wrist-hand orthosis or tenodesis splint). Cumbersome, heavy upper extremity orthoses are often discarded and are now less frequently prescribed. Table 28.3 lists commonly used orthoses for different levels of tetraplegia.

Surgical Interventions to Restore Upper Extremity Function
Surgical procedures to increase function of the upper extremities include procedures to relieve disabling contractures (e.g., release of elbow flexion contractures or radial osteotomy to counter supination contractures), and surgery to restore upper extremity function through tendon transfers and related procedures.

Tendon transfer surgery involves detachment of a functioning muscle and its tendon from its normal insertion and rerouting it into a different muscle to help restore the desired function. Surgical reconstructive procedures could also involve joint immobilization and/or attaching tendons to bone to create passive tightening of the anchored tendon to move a distal joint (surgical tenodesis). Table 28.4 summarizes surgical procedures for functional restoration of the upper extremity.

Goals of Reconstructive Upper Extremity Surgery
Goals of reconstructive upper extremity surgery, in general order of priority (if that function is not already available) are to restore: elbow extension, wrist extension, lateral pinch and release, and palmer grasp and release.

Candidates for Upper Extremity Surgery
Identifying and matching appropriate candidates for various upper extremity reconstructive procedures is critical. In view of lack of available muscles to transfer in those with C4 or higher levels of injury, this option is generally only available for those with C5 or lower LOI. Neurological stability should be established before proceeding with surgery; waiting till after one year or

Table 28.3

Upper Extremity Orthoses to Improve Function in Tetraplegia

Orthosis	Level of Injury (LOI)	Purpose/Description
Resting hand splint	C1–C4	Maintains hand in a functional position (wrist at ~20°–30° extension, metacarpophalangeal joints at ~70° flexion, extended interphalangeal joints, and thumb in abduction), prevents contracture
Balanced forearm orthosis (mobile arm support)	C4 with weak C5 function	Allows horizontal motion of shoulder and elbow to compensate for weak elbow flexion, allowing hand to be positioned for performing activities or close to face for feeding and grooming
Universal cuff	C5, C6, C7	Provides a slot in which utensils and other objects can be inserted; (with C5 LOI universal cuff is often combined with an orthosis that supports the wrist in a functional position)
Long opponens splint	C5	Positions thumb in a functional key pinch position, stabilizes the wrist
Short opponens splint	C6	Holds thumb in functional pinch position in the presence of preserved wrist extension and tenodesis
Wrist-driven wrist-hand orthosis (tenodesis splint)	C6, C7	Facilitates stronger prehension and pinch in response to wrist extension
Static hand orthosis with metacarpophalangeal block (lumbrical bar)	C8	Goal is to prevent clawing of hand and improve hand opening, but it is often discarded

longer postinjury is typical though in some cases where recovery has clearly plateaued, it may be considered a little earlier. Considerations of the individuals goals, expectations, status and satisfaction with current function, overall medical stability, secondary upper limb complications such as contractures and spasticity, available support, cognition, and ability to participate in the involved postoperative rehabilitation and motor relearning are all important in candidate selection.

Table 28.4

Surgical Options to Restore Upper Extremity Function in Tetraplegia

Level of Injury (INSCSCI)	ICSHT Group	Procedure (Tendon Transfers, Tenodesis)	Goal of Functional Restoration
C5	1	BR to ECRB	Active wrist extension
		FPL tenodesis	Static thumb pinch
		Biceps to triceps (or posterior deltoid to triceps)	Active elbow extension
C6	1 or 2	Br to FPL	Active thumb pinch
		EPL tenodesis	Static thumb extension
		Biceps to triceps (or posterior deltoid to triceps)	Active elbow extension
			Active thumb pinch
			Active finger flexion
	3	Br to FPL	Static thumb extension
		ECRL to FDP	Static finger extension
		EPL tenodesis	Active elbow extension
		EDC tenodesis	
		Biceps to triceps (or posterior deltoid to triceps)	
C7	4 or 5	Br to FPL	Active thumb pinch
		EPL tenodesis	Static thumb extension
		ECRL to FDP	Active finger flexion
		PT to EDC	Active finger extension
	6	Br to FPL	Active thumb flexion
		PT to EPL (or)	Active thumb extension
		Opponensplasty via PT	Active thumb opposition
		ECRL to FDP	Active finger flexion
	7	BR to FPL	Active thumb flexion
		Opponensplasty via PT	Active thumb opposition
		ECRL-FDP	Active finger flexion
C8	8 or 9	Zancolli lasso procedure	Prevents MP hyperextension

Abbreviations: INSCSCI, International Standards for Neurological Classification of Spinal Cord Injury; ICSHT, International Classification for Surgery of the Hand in Tetraplegia; Br, brachioradialis; ECRB, extensor carpi radialis brevis; ECRL, extensor carpi radialis longus; EDC, extensor digitorum communis; EPL, extensor pollicis longus; FDP, flexor digitorum profundus; FPL, flexor pollicis longus; MP, metacarpophalangeal joint; PT, pronator teres.

Surgical Planning

Certain principles underlie surgical planning and selection of appropriate procedures. The donor muscle must have sufficient motor strength (grade of ≥4). Ideally the loss of donor muscle should not compromise existing function. For example the extensor carpi radialis longus (ECRL) can only be considered for transfer to restore palmer grip if a strong extensor carpi radialis brevis (ECRB) is present so that wrist extension is not compromised with the procedure. Multiple procedures may be carried out in the same sitting or be performed in a staged manner. Preoperative strengthening, conditioning, and, if/as needed, management of spasticity or contractures is important.

Choice of Surgical Procedures (Table 28.4)

Elbow extension can be provided to those with C5 or C6 LOI (ICHST 1, 2, or 3) with a posterior deltoid to triceps transfer or with a biceps to triceps tendon transfer. While there can be some loss of elbow flexion with biceps transfer, it is often of limited functional significance, and the procedure typically leads to a stronger elbow extension than a posterior deltoid to triceps transfer, so is often the preferred option.

Wrist extension can be provided to patients with C5 LOI, ICHST 1, through a brachioradialis (Br) to ECRB tendon transfer.

Pinch may be provided either as a static thumb pinch or an active lateral pinch based on available muscles. Static thumb pinch may be provided through tenodesis of the flexor pollicis longus (FPL) to the radius (often combined with restoration of wrist extension in those with C5 LOI) so that greater pinch force is generated with wrist extension than would naturally occur (although this is often of limited strength and functional utility, so is not often performed). Active thumb pinch is much more functionally useful and is an option for those with C6 or C7 LOI through a Br to FPL transfer. Tenodesis of the thumb extensors and arthrodesis of the first carpometacarpal joint is sometimes performed concomitantly with this procedure to place the thumb in a more functionally stable position for a stronger pinch.

Palmer grasp and release may be an option in the presence of sufficient donor muscles. Active finger flexion can be accomplished by ECRL to flexor digitorum profundus transfer. Active finger extension can be accomplished with a pronator teres (PT) to extensor digitorum communis transfer or active thumb extension through PT to extensor pollicis longus transfer. Patients with C8 LOI often have good hand function despite reduced grip strength and claw hand deformity, and may not need, or be interested in, surgical options. The Zancolli lasso procedure is an option that involves tendon transfer to prevent hyperextension of the metacarpophalangeal joints.

Postoperative Care and Rehabilitation

Postoperative care after reconstructive upper extremity surgery is typically quite involved and requires considerable patient cooperation and participation. Depending on the procedure, there is usually a period of immobilization during which functional independence is reduced. Rehabilitation includes edema prevention, scar management, gradual mobilization, muscle reeducation, and functional skills training. Close cooperation between the surgeon and rehabilitation team with specific expertise and experience in this postsurgical rehabilitation is essential for success.

Functional Electrical Stimulation of the Upper Extremity
Electrical stimulation can be used to stimulate paralyzed muscles of the hand and upper extremity. Stimulation is applied with surface or implanted electrodes. The control signal is typically elicited from a movement under voluntary control. Lower motor neuron paralysis will not respond to electrical stimulation, so that distinction is important to make for muscles at and around the zone of injury. A transcutaneous neuroprosthesis to provide grasp for patients with C5 or weak C6 tetraplegia is commercially available, though it is more often used for muscle conditioning than for long-term functional use. The bionic glove is neuroprosthesis that utilizes electrical stimulation of the finger flexors, extensors, and thumb flexors to produce a functional grasp through tenodesis action at the wrist. Commercial marketing of a previously available implanted functional electrical stimulation system with multiple upper extremity electrodes was discontinued a few years ago based on limited demand, but newer systems are being developed.

KNOWLEDGE GAPS AND EMERGING CONCEPTS

Ongoing advances in rehabilitation technology are creating additional avenues to increase function for individuals with spinal cord injury. As technology to control the environment becomes increasingly available to the general population, the same technology has the potential to greatly improve environmental access and function for people with tetraplegia, and often at a lowered cost due to widespread commercial availability.

Current research in implanted upper extremity neuroprostheses is ongoing with development and trials of myoelectrically-controlled second-generation implanted neuroprostheses.

Brain–computer interface is an emerging and exciting area of research where neural signals from the cerebral cortex are recorded and used to control movement of a computer cursor or other external device. This technology needs considerable development and testing, but creates the possibility of developing systems that can bypass the injured spinal cord to control paralyzed extremities.

SUGGESTED READING

Anderson KD. Targeting recovery: priorities of the spinal cord–injured population. *J Neurotrauma*. 2004;21:1371-1383.

Bryden AM, Peljovich AE, Hoyen HA, Nemunaitis G, Kilgore KL, Keith MW. Surgical restoration of arm and hand function in people with tetraplegia. *Top Spinal Cord Inj Rehabil*. 2012;18(1):43-49.

International SCI Standards and Data Sets Executive Committee. International Spinal Cord Society (ISCoS) and American Spinal Injury Association (ASIA). International Spinal Cord Injury Upper Extremity Basic Data Set (Version 1.0) July 7, 2013.

Mulcahey MJ, Hutchinson D, Kozin S. Assessment of upper limb in tetraplegia: considerations in evaluation and outcomes research. *J Rehabil Res Dev*. 2007;44(1):91-102.

Paralyzed Veterans of America Consortium for Spinal Cord Medicine. Preservation of upper limb function following spinal cord injury: a clinical practice guideline for health-care professionals. *J Spinal Cord Med*. 2005;28(5):434-470.

CHAPTER 29

Wheelchair Prescription and Wheelchair Mobility After SCI

GENERAL PRINCIPLES

The wheelchair is one of the most important therapeutic devices for individuals with spinal cord injury (SCI). Wheelchair mobility is central to independence for those who are unable to walk as their primary mode of locomotion. Provision of an appropriate wheelchair and wheelchair skills training are key aspects of rehabilitation after SCI.

There are several choices for wheeled mobility for persons with SCI. These include manual wheelchairs, power wheelchairs, power-assisted manual wheelchairs, and scooters. An increasing number of options are available for various components and features. Some features are critical for safety, comfort, and maneuverability while other options might be based on personal preference.

Manual Wheelchairs

Table 29.1 summarizes the different features of manual wheelchairs and considerations in choosing between various options for wheelchair weight, frame, seat, backrest, armrests, leg rests and footplates, wheels, tires, pushrims, wheel locks, casters, and accessories. Standard wheelchairs are made of steel and weigh typically between 40 and 65 pounds. Lightweight wheelchairs are made of stainless steel and weigh less than 36 pounds. Ultralight wheelchairs weigh less than 30 pounds and are most often made of high-grade aluminum, but can also be titanium or composite material. In general, chairs made of the lightest, strongest material are preferable for long-term use and should be customizable to optimize mobility and ensure good fit. Heavy duty chairs are indicated for individuals weighing over 250 pounds and have reinforced frames.

Pushrim-Activated Power-Assisted Wheelchairs

Power-assist pushrims can be mounted on certain manual wheelchair bases to convert them to pushrim-activated power-assisted wheelchairs (PAPAWs). The system amplifies the propulsion power supplied by the user through force-sensitive pushrims that are connected to motors. Power-assist devices

Table 29.1

Manual Wheelchair Options and Considerations

Wheelchair Feature/ Options	Considerations
Weight Standard >36 lbs. Lightweight <36 lbs. Ultralightweight <30 lbs. Heavy duty Extra-heavy duty	In general, ultralight wheelchairs require less force to propel, are made of stronger components, and are more durable. So, even if they are more expensive upfront, they cost less to operate over the long term than heavier chairs Heavy duty chairs support persons weighing >250 lbs; extra-heavy duty chairs support weight >300 lbs
Frame Rigid or folding	Rigid frames are lighter, sturdier, more adjustable, and more responsive Folding frames are easier to transport, but less durable and do not always provide as comfortable a ride
Seat Flexible (sling) or rigid	Most manual chairs have a sling seat which is lighter and allows chair to be collapsed Sling seats sag with time; if problematic, a rigid removable base can be placed on a sling seat.
Backrest Sling, solid, tension-adjustable, or custom-molded	Most manual chairs have a flexible backrest. Tension-adjustable and solid backrests are options for those who need more trunk support Custom molded backrests may be needed for those with significant back deformities, which adds weight and cost
Armrests Fixed or adjustable height Desk-length or full-length	Adjustable arms rests are often desirable to permit activities at tables of different heights Full-length armrests are indicated for those who use them for leverage to transfer or stand; for most others, desk-length arms rests are preferred to enable greater access to tabletops and desks Offset armrests reduce chair width Armrests can be omitted altogether for active users with good trunk control
Footplates and leg rests Swing-away or fixed Elevating	If patients can stand up, they require footplates that can be lifted up or swung away Elevating leg-rests can be used to manage orthostatic hypotension or leg edema, although they add weight and length to the chair
Wheels Mag, spoke, or X-core wheels Vertical or cambered	Standard size of wheels is 24", other sizes available from 20" to 26" Cambered wheels (i.e., tilted with more distance between bottoms of the wheels than the tops) provide easier turning and lateral stability, but add width to the chair

(continued)

Table 29.1

Manual Wheelchair Options and Considerations (*continued*)

Wheelchair Feature/ Options	Considerations
Tires Pneumatic, airless or solid	Treaded tires with option of either air or airless inserts provide good traction on regular terrain and are commonly used; airless require less maintenance High-performance tires are available for sports and activities on level surfaces but don't work well on wet surfaces or rough terrain
Pushrims (handrims) Aluminum or plastic-coated	Located just lateral to the wheel to enhance propulsion Plastic-coated pushrims, used in conjunction with gloves, allow better control of wheels (e.g., in those with C6 tetraplegia); knobs or projections can provide the same purpose but are used less often since they increase risk of injury and width of chair Aluminum pushrims are preferred by those who are able to push without coating, since they are more durable and don't cause hand burn while propelling
Front casters Large (6–8″) or small (2–5″)	Smaller casters provide greater agility but are more apt to get stuck and may offer more resistance to rolling
Wheel locks ("brakes") Push/pull or scissors	Push/pull are easier to operate even with limited hand function than scissors type Scissors brakes remain out of the way during propulsion, so maybe preferred in those with good hand function Grade aids are special types of wheel locks that can be added to help push up slopes without rolling back
Miscellaneous	Belts are used to maintain stability and pelvic position while seated in the chair Antitip bars are an option to prevent the chair from tipping backwards (but make it difficult to ascend curbs or pop a wheelie, and advanced users often remove them) Wheel-guards to cover wheel spokes to prevent injury to the hand
Sports wheelchairs	There are numerous types of sport wheelchairs that are unique for each sport, e.g., wheelchair racing, basketball, and rugby, and often customized for the individual participant. The common factor is that they are generally very rugged, durable, light, and cambered

have been shown to require considerably less energy expenditure to propel than a manual wheelchair, and reduce the amount of effort that the patient must exert. However, the weight of the wheels, range on a single charge, and expense are a few of the challenges that should be kept in mind when considering a power add-on or power-assist unit.

Power Wheelchairs

There are three different power wheelchair drive bases: rear wheel drive, mid wheel drive, and front wheel drive. Mid-wheel drive wheelchairs provide good maneuverability and are commonly prescribed for general use. Rear-wheel power chairs are easier to control in difficult terrains.

Several of the general principles and components applicable to manual wheelchairs are also applicable to powered wheelchairs. The type of headrest can vary with the extent of support needed.

Various control mechanisms options are available including hand-control with a joystick, or chin, head, or breath (sip and puff) control. Selection is based on the present and anticipated function. The electronic set-up for the joystick controls can be proportional (where both speed of movement and direction are controlled) or nonproportional which only controls direction.

Power wheelchairs have batteries that need to be charged daily. Accessories include ventilator tray and battery box.

Powered Seating Options

Power chairs often incorporate a tilt-in space or recline feature to allow for pressure relief, and as an option for orthostatic hypotension in the upright position. Other powered seating options may include standing or seat elevation. Providing seat elevation or possibly a standing position to people with SCI who use power wheelchairs and have arm function should be considered as a measure to protect the shoulder from overuse and impingement with repeated overhead activity. These allow individuals to remain seated but elevate or lower the seat to meet activity of daily living requirements such as reaching for objects on high shelves. The height of the seat can be adjusted to make eye contact with individuals while interacting, thereby having a tremendous social impact. A standing wheelchair allows the patient to sit or stand and may provide increased accessibility to surfaces out of reach from a seated position in a home or work environment. An assessment of the patient's range of motion and trunk balance, to determine the external support that will be necessary, is important to assess when considering a standing chair.

Cushions and Seating Surface

Commercially available wheelchair cushion types include air, foam, gel, and hybrid cushions. These are also discussed in Chapter 37. There is insufficient evidence to categorically recommend one cushion over another, and decisions are based on clinical reasoning and rationale. Pressure mapping may be used to measure skin-interface pressures. Effectiveness of air-based cushions depends on appropriate inflation. Gel-based cushions dissipate pressure by allowing gel to move from areas of high to low pressure. Effectiveness of foam-based cushions to redistribute pressure depends on cut and compressibility.

Other considerations in choice of cushion include ease of maintenance, effect on seating stability, mobility, and posture, weight, and cost considerations. Air-based cushions need to be regularly checked for proposer inflation and for any punctures. All cushions need to be replaced after a period of use. Foam cushions often need replacement every year while air and gel cushions need replacement every few years. Gel cushions are heavier than air or foam cushions. Foam cushions are typically the least expensive.

CLINICAL CONSIDERATIONS

Wheelchair Prescription

A team approach generally works best, including input from the individual with SCI. Specialized centers often have seating teams with individuals from different backgrounds that could include physicians, therapists, assistive technology specialists, rehabilitation engineers, wheelchair technicians, case managers, and vendors. Input from others on the SCI team, for example vocational specialists, can be invaluable.

The neurological level and completeness of SCI and the current and projected functional status are the primary factors in determining choice of wheelchair and seating (Table 29.2). Factors such as spasticity and contractures can also be important considerations. In addition, an evaluation of the whole person including cognitive function, lifestyle, goals, and preferences are all important to consider in prescribing a wheelchair.

Choosing Between Manual and Power Mobility Options
For many people with high cervical SCI, a power wheelchair is an absolute necessity. However, even if for a lower injury, a power chair might sometimes be appropriate for those that have an upper extremity overuse injury. Time in chair, age, weight, prior injury, and environmental factors (such as steep hills or rough terrain) may make individuals more susceptible to repetitive strain injuries to upper limb joints.

For people with good arm strength, the convenience and versatility of a manual chair is the clear choice. For people with weak arms or a painful arm condition, deciding whether to go with a manual or power chair involves many factors. For most people, the chair that supports the most independence is the right chair. This is an area of some controversy, and different practitioners having differing thresholds for when they consider a power chair to be appropriate.

The advantages of power wheelchairs include:

- Reduced propulsion-related repetitive strain.
- Conserved energy and therefore reduced fatigue.
- Increased speed.
- Increased ease of traversing uneven terrain and inclines.

Table 29.2

Typical Wheelchair Needs Based on Neurological Level of Injury	
Level of Injury[a]	Typical Wheelchair
C1–C4 tetraplegia	Power recline and/or tilt WC, with head, chin, or breath control and manual recliner, vent tray (for those requiring assisted ventilation); back-up manual WC (pushed by others)
C5 tetraplegia	Power recline and/or tilt WC with arm-drive control; lightweight manual WC with hand rim modifications (which they can propel by self on flat smooth surfaces, but will need assistance elsewhere)
C6 tetraplegia	Lightweight manual WC, with hand rim modifications, often need power WC for long distances and/or for difficult or uneven terrain
C7–C8 tetraplegia	Manual rigid or folding lightweight WC, or folding WC with modified rims
Paraplegia	Manual rigid or folding lightweight wheelchair

[a] This table refers to motor complete SCI; for incomplete SCI wheelchair needs depend on the extent of motor impairment.
Abbreviation: WC, wheelchair.

The disadvantages include:

- Decreased transportability.
- Increased maintenance.
- Increased cost.
- Possible weight gain.
- Possible decreased fitness.

Alternatives for Powered Mobility
In addition to power wheelchairs, other alternatives to manual mobility include scooters, and power-assist and add-on devices. To consider a scooter, the patient must have good sitting balance, proximal stability, and shoulder mobility to steer the scooter. Good hand control is necessary to operate the accelerator. While scooters may be used by some patients with paraplegia with good trunk control, or incomplete SCI, power chairs offer more options and are often the preferred option when powered mobility is indicated for those with SCI. PAPAW may be a useful alternative to an electric-powered wheelchair or an intermediate option for those for whom a manual wheelchair is no longer meeting needs optimally.

People with power wheelchair should have a back-up manual wheelchair to use, with assistance as needed, for example when the power chair is being repaired or when visiting a location that is not accessible for the power chair.

Medical Justification

Medical justification for wheelchairs, especially the more expensive ones, is often needed for funding and policy reasons. It should document reasons why less expensive alternatives are not adequate and reasoning behind the proposed choice, addressing issues such as ability or inability to propel due to neurological or musculoskeletal impairments and limitations, ability or inability to maintain an upright posture without the needed support, postural deformities, endurance, pain, and needs related to vocational or educational participation.

Wheelchair Set-Up

Wheelchair prescription not only includes choosing the appropriate product and features, but also ensuring proper fitting and set-up. Certain seating principles are universally applicable, regardless of the type of wheelchair and the technology used. Proper positioning of the pelvis and trunk provides a stable base of support for upper extremities. The wheelchair position should allow patients to sit comfortably, with proper pressure distribution and adequate upright stability, and support efficient propulsion. Wheelchair set-up includes fitting and adjustment of seat height, depth, width, and slope, and of backrest height, width, and recline.

Given the repetitive nature of wheelchair propulsion, attention to measures that reduce abnormal force transmission to the upper limb are crucial considerations in manual wheelchair set-up. The rear wheel axle position has a significant impact on efficiency of propulsion, forces transmitted to the upper limb, and wheelchair stability (Table 29.3).

Table 29.3

Importance of Wheelchair Rear Axle Position for Minimizing Upper Extremity Overuse Injury

Vertical Adjustment

-The rear axle should be positioned so that when the hand is placed at the top center position of the pushrim, the angle between the upper arm and forearm is between 100° and 120°.

-If the angle is larger (i.e., the seat is too high relative to the wheel), it decreases propulsion efficiency. If the angle is smaller (because the seat is too low) the wheelchair user will be forced to push with abducted arms, which could increase shoulder impingement.

-Another way to determine correct seat position is to have the individual sit with arms hanging down the side. Fingertips should be level or just past the axle of the wheel.

Horizontal Adjustment

-The rear wheel axle should be adjusted as far forward as feasible without compromising wheelchair user stability.

-A more forward axle position increases propulsion efficiency, decreases stroke frequency, and lowers peak forces and loading of the upper limb. However, this has to be balanced with decreased stability and increased tendency for the chair to tip backward if the rear axle position is too far forward.

The optimal set-up for a wheelchair for an individual patient often changes over the first few months as function and mobility evolve. For this reason the prescription of a permanent wheelchair may be delayed and a loaner or temporary wheelchair provided in the interim, or a highly adjustable chair may be provided as the initial wheelchair. Individuals with new injuries may initially need the wheelchair setup for more stability and safety, and as they gain wheelchair skill proficiency, the wheelchair components can be adjusted for maximum performance and efficiency.

Wheelchair Skills Training

Wheelchair skills include basic and advanced activities. Basic skills' training includes wheelchair propulsion on different surfaces and terrains, transfers to and from wheelchairs to different surfaces including bed, toilet, and car, and negotiating low curbs and inclines. Patients with mid- or lower-thoracic paraplegia should be able to learn more advanced skills as well, including propelling on uneven terrain, performing wheelies, and negotiating higher curbs and steps. Fall safety should be stressed, especially during transfers from wheelchairs. Wheelchair folding or disassembly and transportation should be addressed as part of wheelchair skills training and education. Standardized wheelchair skills testing has been developed to allow for testing both basic and advanced skills.

Caregivers should be trained in providing needed assistance, for example, to negotiate environmental obstacles that the individual is unable to negotiate independently.

Wheelchair Access

Wheelchair access in the home and community environment is necessary to evaluate and address. Some important requirements for wheelchair access include: ramps that provide at least 12" of length for every 1" in rise (i.e., are not too steep), doorways that are a minimum of 32–36" in width depending on the type of wheelchair (32" for manual, 34" for power, and 36" if a turn is involved), and light switches at 36" or lower height.

Wheelchair Transportation

Manual wheelchairs can be transported in a car by folding or disassembling. Power chairs often require a van, with a built-in lift or ramp. When selecting a wheelchair and vehicle, it is critical to ensure that the two devices are compatible. If patients remain seated in the wheelchair while travelling, it needs to be secured to the vehicle. Special tie-downs are available to secure the chair during transportation in a van.

Follow-Up

Periodic follow-up and review is needed, both to make sure that the wheelchair is continuing to meet the needs of the individual and for ongoing maintenance and needed repair/replacement.

KNOWLEDGE GAPS AND EMERGING CONCEPTS

Advances in materials and new technologies have progressively improved wheelchair design to meet the needs of people with SCI.

Emerging trends in wheelchair-related technologies include computer interfaces that enable wheelchairs to conform to individual needs, and intelligent systems incorporated into wheelchairs that learn from the user's behavior and environmental input and adapt accordingly. Other examples of emerging technology include robotic obstacle-climbing wheelchairs to negotiate curbs and steps.

SUGGESTED READING

Boninger M, French J, Abbas J, et al. Technology for mobility in SCI 10 years from now. *Spinal Cord*. 2012;50(5):358-363.

Fliess-Douer O, Vanlandewijck YC, Lubel Manor G, Van Der Woude LH. A systematic review of wheelchair skills tests for manual wheelchair users with a spinal cord injury: towards a standardized outcome measure. *Clin Rehabil*. 2010;24(10):867-886.

Hastings JD. Seating assessment and planning. *Phys Med Rehabil Clin N Am*. February 2000; 11(1):183-207.

Oyster ML, Smith IJ, Kirby RL, et al. Wheelchair skill performance of manual wheelchair users with spinal cord injury. *Top Spinal Cord Inj Rehabil*. 2012;18(2):138-139.

Sisto SA, Forrest GF, Faghri PD. Technology for mobility and quality of life in spinal cord injury. *IEEE Eng Med Biol Mag*. 2008;27(2):56-68.

CHAPTER 30

Walking After Spinal Cord Injury

GENERAL PRINCIPLES

Being able to walk again is a goal of the majority of people following spinal cord injury (SCI). However, it is not a feasible long-term ambulation option for many of those individuals. While walking does have several potential medical, psychological, and practical benefits, the high energy requirements and excessive demands on the upper extremities for weight bearing are primary factors that limit its utilization for long-term functional ambulation after SCI even with the use of orthoses and assistive devices. Wheelchair propulsion, on the other hand, has similar energy costs and speed as normal walking.

Patient Selection for Trial of Walking

The selection of patients for a trial of walking is an area of controversy. Ideally all people who have the potential to walk should be given the opportunity to try it should they wish to do so, in the absence of any medical or orthopedic contraindications (even with the knowledge that it will not be a viable long-term option for many). At the same time, however, unrealistic expectations can be counter-productive. Gait training should not supersede other aspects of rehabilitation that are crucial for improving function and independence such as transfers, mat activities, wheelchair skills, and activities of daily living.

Factors Affecting Ability to Walk After SCI

As discussed in Chapter 26 and Table 26.2, available motor function based on the level and completeness of SCI is the primary determinant of walking ability.

Several other factors including muscle tone, range of motion, proprioception, endurance, age, and additional impairments or comorbidities are also important in determining the options available for walking after SCI (Table 30.1).

CLINICAL CONSIDERATIONS

Assessment

It is important to quantify the principal elements of walking to make meaningful functional assessments and measure changes in walking ability and function.

222

IV. *Physical Function and Rehabilitation*

Table 30.1

Factors Affecting Options for Walking After SCI

Muscle strength	- Primary determinant of walking ability. Muscle strength, including trunk/pelvic control and LEMS (see Table 26.2), is key in determining ability and options for walking - People with complete SCI at or above T9 are unlikely to become community ambulators - LEMS for walking needs to be higher in those with tetraplegia than with paraplegia in order to compensate for upper extremity weakness
Endurance	- High energy requirement of walking with assistive devices and lower extremity orthoses is a primary limiting factor for sustained walking - The significantly higher energy requirements for those who require an HKAFO or bilateral KAFOs for walking than those who can use an AFO at least on one leg make the former much less likely to become community ambulators - Older age and comorbidities (e.g., cardiovascular) that limit endurance may preclude walking as an option
Spasticity	- Mild to moderate spasticity may be helpful, e.g., knee extensor and ankle plantar flexor spasticity may provide stability in single limb stance while walking - However, more severe spasticity impairs forward progression and ambulatory function - The degree and pattern of spasticity may guide options and orthotic needs
ROM	- Preserved ROM at the hip, knee, and ankle are important for biomechanical stability and bracing, especially for those needing KAFOs. - While mild contractures may be accommodated, moderate to severe contractures are destabilizing
Proprioception	- Proprioception at the hip has been shown to be an important determinant for separating walkers from non-walkers - The inability to perceive where one's limb is in space results in loss of sense of stable vs. unstable postures and ability to make useful muscle substitutions
SCI-related comorbidities	- Effect of SCI on skin integrity, autonomic function, upper extremity overuse, and bone density may affect walking options
Preference and motivation	- Individual preference is an important factor in making an informed choice between viable options for ambulation based on level and completeness of injury with consideration of pros and cons of various options - Many individuals give up walking in favor of the efficiency and low energy cost of wheelchair ambulation

Abbreviations: AFO, ankle-foot-orthosis; HKAFO, hip-knee-ankle-foot-orthosis; KAFO, knee-ankle-foot-orthosis; LEMS, lower extremity motor score; ROM, range of motion; SCI, spinal cord injury.

Table 30.2 lists some of the primary assessment tools that are used to measure various aspects of walking ability and outcomes.

Gait analysis can be helpful to assess gait deviations during the gait cycle (stance and swing phases) and the functional tasks of weight acceptance, single limb support, and limb advancement, and provides useful information to determine orthotic needs.

Therapeutic Strategies for Ambulation After SCI

Approaches to facilitate ambulation after SCI can be broadly grouped into two main categories:

- Compensatory strategies, which include use of assistive devices and lower extremity orthoses, functional electrical stimulation (FES), or a combination of the two to compensate for the loss of muscle strength for walking.
- Locomotor training (LT), utilizing techniques towards a goal to facilitate restoration of walking by promoting plasticity in the central nervous system.

Available compensatory therapeutic options for walking based on level of injury are summarized in Table 30.3 for those with complete SCI. For incomplete SCI,

Table 30.2
Tools to Assess Walking Function After SCI

Walking Assessment	Description
Walking Index for Spinal Cord Injury–II (WISCI-II)	Characterizes walking function based on the extent of bracing, assistive device use, and assistance required. It is a 21-level scale, ranging from 0 (unable to stand and/or participate in assisted walking) to 20 (ambulates 10 meters with no devices, no braces, and no physical assistance)
Spinal Cord Injury Functional Ambulation Inventory (SCI-FAI)	Addresses three separate domains: Gait, Assistive Device Use, and Walking Mobility. Each domain is scored separately. It, therefore, measures the level of independence in walking, as well as the quality of gait and the use of assistive devices
6-minute walk test[a]	This assessment measures the distance walked after asking the individual to walk as far as possible for duration of 6 minutes
10-meter walk test[a]	This is a measure of walking speed with the individual being instructed to walk as fast as he/she can along a straight walkway
Timed Up and Go (TUG)[a]	Measures the time required for an individual to stand up, walk 3 meters, return to a chair, and sit down

[a]Excellent correlation has been demonstrated between the three timed tests, but the correlation of these tests with WISCI is good only for those with relatively good walking ability (WISCI score of 11–20); these timed tests should be interpreted with caution in those with poor walking ability.

the options for walking will vary depending on the extent and distribution of muscle weakness.

Lower Extremity Orthoses
Considerations in Orthotic Prescription
The purpose of an orthosis to aid in ambulation is to provide stability during stance, enhance swing, or do both. Many of the factors listed in Table 30.1 may influence the choice of orthotic prescription. Additional considerations include weight of the orthosis, adjustability (especially important in the initial period), potential for skin damage, ease of donning and doffing, cosmesis, durability, and cost.

Ankle-Foot-Orthoses
These are used for people who have enough quadriceps strength to stabilize their knee during stance but need the orthosis for control at

Table 30.3
Ambulation Options Following Complete SCI[a]

LOI	Therapeutic Options for Walking
C1–C8	- Functional walking is not feasible
T1–T9	- May walk for exercise only with forearm crutches or walker using bilateral KAFOs or HKAFOs; unlikely to walk functionally - A neuroprosthetic system that uses FES (Parastep) is available as an option (for those with T4–T12 complete SCI) but is cumbersome and has excessive energy requirements so is primarily useful for exercise only; other hybrid systems that combine FES with an HKAFO are also available - Powered exoskeletons may be a viable option that require lesser energy consumption, though their use is currently investigational
T10–L2	- May walk in the house and limited distances in the community using forearm crutches or walker in conjunction with bilateral KAFOs using swing-to or swing-through gait (or HKAFO may be used for those with T10–T12 LOI) - Powered exoskeletons may be a viable option for some, though their use is currently investigational
L3–L4	- Potential for community ambulation with AFOs (with plantar flexion stop or dorsiflexion assist to allow for toe clearance during swing) and assistive device: forearm crutches, or (for L3) walker, or (for L4) canes - A neuroprosthetic FES system that provides electric stimulation during the appropriate gait phase to counteract foot drop due to weak ankle dorsiflexors may be an option in some cases
L5–S1	- Community ambulation with standard canes and AFOs with dorsiflexion stop to prevent excess dorsiflexion during late stance (S1 may or may not need cane or AFO)
S2	- Community ambulation without any assistive device or orthosis

Abbreviations: AFO, ankle-foot-orthosis; FES, functional electrical stimulation; HKAFO, hip-knee-ankle-foot-orthosis; KAFO, knee-ankle-foot-orthosis; LOI, level of injury.
[a]For incomplete SCI, the options for walking will vary depending on the extent and distribution of muscle weakness.

their ankle. The control needed at the ankle depends on the available motor function.

- When dorsiflexors are weak, a dorsiflexion assist (or a posterior leaf-spring ankle-foot-orthosis [AFO]) will prevent excess plantar flexion during swing and prevent toe drag.
- With increased tone in the planter flexors, a plantar flexion stop should be used instead of a dorsiflexion assist since the latter may be over-powered by the spastic plantar flexors and may trigger spasticity by providing a rapid stretch to plantar flexors. A plantar flexion stop may, however, increase the flexion moment at the knee during early stance, increasing the demand on the quadriceps.
- Weakness in plantar flexors may require a dorsiflexion stop (e.g., limiting dorsiflexion to 10°) to prevent excess ankle dorsiflexion and the resulting knee flexion during stance.
- In addition to controlling ankle motion, an AFO can also be used to provide control at the knee. An AFO that limits dorsiflexion can help prevent knee flexion during stance (called a ground reaction AFO) and partly compensate for weak quadriceps. An AFO that limits plantar flexion has the opposite effect on the knee and can be used to limit genu recurvatum.

In case of a metal orthosis with a double-action ankle joint, dorsiflexion stop can be provided by pins in the anterior channel of the joint, plantar flexion stop by pins in the posterior channel of the joint, and a dorsiflexion assist by springs in the posterior channel. The pins can be adjusted to control the motion allowed. For plastic AFOs, ankle control can be provided either with an articulating ankle or is based on trim lines and materials of the AFO.

Knee-Ankle-Foot-Orthoses

Knee-ankle-foot-orthoses (KAFOs) are used when orthotic stabilization for walking is needed both at the knees and ankles. A Scott-Craig KAFO is a type of KAFO with metal uprights that is designed to provide stability at the ankle and foot, making it feasible to balance in standing without needing upper limb support. It has offset knee joints with a bail knee lock, adjustable ankle joint set at 5° to 10° of dorsiflexion, an extended foot plate that is embedded in the sole of the shoe, and a cushioned heel. KAFOs can be metal or thermoplastic. Advances in orthotic material have allowed fabrication of lighter KAFOs. Absence of significant lower limb contractures and good upper extremity strength are needed for walking with bilateral KAFO's. The high energy cost of walking with two KAFO's limits this as an option for long-distance ambulation, and a high rate of abandonment of its use.

Hip-Knee-Ankle-Foot-Orthosis

Hip-knee-ankle-foot-orthoses (HKAFOs) incorporate orthotic control at the hip in addition to the more caudal lower limb joints. An assistive device is needed for ambulation with HKAFOs. They are more difficult and cumbersome for transfers or curb/step negotiation and have high energy costs that make them unpractical for community ambulation for adults with SCI. A variant of the HKAFO is the hip guidance orthosis, also called the Parawalker, which has been used in children with spina bifida.

Reciprocating Gait Orthosis

A reciprocating gait orthosis (RGO) is a specialized type of HKAFO that allows reciprocal motion of the hips during ambulation through cables that link the two hip joints so that extension of one hip results in flexion of the other and a reciprocating gait is possible. A pelvic band with thoracic extensions provides trunk stability. All variants of the RGO are slow and have high energy costs, which limits their potential for long-term use.

Functional Electrical Stimulation and Hybrid Systems to Facilitate Gait

Lower limb electric stimulation, provided during the appropriate phase of gait, has been used to facilitate ambulation in people with SCI, either used alone or in a hybrid system in combination with orthoses.

Such systems may target just one movement, for example, electrical stimulation to counteract foot-drop in patients with ankle dorsiflexor weakness, or the system could be more complex. An example of the latter is the Parastep system which is a Food and Drug Administration approved neuroprosthetic system for people with T4 to T12 complete paraplegia. It uses electrical stimulation at multiple sites including the quadriceps, glutei, and peroneal nerves. Used in conjunction with a rolling walker that has finger-activated control switches, it allows independent standing and ambulation. However, the system is cumbersome and inefficient, and is more suitable for exercise than as a primary mode of ambulation.

When applying electrical current to contract muscles, large diameter (type II) muscle fibers, which are easily fatigable, are preferentially stimulated. This is in contrast to normal activation of motor units by the central nervous system, where the smaller fibers (type I) that are less prone to fatigue are stimulated first. Muscle fatigue is, therefore, a significant limiting factor of these FES systems. Other potential side effects and/or limitations of some of these systems include excessive energy expenditure, electrode failure, autonomic dysreflexia, spasticity, cumbersome electrical hardware, and the need for considerable preparatory training.

Locomotor Training for Restoration of Walking

LT, with a goal to restore walking by promoting plasticity in the central nervous system, has been gaining popularity in the past few years. The theory behind LT is that repetitive task-specific training has the potential to activate neural circuits (central pattern generator) in the spinal cord and enhance neural plasticity.

Various modes of providing LT include manual assisted body weight-supported treadmill training (BWSTT), robotic BWSTT, and LT in conjunction with FES. Guiding principles for LT that have been suggested include (1) maximize weight-bearing on the legs (and minimize or eliminate weight-bearing through the arms), (2) optimize sensory cues consistent with standing or walking, (3) promote postural control and optimize trunk, limb, and pelvic kinematics for walking and associated motor tasks, and (4) maximize recovery and use of normal movement patterns and minimize use of compensatory movement strategies.

The emerging evidence to support the concept behind such LT in humans, while promising, is currently not conclusive or universally accepted. Improved endurance, balance, and posture also contribute to the benefits of LT. Current evidence from randomized controlled trials has not demonstrated significant differences in walking outcomes between LT with BWSTT and conventional over-ground gait training. These trials do suggest, however, that early intensive weight bearing with repetitive standing and stepping, whether provided by BWSTT or by over-ground training, can improve functional outcomes related to walking in people with incomplete SCI.

KNOWLEDGE GAPS AND EMERGING CONCEPTS

Ongoing collaborative efforts between clinicians and engineers are needed to develop technologies for ambulation that are more effective, easier to use, and cost-effective.

Additional trials are needed to establish the effectiveness of LT, and to determine optimal parameters to deliver such training.

There have been exciting developments in the field of LT. A case study published by Harkema and others in 2011 demonstrated that epidural stimulation of the lumbosacral spinal cord distal to the site of SCI in an individual with motor complete tetraplegia, with ongoing LT and repetitive standing and stepping, was associated with improved standing and locomotion and some return of leg movements. These findings support the hypothesis that epidural stimulation might reactivate previously silent spared neural circuits or promote plasticity in the spinal cord. Further research is awaited in this regard.

SUGGESTED READING

Ditunno JF Jr, Ditunno PL, Graziani V, et al. Walking index for spinal cord injury (WISCI): an international multicenter validity and reliability study. *Spinal Cord.* 2000;38(4):234-243.

Dobkin B, Barbeau H, Deforge D, et al. The evolution of walking-related outcomes over the first 12 weeks of rehabilitation for incomplete traumatic spinal cord injury: the multicenter randomized Spinal Cord Injury Locomotor Trial. *Neurorehabil Neural Repair.* 2007;21(1):25-35.

Esquenazi A, Talaty M, Packel A, Saulino M. The ReWalk powered exoskeleton to restore ambulatory function to individuals with thoracic-level motor-complete spinal cord injury. *Am J Phys Med Rehabil.* 2012;91(11):911-921.

Giszter SF. Spinal cord injury: present and future therapeutic devices and prostheses. *Neurotherapeutics.* 2008;5(1):147-162.

Harkema S, Gerasimenko Y, Hodes J, et al. Effect of epidural stimulation of the lumbosacral spinal cord on voluntary movement, standing, and assisted stepping after motor complete paraplegia: a case study. *Lancet.* 2011;377(9781):1938-1947.

Harvey L, Wyndaele JJ. Are we jumping too early with locomotor training programs? *Spinal Cord.* 2011;49(9):947.

Hussey RW, Stauffer ES. Spinal cord injury: requirements for ambulation. *Arch Phys Med Rehabil.* 1973;54(12):544-547.

Morawietz C, Moffat F. Effects of locomotor training after incomplete spinal cord injury: a systematic review. *Arch Phys Med Rehabil.* 2013;pii:S0003-9993(13)00515.

Quintero HA, Farris RJ, Hartigan C, Clesson I, Goldfarb M. A powered lower limb orthosis for providing legged mobility in paraplegic individuals. *Top Spinal Cord Inj Rehabil.* 2011;17(1):25-33.

Sisto SA, Forrest GF, Faghri PD. Technology for mobility and quality of life in spinal cord injury. *IEEE Eng Med Biol Mag.* 2008;27(2):56-68.

Swinnen E, Duerinck S, Baeyens JP, Meeusen R, Kerckhofs E. Effectiveness of robot-assisted gait training in persons with spinal cord injury: a systematic review. *J Rehabil Med.* 2010;42(6):520-526.

V. Medical Consequences and Complications of SCI

CHAPTER 31

Medical Complications and Consequences of SCI: Overview

GENERAL PRINCIPLES

Spinal cord injury (SCI) can result in a multitude of secondary conditions and associated problems. All body systems can be affected. The chapters in this section cover each body system and related conditions.

CLINICAL CONSIDERATIONS

Presentation may be vague and nonspecific. Sensory and autonomic impairments can result in absent or atypical symptoms in people with SCI. For example, urinary tract infections may not manifest with classic symptoms of urgency and dysuria but with increased spasticity, increased frequency of spontaneous voiding, and lethargy. The patient with pneumonia may present with fever, shortness of breath, or with non-specific complaints of lethargy or increasing anxiety. Headache may be indicative of autonomic dysreflexia and may be the primary or only presentation of a variety of pathologic processes ranging from bladder distention, urinary infection, constipation, or ingrown toenail to myocardial infarction or acute abdominal emergencies.

Because symptoms can reflect a variety of underlying conditions, these need to be evaluated carefully. The differential diagnosis of common presenting systems is included in Table 31.1, illustrating the wide diversity of conditions that can have similar or overlapping presentation for people with SCI.

Table 31.1

Differential Diagnosis of Common Symptoms in SCI

Symptom	Possible Cause
Fever	Infectious Urinary tract infection Pneumonia Infected pressure ulcer, cellulitis, osteomyelitis Intra-abdominal or pelvic infection Hot environment (due to poikilothermia) Deep venous thrombosis Heterotopic ossification Pathologic limb fracture Drug fever (e.g., from antibiotics or anticonvulsant pain medications)
Fatigue	Nonspecific, but could be the only symptom of serious illness Infection Respiratory or cardiac failure Side effect of medications Depression (inquire about associated dysphoric symptoms)
Daytime drowsiness	Side effect of medications (e.g., narcotics, antispasticity agents) Nocturnal sleep apnea Ventilatory failure with carbon dioxide retention Depression
Shortness of breath	Pneumonia Abdominal distension (e.g., postprandial, obstipation) Pulmonary embolus Ventilatory impairment (can be postural with sitting up if borderline) Cardiac causes
Diarrhoea	Altered bowel management schedule *Clostridium difficile* infection Spurious diarrhoea with bowel impaction Side effect of medications (antibiotic, excess laxative or stool softener)
Rectal bleeding	Haemorrhoids Trauma from bowel care Colorectal cancer

(continued)

Symptom	Possible Cause
Haematuria	Urinary tract infection Urinary stones Traumatic bladder catheterization Bladder cancer
Headache	Autonomic dysreflexia; may be associated with any noxious stimulus below injury level Consider other causes in absence of increased blood pressure
Increased spasticity	Urine infection Pressure ulcer Bowel impaction Any noxious stimulus Syringomyelia
Shoulder pain	Rotator cuff/subacromial pain syndrome Tendinitis Cervical radiculopathy Posttraumatic syringomyelia Referred visceral pain in absence of abdominal discomfort
Unilateral leg swelling	Osteoporotic fracture of the lower extremity Deep venous thrombosis Heterotopic ossification Cellulitis Hematoma Invasive pelvic cancer
New weakness or numbness	Syringomyelia Entrapment neuropathy (median at wrist, ulnar at elbow)

SUGGESTED READING

Bauman WA, Korsten MA, Radulovic M, Schilero GJ, Wecht JM, Spungen AM. 31st g. Heiner sell lectureship: secondary medical consequences of spinal cord injury. *Top Spinal Cord Inj Rehabil*. 2012;18(4):354-378.

Burns S. Review of systems. In: Hammond MC, ed. *Medical Care of Persons with Spinal Cord Injury*. Washington, DC: Department of Veterans Affairs; 1998:17-22.

Gorman PH. The review of systems in spinal cord injury and dysfunction. *Continuum (Minneap Minn)*. 2011;17(3 Neurorehabilitation):630-634.

Hammond FM, Horn SD, Smout RJ, et al. Acute rehospitalizations during inpatient rehabilitation for spinal cord injury. *Arch Phys Med Rehabil*. 2013;94(4 suppl):S98-S105.

CHAPTER 32

Respiratory Issues in Spinal Cord Injury

Respiratory problems are a significant cause of morbidity, and the most common cause of death in people with spinal cord injury (SCI).

GENERAL PRINCIPLES

Anatomy and Physiology

Muscles involved in respiration include the diaphragm, abdominal muscles, intercostal, and accessory muscles (sternocleidomastoid, scalene, and trapezius).

Ventilation is primarily due to action of the diaphragm and secondarily due to cervical accessory muscles and the external intercostal muscles. Cough is primarily due to contraction of abdominal muscles, aided by internal intercostal muscles.

Innervation of respiratory muscles is as follows:

- Diaphragm: C3–C5, predominantly C4 (phrenic nerve)
- Intercostal: T1–T11 (intercostal nerves)
- Abdominals: T6–12
- Accessory muscles
  - Trapezius, sternocleidomastoid—Cranial nerve X1, C2–C4
  - Scalene: C4–C8

Pathophysiology of Respiratory Dysfunction after SCI (Tables 32.1 and 32.2)

Respiratory impairment after SCI includes: (a) impaired ventilation in those with paralysis of the diaphragm, (b) impaired cough due to expiratory muscle weakness—leading to retained secretions, mucus plugging, and pneumonia.

Table 32.1
Contributors to Respiratory Impairment After SCI

Hypoventilation due to diaphragm paralysis

Ineffective cough due to abdominal muscle paralysis

Paradoxical respiration due to intercostal paralysis

Inadequate expansion of alveoli due to respiratory muscle weakness leading to atelectasis

Loss of spontaneous sigh

Increased mucus secretion and airway hyperactivity due to parasympathetic predominance

Abdominal distension due to paralytic ileus

Associated chest wall or abdominal injury or surgery

Dysphagia and aspiration risk (e.g., with tracheostomy, restrictive cervical orthoses, anterior spinal surgery, vocal cord paralysis)

Abbreviation: SCI, spinal cord injury.

Table 32.2
Respiratory Complications in SCI

Pneumonia

Atelectasis and mucus plugs

Ventilatory failure

Sleep-disordered breathing

Pulmonary embolism

Neurogenic pulmonary edema

Abbreviation: SCI, spinal cord injury.

Paradoxical breathing (i.e., absence of chest wall expansion during inspiration due to intercostal muscle paralysis) adds to ventilatory impairment and lowered vital capacity.

Impaired sympathetic function and relative parasympathetic predominance contribute to increased bronchial mucus secretion and bronchoconstriction.

Vocal cord paralysis, tracheostomy, restrictive neck orthoses, and/or anterior cervical spinal surgery may result in impaired swallowing (primarily in the acute phase) that can lead to aspiration.

Abdominal distention due to paralytic ileus or associated chest or abdominal injuries can add to respiratory impairment in the acute stage.

There is a higher incidence of respiratory complications with older age, higher level of injury, and complete injuries.

Respiratory Impairment Correlation With Injury Level

At T12 and below: There is essentially no impairment.

T12 through T5: There is progressive loss of abdominals with impaired cough and forceful expiration. Also begin to lose intercostal (I/C) function.

T5 through T1: Remainder of I/C function lost with further impairment of respiratory effort.

C8 through C4: No I/C or abdominal function is present. There is dramatically impaired cough.

Loss of vital capacity is mainly due to lost expiratory reserve volume. Paradoxical respiration may be seen (upper chest caves in as abdomen expands). Vital capacity may double in 3 to 6 months as paradoxical respiration decreases with development of intercostal and abdominal spasticity.

C3 and above: Ventilatory failure results from diaphragm weakness. At C3 accessory muscles still largely functioning, and can generate tidal volumes of several hundred cc, but that is not sustained due to fatigue. Individuals with complete injury at or above the C2 level maybe apneic.

Preventive Care and Health Maintenance
Smoking cessation should be stressed. Annual influenza vaccination is recommended, and has been shown to produce an immunological response similar to the general population. Pneumococcal vaccination is recommended since *Streptococcus pneumoniae* is the most commonly identified pathogen of community-acquired pneumonia. Those who received the pneumococcal polysaccharide vaccine before age 65 years should receive another dose at 65 years or later, if at least 5 years have passed since their previous dose.

Effect of Position on Vital Capacity
Vital capacity in people with tetraplegia improves in the supine position. The diaphragm is pushed up by abdominal contents into a domed configuration in the chest (with improved length-tension relation). Loss of vital capacity in upright position can be partially corrected with an abdominal binder.

CLINICAL CONSIDERATIONS

Assessment

In the acute setting, patients with SCI should be carefully monitored for signs of respiratory infection.

Serial determination of vital capacity, oximetry, peak expiratory flow, and negative inspiratory force, especially in those with high tetraplegia, are helpful in monitoring patients for deterioration in the acute phase (chapter 32B).

Management

Intubation is indicated in the presence of intractable respiratory failure or with demonstrable or high risk of aspiration in the setting of respiratory compromise.

Management of ventilatory impairment is discussed in Chapter 32B. Increased ventilator tidal volumes may decrease occurrence of atelectasis as may the use of intermittent positive pressure breathing (IPPB), bi-level positive airway pressure, or continuous positive airway pressure. However, the evidence for this is not consistent in different studies.

Secretion Management
Secretion management is critical for prevention and treatment of respiratory complications in SCI (Tables 32.3 and 32.4).

Deep breathing and voluntary coughing are encouraged if the patient is able to perform those.

Suctioning may be performed through a tracheostomy or endotracheal tube. Angulation of the left main bronchus makes suctioning in that region more challenging, and directional catheters may be useful in such instances.

Assisted cough (or Quad cough) is helpful with postural drainage and to clear secretions, and may be used in association with insufflator treatment or with use of IPPB. Manually assisted coughing involves providing an upwardly directed thrust, delivered with an open palm, placed hands down just below the lower end of the sternum in coordination with expiratory efforts, and preceded by a deep breath by the patient, or delivered via a bag-valve mask or ventilator.

Table 32.3

Secretion Management and Preventive Measures in the Inpatient Setting

Aggressive assisted pulmonary toileting, chest clapping

Positioning, postural drainage, regular turning

Chest vibration with hand or mechanical device

IPPB with nebulized bronchodilator

Endotracheal suctioning

Adequate hydration

Mucolytic medications

Assisted cough

Insufflation-exsufflation treatment

Fiberoptic bronchoscopy

Incentive spirometry

Abbreviation: IPPB, intermittent positive pressure breathing.

Table 32.4

Ongoing Secretion Management and Preventive Measures

Smoking cessation

Influenza vaccine yearly, pneumococcal vaccine

Weight loss for obese

Prompt identification and treatment of complications

Respiratory muscle training

Assisted cough

Possible methods to improve cough effectiveness (e.g., strengthening of clavicular
    portion of pectoralis major, use of functional electrical stimulation)

Insufflation-exsufflation treatment is given through a machine that provides a deep breath followed by exhalation assist through alternately delivering positive and negative pressure through the airway. It has been documented to improve airflow and assist with clearance of mucus. The positive and negative pressures can be adjusted on the machine. Pressure is typically set at around 10 cm H_2O to begin with and increased to 40 cm H_2O of positive and negative pressure as tolerance improves. Insufflation with positive pressure is provided for around 3 seconds, followed by exsufflation with negative pressure for around 2 seconds, and repeated as needed. This treatment is contraindicated in the presence of pneumothorax, pneumomediastinum, or bullous emphysema.

Chest clapping, performed vigorously with a cupped hand, can be done in conjunction with positioning to aid in postural drainage. Some positions, such as head down position to aid in drainage of the lower lobes may not be well tolerated in the presence of respiratory impairment or gastro-esophageal reflux, but combination of positions to allow drainage of all lobes should be attempted.

Rotating beds can help with postural drainage in the acute setting.

Nebulized medications such as acetylcysteine or sodium bicarbonate in conjunction with adequate hydration may help loosen secretions.

Bronchoscopy may be needed to remove mucus and tenacious secretions in conjunction with other measures in resistant cases.

Practice Pearls

Positioning patients with tetraplegia in the supine or trendelenburg position improves ventilation. Use of abdominal binders is helpful in minimizing postural worsening and fall in vital capacity when patients first start sitting up.

KNOWLEDGE GAPS AND EMERGING CONCEPTS

Evidence of effectiveness for several measures for prevention and treatment of atelectasis is inconclusive.

Epidural electrical stimulation of the lower thoracic cord is being studied as a technique to generate cough with an effective peak expiratory pressure through activation of abdominal and internal intercostal muscles.

SUGGESTED READING

Biering-Sørensen F, Krassioukov A, Alexander MS, et al. International spinal cord injury pulmonary function basic data set. *Spinal Cord.* 2012;50(6):418-421.

Consortium for Spinal Cord Medicine. *Respiratory Management Following Spinal Cord Injury. Clinical Practice Guidelines for Health Care Professionals.* Washington, DC, Paralyzed Veterans of America; 2005.

Mueller G, Hopman MT, Perret C. Comparison of respiratory muscle training methods in individuals with motor complete tetraplegia. *Top Spinal Cord Inj Rehabil.* 2012;18(2): 118-121.

Reid WD, Brown JA, Konnyu KJ, Rurak JM, Sakakibara BM. Physiotherapy secretion removal techniques in people with spinal cord injury: a systematic review. *J Spinal Cord Med.* 2010;33(4):353-370.

Wong SL, Shem K, Crew J. Specialized respiratory management for acute cervical spinal cord injury: a retrospective analysis. *Top Spinal Cord Inj Rehabil.* 2012;18(4):283-290.

Pneumonia

GENERAL PRINCIPLES

Pneumonia is among the most common causes of hospitalization in people with tetraplegia, and the leading cause of death in this population.

The reported incidence of pneumonia depends on the population being studied. The incidence is higher in the first few weeks of the immediate postinjury period. People with tetraplegia are at a higher risk than those with lower levels of injury. As discussed in Chapter 32, factors contributing to risk of respiratory infections include respiratory muscle paralysis, ineffective cough with inability to clear bronchial secretions, and increased mucus production.

Use of high dose methylprednisolone for treatment of acute spinal cord injury (SCI) is associated with a higher incidence of respiratory infections in the acute phase.

Aspiration pneumonia may occur, especially in the presence of altered consciousness (e.g., due to associated brain injury or sedating medications) or with impaired swallowing.

Patients who require mechanical ventilation are susceptible to ventilator-associated pneumonia (see Chapter 32B). The presence of tracheostomy or endotracheal tube may increase risk of infection with methicillin-resistant *Staphylococcus aureus* (MRSA) or *Pseudomonas aeruginosa*.

Community acquired pneumonia (CAP) is most often caused by *Streptococcus pneumonia* in people with SCI, as it is in the general population. Other pathogens include *Haemophilus influenzae*, and a significant proportion with pseudomonas infections (which is an uncommon pathogen for CAP in the general population).

CLINICAL CONSIDERATIONS

Assessment

History and Examination
Presentation may be subtle; for example the initial manifestation may only be an increased respiratory rate (Table 32A.1). Patients may not experience dyspnea

Table 32A.1

Challenges in Diagnosing Respiratory Infections in People With SCI
Patients with tetraplegia may have absent or altered sensations of dyspnea or chest pain
Purulent secretions may not be obvious because of inadequate cough
May be confused with other causes of shortness of breath in these patients (Table 32A.2)
Chest examination may be inadequate due to difficulty in positioning
Adequate sputum sample for culture may be difficult to obtain in presence of ineffective cough

Abbreviation: SCI, spinal cord injury.

or chest discomfort. On the other hand, disease presentation and course of pneumonia in people with SCI can be fulminant because of inability to clear the increased secretions associated with the respiratory infection and/or due to worsening of borderline ventilation.

Symptoms of pneumonia may include shortness of breath, rising temperature, increased anxiety or increased volume, and tenacity of secretions.

On examination patients may be febrile, with increased respiratory rate, increased pulse rate, decreased breath sounds, and rhonchi and/or crackles on chest auscultation.

It is important to do a thorough chest examination including careful auscultation of the left lower lobe, which is a common site for pneumonia and atelectasis. Shortchanging the examination due to difficulty in positioning the patient or failing to roll or sit them up to complete the examination can result in missing the diagnosis.

Differential diagnosis: While pneumonia and atelectasis are common causes of shortness of breath in this population, other causes should also be considered in evaluating dyspnea and/or a fall in oxygen saturation in people with SCI (Table 32A.2). These include:

- Mucus plugging
- Abdominal distension (e.g., obstipation, paralytic ileus)
- Pulmonary embolus
- Ventilatory impairment
- Cardiac causes

Diagnostic Tests
Chest radiographs should be performed to look for infiltrates, and to distinguish pneumonia from acute bronchitis. However these may be inadequate if

Table 32A.2

Differential Diagnosis of Shortness of Breath in SCI

Pneumonia

Mucus plugging

Atelectasis

Abdominal distension (e.g., obstipation, paralytic ileus)

Pulmonary embolus

Ventilatory impairment

Tracheal stenosis

Cardiac causes

Abbreviation: SCI, spinal cord injury.

only done in the supine position. If unable to obtain adequate plain films, computed tomography scan or magnetic resonance imaging should be considered.

Laboratory testing includes complete blood count with differential, serum chemistry panel, and blood cultures. Sputum gram stain and culture (and blood cultures as needed) should be obtained prior to starting antibiotics whenever feasible. Patients may need respiratory assistance in order to produce an adequate sample because of ineffective cough.

Pulse oximetry is monitored. Serial determination of vital capacity, peak expiratory flow, and negative inspiratory force, especially in those with high tetraplegia in the acute phase, are helpful in monitoring patients for deterioration.

Management

Antibiotics
Given the potential for a fulminant course, antibiotic treatment should be expeditiously initiated once cultures are obtained. Given the high case fatality, increased possibility of resistant organisms, and potential for inadequate clearance of secretions, hospitalization is usually indicated.

Initial empiric antibiotic treatment is chosen based on knowledge of likely organisms and subsequently adjusted based on results of culture and antibiotic sensitivity. A quinolone or combination of a cephalosporin and a macrolide may be initiated for community-acquired pneumonia. Hospital-acquired aspiration pneumonia warrants antibiotic coverage for anaerobes and gram-negative organisms. Patients with respiratory devices should be empirically covered for MRSA and pseudomonas pending culture results. Antibiotic treatment for pneumonia is typically continued for 10 to 14 days. The management of ventilator-associated pneumonia is also discussed in Chapter 32B.

Secretion management is a crucial component of treatment (Chapter 32 and Table 32.3).

Patient Education

Educating patients and caregivers about early recognition and treatment of respiratory infections is a key aspect of management. As discussed in Chapter 32, key prevention measures include smoking cessation, pneumococcal and yearly influenza vaccination, and measures to ensure adequate clearance of respiratory secretions (Table 32.4).

Practice Pearls

Nonspecific malaise, tachypnea, or tachycardia may be the only clues to the presence of pneumonia in patients with tetraplegia. Given the frequency of this complication, a low threshold for suspicion is warranted.

SUGGESTED READING

Burns SP. Acute respiratory infections in persons with spinal cord injury. *Phys Med Rehabil Clin N Am.* May 2007;18(2):203-216.

Consortium for Spinal Cord Medicine. *Respiratory Management Following Spinal Cord Injury. Clinical Practice Guidelines for Health Care Professionals.* Washington, DC: Paralyzed Veterans of America; 2005.

Evans CT, Weaver FM, Rogers TJ, et al. Guideline-recommended management of community-acquired pneumonia in veterans with spinal cord injury. *Top Spinal Cord Inj Rehabil.* 2012;18(4):300-305.

Ventilatory Impairment

GENERAL PRINCIPLES

Etiology

Patients with injuries at or above C3, and some with lesions at C4 and below with associated pulmonary or traumatic brain injuries require assisted ventilation.

Epidemiology/Pathophysiology

Many people with spinal cord injury (SCI) can be weaned from ventilator as diaphragm function improves, others need lifelong mechanical ventilation.

Late onset ventilatory failure may occur in people with tetraplegia who were previously ventilator-free. Contributing factors may include: age-related decrease in chest wall and lung compliance, decreased number of alveoli, and decreased vital capacity that may decompensate borderline ventilators; progressive spinal deformity with thoracic kyphoscoliosis; excess weight gain and obesity; or neurological deterioration due to progressive posttraumatic syringomyelia.

CLINICAL CONSIDERATIONS

Assessment

Clues to impaired ventilation (Table 32B.1) may include shortness of breath, impaired or fluctuating mental alertness, daytime drowsiness, sleep dysfunction, morning headaches, irritability or anxiety, tachypnea, increased respiratory effort, increased postural influences on breathing, or unexplained erythrocytosis.

Indications for mechanical ventilation (Table 32B.2) include apnea, signs of respiratory distress (accessory muscle use, tachypnea, tachycardia, cyanosis, altered mental status), respiratory failure (defined as PaO_2 less than 50 mmHg, or $PaCO_2$ over 50 by arterial blood gas testing while on room air), severe hypoxemia that is unresponsive to oxygen administration, forced vital capacity less than 10 mL/kg or 25% predicted, or intractable and worsening atelectasis.

Table 32B.1

Symptoms and Signs of Impaired Ventilation
Shortness of breath
Impaired or fluctuating mental alertness
Daytime drowsiness, sleep dysfunction
Irritability, anxiety
Tachypnea
Increased respiratory effort
Increased postural influences on breathing
Unexplained erythrocytosis

Table 32B.2

Indications for Mechanical Ventilation in SCI
Apnea
Signs of respiratory distress, i.e., accessory muscle use, tachypnea, tachycardia, cyanosis, altered mental status)
Respiratory failure—defined as PaO_2 less than 50 mmHg, or $PaCO_2$ over 50 by arterial blood gas testing while on room air
Severe hypoxemia that is unresponsive to oxygen administration
Forced vital capacity less than 10 mL/kg or 25% predicted
Intractable and worsening atelectasis

Abbreviation: SCI, spinal cord injury.

Management

Intubation and positive pressure ventilation are indicated for acute respiratory failure.

Aspiration risk is reduced with head-up position at a 45 degree angle if it can be tolerated.

Tracheostomy is typically performed within a few days of intubation unless extubation is anticipated to be imminent. Some centers report successful use of noninvasive methods to avoid tracheostomies.

Tracheostomy Care and Complications

Scrupulous tracheostomy care and vigilance for signs of tracheostomy or endotracheal tube related problems is important (Table 32B.3). Use of proper sized tubes and avoidance of excess cuff pressures are important preventive measures. Tracheal stenosis may present with exertional dyspnea, stridor, acute respiratory distress, difficulty clearing secretions, cough, or aphonia.

Table 32B.3

Complications of Tracheostomy
Stoma infection
Tracheal stenosis, granuloma
Tracheomalacia
Tracheitis
Tracheo-esophageal fistula
Hemorrhage
Aspiration
Swallowing dysfunction
Obstruction with secretions

Imaging and laryngoscopy are indicated to confirm the diagnosis, and surgical intervention is often needed.

Secretion Management
Ongoing respiratory care including positioning, chest percussion, and secretion management is essential. Patients should be on scheduled respiratory treatments, typically in conjunction with administration of inhaled bronchodilators. Chapter 32 includes further discussion on various interventions for secretion management.

Ventilator Set-Up and Management
Suggested protocols for ventilator set-up and management have been published by the Consortium for Spinal Cord Medicine *(Respiratory Management Following Spinal Cord Injury, 2005).*

Vital capacity, negative inspiratory pressure, and arterial blood gases are monitored to ensure that ventilation is adequate.

Ventilator settings in people with SCI remain controversial with lack of uniform agreement about the optimal tidal volume. Some centers advocate higher tidal volumes on the basis of experience with reduced atelectasis and increased success in weaning. Some studies have found significantly increased mortality and complications with high compared to low tidal volumes, but these did not include patients with neuromuscular disease such as SCI. Several SCI Centers follow a protocol of gradually increasing tidal volume by 50–100 mL/day with a goal of reaching 15–20 mL/kg.

Ventilation is initiated in the supine position; as mentioned in Chapter 32, vital capacity increases in this position in people with tetraplegia. If not anticipated to be rapidly weaned off the ventilator, patients are often switched to a portable ventilator based on medical status and ability to tolerate upright position, which allows fuller participation in rehabilitation. An abdominal binder is helpful in maintaining vital capacity when patients start sitting up.

Assessment and Management of Ventilator-Associated Pneumonia (VAP)
Diagnosis of VAP can be challenging due to non-specific signs and symptoms, especially in the acute setting. Often applied clinical criteria for diagnosis of VAP are the presence of a new infiltrate on chest radiography, plus at least two of the following: fever greater than 38°C, leukocytosis or leukopenia, and purulent secretions. Cultures of respiratory secretions may be helpful. Blood cultures should also be performed before starting antibiotics, if feasible, though are often negative. Prompt initiation of antibiotics is the cornerstone of treatment. Initial therapy should be broad (including coverage for methicillin-resistant *Staphylococcus aureus* (MRSA) and *Pseudomonas aeruginosa*), and modified as appropriate when culture results are available.

Addressing Communication During Mechanical Ventilation (Table 32B.4)
It is important to address communication during mechanical ventilation. Table 32B.4 lists mechanisms that patients may use to communicate while ventilated. Vocalization can be immensely helpful from a communication, as well as psychological, viewpoint. Inspired tidal volume can be increased as needed to compensate for loss of tidal volume that occurs with cuff deflation or use of a fenestrated tube. Minor ventilator adjustments such as decreased inspiratory flow rate and addition of positive end-expiratory pressure may significantly improve speech quality and volume.

Glossopharyngeal Breathing
Glossopharyngeal breathing ("frog-breathing") is a helpful skill to teach patients who require assisted ventilation. It can provide periods of ventilator free time, and also serve as an emergency back-up. The technique involves use of oropharyngeal muscle forcing air into lungs with 10 to 14 gulping maneuvers per breath, followed by passive exhalation.

Ventilator Weaning
Parameters for readiness to wean and those to discontinue weaning are listed in Tables 32B.5 and 32B.6.

Table 32B.4

Communication During Mechanical Ventilation
Lip speaking/mouthing, eye blinks, tongue clicks
Communication board
Passey Muir valve
Cuff deflation (or uncuffed tube)
Cuffed fenestrated tubes, talking trach
Electrolarynx

Table 32B.5
Criteria for Ventilator Weaning in SCI[a]

Patient agrees and is willing to participate in the procedure

Afebrile with stable vital signs for more than 24 hrs

Chest x-ray is clear or improving

Secretions are manageable

Vital capacity at least 10–15 mL/kg ideal body weight

PaO_2 >75 mmHg, PCO_2 35–45, pH 7.35–7.45

Abbreviation: SCI, spinal cord injury.
[a]The figures in the table are approximate and protocols may vary between centers.

Table 32B.6
Criteria for Discontinuing Weaning Trial[a]

Drop in vital capacity by 25%

Respiratory rate over 25–30/min or increased over 10/min from baseline

O_2 saturation less than 95% despite increase in FIO_2

Heart rate increased by 20 from baseline

Blood pressure change (increase or decrease) of more than 30 mmHg from baseline

Vital capacity decrease by more than 25% from baseline

PaO_2 >75 mmHg, PCO_2 35–45, pH 7.35–7.45

Fever with temperature over 101°F

Marked increase in spasms, sweating, or change in mental status

Unresolved panic, or marked increase in complaints of shortness of breath

[a]The figures in the table are approximate and protocols may vary between centers.

Ventilator weaning is often a high anxiety experience, and it is critical to explain the procedure thoroughly to patients.

Both progressive ventilator-free breathing (PVFB) using a t-piece and synchronized intermittent mandatory ventilation have been used as weaning techniques. Many centers report greater success and preference for the former method. PVFB may begin with as little as 2 minutes off the ventilator three times a day, with weaning time progressively increased at 1 to 3 day intervals based on tolerance and patient cooperation.

Alternatives for Long-Term Assisted Ventilation
In addition to mechanical ventilation, there are noninvasive options for long-term assisted ventilation that may be appropriate for some patients. These include diaphragm and phrenic nerve pacing, use of pneumobelt, and positive pressure ventilation delivered through the nose or mouth.

Phrenic nerve and diaphragm pacing: This allows freedom from ventilator in selected patients. It requires viability of phrenic nerves and healthy lungs, and is an option when injury is above the anterior horn cells of C3 to C5 that constitute the phrenic nerve nucleus. Evaluation includes phrenic nerve conduction studies and fluoroscopy of diaphragm.

Phrenic nerve pacing involves electric stimulation of the phrenic nerve via surgically implanted cuff electrodes, which contracts the diaphragm. These are connected to a radiofrequency receiver which is implanted subcutaneously on the anterior chest wall. An external battery-powered transmitter sends signals to the device by an antenna which is worn over the receiver. Equipment failure (e.g., receiver deterioration) is a potential problem, as is infection or phrenic nerve injury, though these are becoming less common. Diaphragm pacing involves direct placement of electrodes into the diaphragm, which can be performed with laparoscopy. Many patients continue to have tracheostomies and back-up ventilators.

Several weeks of diaphragm reconditioning is typically required in the postoperative period before ventilator can be discontinued.

Pneumobelt: This is rarely used at present but remains a potential option. It consists of an air bladder in a corset form that is connected to a ventilator. In this form of intermittent abdominal pressure ventilation active exhalation occurs in the inflation phase, and passive inhalation occurs with deflation. It is only effective when the individual is reclined to no more than 50 to 60 degrees from vertical.

Noninvasive positive pressure ventilation (NIPPV) through the nose or mouth: Effective use of this technique of noninvasive ventilation has been demonstrated with considerable success in a few centers, though the expertise and experience for consistently using it is not widespread. NIPPV is discussed further in Chapter 25 under the respiratory management of Amyotrophic Lateral Sclerosis.

Follow-Up
Periodic surveillance of lung function should be done especially in those at high risk (high tetraplegia, ventilator dependency, phrenic pacers, concomitant chronic obstructive airway disease).

Studies suggest a higher than predicted quality of life and life-satisfaction reported by individuals with SCI living with long-term assisted ventilation. Appropriate technology, electronic aids, and availability of social support and resources for participation are all important contributing factors.

Patient/Caregiver Education
For patients who are discharged home on ventilators for long-term use, ensuring that caregivers have the needed education, skills, and support is critical (Table 32B.7).

Table 32B.7

Caregiver Skills and Patient/Caregiver Education for Long-Term Mechanical Ventilation

Airway management—Tracheal/stoma care, suctioning, changing the tracheostomy tube

Assisted cough, medication/inhalation therapy administration, safe swallow techniques

Cardio-pulmonary resuscitation

Infection control, safety practices

Early recognition and treatment of infections

Knowledge of health care and community resources

Equipment maintenance

Emergency measures—ventilator failure, power failure, equipment malfunction, hazards, alarms, dislodged tracheostomy tube

Should have a back-up ventilator

KNOWLEDGE GAPS AND EMERGING CONCEPTS

Additional studies are needed to establish optimal tidal volumes for patients with SCI who require mechanical ventilation.

More widespread evaluation of techniques for noninvasive ventilation would be helpful to facilitate broader adoption of these practices.

Newer techniques of diaphragm pacing are becoming less invasive.

SUGGESTED READING

Bach JR. Noninvasive respiratory management of high level spinal cord injury. *J Spinal Cord Med.* 2012;35(2):72-80.

Bach JR, Tilton MC. Life satisfaction and well-being measures in ventilator assisted individuals with traumatic tetraplegia. *Arch Phys Med Rehabil.* 1994;75(6):626-632.

Consortium for Spinal Cord Medicine. *Respiratory Management Following Spinal Cord Injury. Clinical Practice Guidelines for Health Care Professionals.* Washington, DC: Paralyzed Veterans of America; 2005.

Hoit JD, Banzett RB, Lohmeier HL, Hixon TJ, Brown R. Clinical ventilator adjustments that improve speech. *Chest.* 2003;124(4):1512-1521.

Shavelle RM, DeVivo MJ, Strauss DJ, Paculdo DR, Lammertse DP, Day SM. Long-term survival of persons ventilator dependent after spinal cord injury. *J Spinal Cord Med.* 2006;29(5):511-519.

Sleep-Disordered Breathing

GENERAL PRINCIPLES

Sleep disordered breathing involves an abnormal frequency of periods during sleep with cessation (apnea) or reduction (hypopnea) of airflow lasting for 10 or more seconds.

The apnea-hypopnea index (AHI), which is calculated by dividing the number of events by the numbers of hours of sleep, is an index of sleep apnea severity. AHI values are 5 to 15/hr in milder forms and over 30/hr in severe cases.

Etiology

Sleep apnea may be obstructive (associated with upper airway collapse), central (due to reduced respiratory effort, for example, with syringobulbia or associated injury to the brainstem), or mixed.

Patients with spinal cord injury (SCI) spend more time sleeping in the supine position than able-bodied individuals, which may also be a contributing factor to obstructive sleep apnea (OSA).

Epidemiology

OSA is more common in people with tetraplegia than with lower levels of injury or the general population. High prevalence of sleep apnea, over 50% in some studies, has been reported in chronic tetraplegia.

Risk factors for OSA in people with SCI include high neurological level, obesity, increased neck circumference, and possibly baclofen and/or diazepam use.

Complications

In addition to problems associated with disturbed sleep and daytime drowsiness, sleep apnea has been associated with increased cardiovascular mortality and morbidity including stroke, hypertension, and heart disease.

CLINICAL CONSIDERATIONS

Assessment

History and Physical Examination
Patients may present with excessive daytime drowsiness, cognitive dysfunction (attention-concentration), loud snoring, or observed apnea episodes by partner or caregivers during sleep.

Examination may reveal large neck, obesity, or retrognathia, but is often unremarkable.

Diagnostic Testing
Nocturnal pulse oximetry can be of some but limited value. It may detect nocturnal arterial desaturation.

Polysomnography (sleep study) is typically needed for diagnosis and helps to establish severity. It is commonly performed in a sleep lab but can also be performed at home.

Management

Positive airway pressure therapy is indicated for significant sleep disordered breathing. Continuous positive airway pressure (CPAP) or bi-level positive airway pressure (BiPAP) is administered through nasal or oropharyngeal mask. Side effects include nasal congestion, skin irritation, and inability to tolerate or discomfort with the mask (though this often improves with time). Custom-fit oral appliances to adjust lower jaw and tongue position during sleep may help in some instances

Weight reduction for obese or overweight individuals may be helpful.

Avoidance of alcohol and sedating medications should be considered. Smoking cessation is recommended.

Surgical procedures may be considered for those who don't respond to conservative measures although experience or literature in those with SCI is sparse. These include uvulopalatopharyngoplasty, palatal implants, tracheostomy, and, especially in children or adolescents, removal of enlarged tonsils and adenoids.

Practice Pearls

In addition to sleep apnea, there are several common causes of sleep dysfunction in people with SCI including sedating medications, sleep disruption due to nursing care, or depression.

However, OSA should be considered in the differential diagnosis of people with tetraplegia who present with disturbed sleep or daytime somnolence.

KNOWLEDGE GAPS AND EMERGING CONCEPTS

OSA is being increasingly recognized as an issue in people with tetraplegia, but precise incidence and risk factors needs to be established.

Additional studies are needed to determine the relationship between medications used for spasticity and OSA.

SUGGESTED READING

Biering-Sørensen F, Jennum P, Laub M. Sleep disordered breathing following spinal cord injury. *Respir Physiol Neurobiol.* 2009;169(2):165-170.
Fuller DD, Lee KZ, Tester NJ. The impact of spinal cord injury on breathing during sleep. *Respir Physiol Neurobiol.* 2013 Sep 15;188(3):344-354.
LaVela SL, Burns SP, Goldstein B, Miskevics S, Smith B, Weaver FM. Dysfunctional sleep in persons with spinal cord injuries and disorders. *Spinal Cord.* 2012;50(9):682-685.

CHAPTER 33

Cardiovascular and Autonomic Consequences: Overview

GENERAL PRINCIPLES

Cardiovascular and autonomic function is altered in individuals with spinal cord injury (SCI). Cardiovascular and autonomic dysfunction is an important cause of morbidity and mortality in SCI.

Pathophysiology

Autonomic innervation of major organs of the body is summarized in Table 33.1. As discussed in Chapter 1, descending autonomic pathways from the brain travel in the spinal cord and terminate on the preganglionic sympathetic neurons in the spinal cord that are located at T1 to L2. Preganglionic parasympathetic neurons to the bladder, reproductive organs, and the lower part of the gut are located at S2 to S4; the rest of the parasympathetic innervation to thoracic and abdominal viscera is via the vagus nerve (cranial nerve X).

Impairment of autonomic function after SCI is a major contributory factor to cardiovascular impairments. In cervical and high thoracic injuries in particular, interruption to the sympathetic outflow plays a key role in cardiovascular dysfunction.

Loss of supraspinal regulatory control of the sympathetic nervous system results in reduced overall sympathetic activity below the level of injury and causes problems such as hypotension, bradycardia, and a blunted cardiovascular response to exercise.

Morphologic changes occur in sympathetic preganglionic neurons distal to the injury. Peripheral alpha-adrenergic hyper-responsiveness may occur, and probably contributes to the excessive pressor response seen in autonomic dysreflexia.

In addition to autonomic abnormalities, there are indirect effects of reduced physical activity, altered metabolic function, and other SCI-related conditions on cardiovascular function.

Table 33.1
Autonomic Innervation of Major Organs

Organ	Sympathetic Innervation	Parasympathetic Innervation
Heart	T1-T5	Vagus (CN X)
Blood vessels	T1-L2	None (exceptions include genital erectile tissue via S2-S4)
Sweat glands	T1-L2	None
Broncho-pulmonary system	T1-T5	Vagus (CN X)
Lower urinary tract	T10-L2	S2-S4
Gastro-intestinal	T1-L2	Vagus (CN X) to splenic flexure, S2-S4 from splenic flexure to anal sphincter
Genitalia and reproductive organs	T10-L2	S2-S4

Abbreviation: CN, cranial nerve.

CLINICAL CONSIDERATIONS

Cardiovascular concerns in SCI occur throughout the care continuum, and are important causes of morbidity and mortality. Major issues are summarized in Table 33.2 below and discussed in further detail in the subsequent sections.

Non-cardiovascular effects of autonomic impairment include bladder, bowel, and sexual dysfunction, and impaired thermoregulation and sweating. These are discussed in Chapters 34A, 36A, 35, and 33F respectively.

Table 33.2
Cardiovascular Issues in SCI

Hypotension (Chapter 33B)

  Low baseline blood pressure

  Orthostatic hypotension

Bradycardia, arrhythmias, cardiac arrest (Chapter 33A)

Autonomic dysreflexia (Chapter 33C)

Reduced cardiovascular fitness and altered exercise capacity (Chapter 43)

Influence on coronary and peripheral artery disease (Chapters 33D and 33E)

  Impact on risk factors

  Silent ischemia, atypical presentations

  Special diagnostic and treatment considerations

Venous thromboembolism (Chapter 8)

Cardiovascular effects of medications in SCI

SUGGESTED READING

American Spinal Injury Association. International standards to document remaining autonomic function after spinal cord injury (ISAFSCI). 2012; Atlanta, GA.

Dhall SS, Hadley MN, Aarabi B, et al. Deep venous thrombosis and thromboembolism in patients with cervical spinal cord injuries. *Neurosurgery.* 2013;72(suppl 2):244-254.

Furlan JC, Fehlings MG. Cardiovascular complications after acute spinal cord injury: pathophysiology, diagnosis, and management. *Neurosurg Focus.* 2008;25(5):E13.

Sabharwal S. Cardiovascular dysfunction in spinal cord disorders. In: Lin V, ed. *Spinal Cord Medicine.* 2nd ed. New York, NY: Demos Publishing; 2010:241-255.

Teasell RW, Arnold MO, Krassioukov A, et al. Cardiovascular consequences of loss of supraspinal control of the sympathetic nervous system after spinal cord injury. *Arch Phys Med Rehabil.* 2000;81(4):506-516.

Teasell RW, Hsieh JT, Aubut JA, Eng JJ, Krassioukov A, Tu L. Venous thromboembolism after spinal cord injury. *Arch Phys Med Rehabil.* 2009;90(2):232-245.

Bradycardia

GENERAL PRINCIPLES

Etiology and Epidemiology

Bradycardia is a particular problem with cervical injuries in the acute stage and may even be life threatening. In patients with complete cervical spinal cord injury (SCI), it occurs almost universally at some point in the initial acute phase. Typically, the severity of bradycardia is directly related to the level and completeness of injury.

The frequency and severity of bradycardia is highest within a 3 to 5 day period following cervical SCI, but it usually resolves after the first 2 to 6 weeks after injury, and rarely lasts beyond 2 months.

While sinus bradycardia is the most common cardiac rhythm problem in the acute stage, other cardiac rhythm abnormalities have also been reported including atrio-ventricular blocks and cardiac arrest.

Pathophysiology

Bradycardia after SCI results from disruption of the sympathetic pathways leading to imbalance in the autonomic nervous system with a decrease in sympathetic activity and a relative predominance of parasympathetic activity.

Other factors can also influence the occurrence of bradycardia and cardiovascular instability in people with tetraplegia. The tracheal stimulation that occurs during suctioning or bronchial toilet can precipitate reflex bradycardia and even cardiac arrest in recently injured patients by increasing the unopposed vagal stimulation. Hypoxia stimulates a vagal response through carotid body chemoreceptor activation, and the normally counter-acting sympathetic response is impaired in SCI.

CLINICAL CONSIDERATIONS

Assessment

Mild bradycardia is often asymptomatic. With heart rate below 40 to 50 beats per minute, patients may experience fatigue or dizziness. In more severe

255

cases, syncope may occur. Onset of severe bradycardia and even asystole may sometimes occur without preceding warning symptoms.

Management

Preventive management consists of ensuring adequate oxygenation, prompt treatment of factors such as respiratory infections that can contribute to hypoxia, and the administration of atropine about 10 minutes prior to tracheal suction, if needed.

Pharmacological management of symptomatic bradycardia includes atropine 0.4 to 0.6 mg administered intravenously. This is typically the first-line treatment for symptomatic bradycardia in this setting. It should be kept readily available at the bedside in those at high risk in the early days after injury.

Inotropes and aminophylline have also been used with reported benefit. Continuous infusion of dopamine at a rate of 2 to 10 mcg/kg/min or epinephrine 0.01 to 0.1 mcg/kg/min have also been used in the acute setting. Aminophylline has been used effectively for management of refractory bradycardia when other agents have failed, given as an initial loading dose of 200 to 300 mg followed by a maintenance dose of 100 mg three times a day for 8 to 12 weeks.

Temporary cardiac pacemakers may be needed in patients with severe recurrent episodes. The indication for a pacemaker is usually severe bradycardia leading to an asystolic cardiac arrest or severe recurrent episodes. There have been reports of permanent pacemaker placement but those are usually not needed, since it is typically a time-limited problem.

KNOWLEDGE GAPS AND EMERGING CONCEPTS

Evidence based literature on the management of bradycardia following SCI is relatively sparse. The role and indications for permanent pacemaker implantation in people with severe SCI-related bradycardia is not clear.

SUGGESTED READING

Franga DL, Hawkins ML, Medeiros RS, Adewumi D. Recurrent asystole resulting from high cervical spinal cord injuries. *Am Surg.* 2006;72(6):525-529.

McMahon D, Tutt M, Cook AM. Pharmacological management of hemodynamic complications following spinal cord injury. *Orthopedics.* 2009;32(5):331.

Moerman JR, Christie B III, Sykes LN, Vogel RL, Nolan TL, Ashley DW. Early cardiac pacemaker placement for life-threatening bradycardia in traumatic spinal cord injury. *J Trauma.* 2011;70(6):1485-1488.

Orthostatic Hypotension

GENERAL PRINCIPLES

Orthostatic hypotension (OH) has been arbitrarily defined as a reduction in systolic blood pressure of at least 20 mmHg or a reduction in diastolic blood pressure of at least 10 mmHg during the first 3 minutes of assuming the upright position or a head-up tilt on a tilt table. However, a smaller drop in blood pressure may be equally important when associated with relevant symptoms that indicate impaired perfusion. Some have defined OH simply as a symptomatic fall in blood pressure in the upright posture.

OH following spinal cord injury (SCI) is common and well documented.

Etiology

The prevalence of OH as well as the degree of fall in blood pressure are higher with cervical than with thoracic SCI. Low plasma volume, hyponatremia, and cardiovascular deconditioning may be additional contributing factors in some instances.

Epidemiology

OH has been reported to be more common after traumatic than nontraumatic SCI. Prevalence in acute SCI has been reported to be as high as 74% though it depends on the population being studied. Symptoms are less likely to occur in SCI below the origin of the major splanchnic outflow at T6 and with incomplete injuries.

Pathophysiology

The major underlying abnormality in SCI related OH is a lack of sympathetically mediated reflex vasoconstriction, especially in large vascular beds, such as those supplying the splanchnic region and skeletal muscle. The gravitational effect of venous pooling in the lower extremities is accompanied by a lack of compensatory changes in other vascular beds, leading to the fall in blood pressure. Venous pooling results in reduced filling pressure at the heart, and decrease in the end-diastolic filling volume and stroke volume. Tachycardia may occur due to reflex vagal inhibition, but is not sufficient to compensate for the reduced sympathetic response.

Course and Natural History

OH following SCI often, but not always, improves over time. Compensatory changes in other vascular beds may contribute to blood pressure homeostasis. Reduced blood flow to the kidneys may activate afferent glomerular dilatation and result in the stimulation of the renin-angiotensin aldosterone system. Other potential mechanisms for improvement over time include vascular wall receptor hypersenstivity, some recovery of postural reflexes at the spinal level, and increased skeletal muscle tone. Tolerance to symptoms of OH often develops over time even with continued evidence of postural reduction in blood pressure in the upright position. It has been suggested that autoregulation of cerebral blood flow, rather than systemic blood pressure, may play a dominant role in the adaptation to OH.

Precipitating Factors

Postural hypotension may be influenced by several factors, many of which are reversible. These include rapid changes in position and prolonged recumbency. Hypotension may be worse in the morning on rising. Heavy meals may exacerbate fall in blood pressure in response to shunting of blood to the splanchnic circulation after a meal. Physical exertion, alcohol intake, or a hot environment can precipitate hypotension by promoting vasodilatation. Sepsis and dehydration can worsen symptoms. Several medications can induce or worsen postural hypotension. Common among these are tricyclic antidepressants, antihypertensives, diuretics, and narcotic analgesics. Deconditioning after prolonged bed-rest exacerbates OH. The late development or worsening of OH months or years after injury may be a sign of posttraumatic syringomyelia (Table 33B.1).

CLINICAL CONSIDERATIONS

Assessment

History
Many of the key manifestations of OH occur as a result of cerebral hypoperfusion. These include dizziness, light-headedness, loss of consciousness, impaired concentration, and visual disturbances such as blurred vision, scotoma, tunnel vision, graying out, and color defects. Pallor or auditory deficits may also occur. Sometimes symptoms may only be nonspecific, for example generalized weakness, lethargy, or nausea. "Coat hanger" headache may be a manifestation of hypoperfusion of continuously active postural muscles of the neck and shoulder. Excess sweating may occur above the level of injury.

OH may hinder functional assessment and participation in rehabilitation therapies due to occurrence of symptoms with sitting up or standing.

Table 33B.1

Reversible Factors Exacerbating Symptomatic Postural Hypotension in SCI
Prolonged recumbency
Rapid position change
Heavy meals
Physical exertion
Hot environment
Dehydration (diarrhea, viral illness)
Sepsis
Medications: Diuretics, antidepressants, alpha blockers, narcotics

The presence of precipitating factors mentioned above that could be causing or worsening OH should be assessed during history taking.

Physical Examination
Blood pressure should be measured when the patient is in the supine position and at least 3 minutes after assuming the upright position.

Diagnostic Testing
Lab studies may be indicated to assess for associated conditions such as sepsis or dehydration with electrolyte imbalance, and to rule out conditions such as hypoglycemia that could present with similar symptoms.

Late occurrence or worsening of OH months or years after SCI should prompt suspicion of posttraumatic syringomyelia, and appropriate diagnostic imaging such as spinal magnetic resonance imaging (MRI) may be indicated.

Autonomic testing may be done in specialized centers but its role in SCI related neurogenic OH is not established. Examples include testing heart rate variability with deep breathing and during Valsalva maneuver, and a head up tilt table test as a tool for evaluation of orthostatic stress.

Prognosis

Frequency and severity of symptoms, time upright before onset of symptoms, influence on activities of daily living, and blood pressure measurements can provide an indication of the severity of OH or response to treatment. Those with incomplete or thoracic injuries are more likely to resolve rapidly, though symptoms improve in most cases irrespective of level and completeness of injury.

Management

No single treatment for OH in SCI is consistently effective. Success may be increased combining and individualizing management. The goal of treatment is to alleviate the disability caused by symptoms, rather than to achieve an optimal target blood pressure reading.

Nonpharmacological Measures

A number of practical nonpharmacologic measures can be taken to minimize the hypotensive effects although evidence of effectiveness in SCI is limited for some.

Small, frequent meals may minimize postprandial symptoms. Limiting alcohol intake with meals may be helpful. Patients may have greater functional capacity before a meal than in the hour following a meal and may be able to adjust their activities accordingly.

If blood pressure is higher later in the day, physical exertion, such as exercise programs or physical therapy, may be better tolerated in the afternoon rather than the early morning. The nocturnal diuresis that sometimes occurs in SCI may lead to inadequate blood volume.

Elevating the head of the bed by 5–10 inches (reverse Trendelenberg position) may reduce nocturnal diuresis, morning postural hypotension, hypovolemia, and supine hypertension, although patients may not be able to tolerate more than a few degrees of head-up tilt during the night. Rapid changes in position should be avoided, as should excessive exertion in hot environments.

A review of patient medications is essential and modification may be indicated to minimize hypotensive side effects. If vasoactive medications are being administered with meals, that may be particularly disabling.

Liberalizing salt and water intake may improve blood volume, although the benefit of salt loading has not been sufficiently proven in people with SCI. Abdominal binders and compressive stockings can be used in an attempt to increase venous pressure and reduce venous pooling through decreased capacitance of leg and abdominal vascular beds. However, donning these may present practical problems for people with SCI and there is conflicting evidence of effectiveness.

Repeated and gradual increase in postural challenges, such as with the use of a tilt-table, may be useful in the acute stages. A tilt-in-space or reclining wheelchair is beneficial for accommodating to a progressive increase in the sitting angle and also allows reclining in response to symptoms.

Evidence for use of body weight-supported treadmill training to improve orthostatic tolerance is currently insufficient. There is some evidence to support a role for functional electrical stimulation (FES) in the treatment of OH in SCI. FES induced contraction of leg muscles may increase venous return, and thus increase cardiac output and stroke volume that can increase blood pressure and decrease hypotension-related symptoms. The response appears to be dose dependent and independent of the site of stimulation. Further research in this area is warranted. Biofeedback has also been tried for the management of OH in SCI.

Pharmacologic Management (Table 33B.2)

Several drugs have been used to treat OH, though effectiveness varies. The drugs for which there has been the most experience in use for SCI-related OH

Table 33B.2

Commonly Used Medications for OH in SCI				
Medication	Mechanism	Dose	Side Effects	Considerations
Fludrocortisone	Renal sodium retention	0.1–0.4 mg daily	Hypokalemia, fluid retention, edema, weight gain, headache, interaction with warfarin	Delayed onset of action so dose increased no faster than biweekly; little glucocorti-coid effect at this dose
Ephedrine	Nonselective sympath-omimetic with direct and indirect effects due to release of norepinephrine	25–50 mg three times a day	Tremulousness, palpitations, anxiety, supine hypertension, urine reten-tion, abuse potential, tachyphylaxis	Often given prn 15–30 min before arising or prior to anticipated therapies or exertion
Midodrine	Alpha 1-adreno-receptor agonist, direct arteriolar and venous constriction	2.5–10 mg two to three times a day	Supine hyper-tension (FDA black box warning on product label), scalp paresthesia, pruritis, uri-nary retention	Giving last dose by mid-afternoon mitigates supine hypertension at night; FDA approved for neurogenic OH

include fludrocortisone, ephedrine, and midodrine (Table 33B.2). Of these, only Midodrine has been approved by the Food and Drug Administration (FDA) for the treatment of neurogenic OH following demonstrated effectiveness in pre-marketing placebo controlled trials.

Other supplementary agents have been used to treat OH with variable success, but there is little to no published experience of their use in SCI related OH. These include physostigmine, recombinant human erythropoietin, the vasopressin analog desmopressin (DDAVP), and the somatostatin analog octreotide. Nonsteroidal anti-inflammatory drugs, such as indomethacin or ibuprofen, act through inhibition of prostaglandin-induced vasoconstriction. Clonidine has been reported to cause a paradoxical beneficial increase in blood pressure in some patients with OH.

Patient and Family Education

Counseling about avoidance of exacerbating factors and measures that patients and caregivers can take is helpful. For example, patients should be advised to move from supine to upright gradually, especially in the morning, and to avoid exertion in hot weather.

Practice Pearls

Patients with co-existing OH and supine hypertension are especially challenging to manage, and require careful titration and trial of medications. Short acting antihypertensive agents at night, for example, a nitroglycerin patch, may help control nocturnal hypertension without exacerbating daytime OH. Raising the head end of the bed may also mitigate supine hypertension.

KNOWLEDGE GAPS AND EMERGING CONCEPTS

Droxidopa, a synthetic amino acid precursor of epinephrine, is being studied for use in SCI related OH.

Given the lack of consistently effective treatment newer therapies need to be developed. Well designed controlled studies for current treatments are very limited. Lack of postmarketing efficacy studies led to threats of withdrawal of FDA approval of Midodrine for neurogenic OH in 2010, but extension was granted contingent on additional studies by the manufacturer.

Further studies are also needed to evaluate long-term consequences of SCI related OH.

SUGGESTED READING

Freeman R. Neurogenic orthostatic hypotension. *NEJM*. 2008;358:615-624.

Gonzalez F, Chang JY, Banovac K, et al. Autoregulation of cerebral blood flow in patients with orthostatic hypotension after spinal cord injury. *Paraplegia*. 1991;29(1):1-7.

Groomes TE, Huang CT. Orthostatic hypotension after spinal cord injury: treatment with fludrocortisone and ergotamine. *Arch Phys Med Rehabil*. 1991;72(1):56-58.

Kaufmann H. L-dihydroxyphenylserine (Droxidopa): a new therapy for neurogenic orthostatic hypotension: the U.S. experience. *Clin Auton Res*. 2008;18(suppl 1):19-24.

Low PA, Singer W. Management of neurogenic orthostatic hypotension: an update. *Lancet Neurol*. 2008;7:451.

Mitka M. Trials to address efficacy of midodrine 18 years after it gains FDA approval. *JAMA*. 2012;307(11):1124-1127.

Nobunaga AI. Orthostatic hypotension in spinal cord injury. *Top Spinal Cord Inj Rehabil*. 1997;4(1):73-80.

Sabharwal S. *Orthostatic hypotension in SCI*. PM&R Knowledge NOW/American Academy of Physical Medicine and Rehabilitation. http://now.aapmr.org/cns/complications/Pages/Orthostatic-Hypotension-in SCI.aspx. October 15, 2012. Modified June 8, 2013.

Teasell RW, Arnold MO, Krassioukov A, et al. Cardiovascular consequences of loss of supraspinal control of the sympathetic nervous system after spinal cord injury. *Arch Phys Med Rehabil*. 2000;81(4):506-516.

Autonomic Dysreflexia

GENERAL PRINCIPLES

Autonomic dysreflexia (AD) is a condition that is unique to people with spinal cord injury (SCI) at T6 or above level of injury. It is characterized by a sudden, massive, uninhibited reflex sympathetic discharge, typically precipitated by a noxious stimulus, which results in a significant and potentially dangerous rise in blood pressure. AD is also referred to by the term autonomic hyperreflexia. It is potentially life threatening.

Etiology

Bladder problems are the most common precipitating cause, accounting for over 75% of episodes, followed by bowel distension or impaction, but any noxious stimulus below the level of injury can precipitate AD (Table 33C.1)

The reported incidence of AD in people with SCI varies between different studies, likely a reflection of differences in the population being studied.

Epidemiology

SCI at the thoracic level T6 or above, that is, above the major splanchnic outflow, predisposes to AD, though occurrence with injuries as low as T8 is described.

AD is more likely to occur in people with complete injuries though can also be seen in those with incomplete SCI.

Pathophysiology

AD results from noxious stimuli below the level of injury, which ascend in the spinothalamic tract and posterior columns. These in turn trigger sympathetic hyperactivity by stimulating neurons in the intermediolateral gray matter in the spinal cord. Inhibitory impulses that arise above the level of injury are blocked so that there is unopposed sympathetic outflow (T6 through L2) with excessive catecholamine release, including norepinephrine, dopamine-beta-hydroxylase, and dopamine.

Table 33C.1

Causes of Autonomic Dysreflexia

Urinary (>75%)

Bladder distension

Blocked catheter

Bladder or kidney stones

Catheterization

Urologic instrumentation

Detrusor sphincter dyssynergia

Lithotripsy

Urinary tract infection

Gastrointestinal

Bowel distension

Bowel impaction

Gastrointestinal instrumentation

Appendicitis

Gallstones

Gastric ulcers

Hemorrhoids

Skin

Ingrown toenail

Constrictive clothing, shoes, leg-bag strap or other appliances

Contact with hard or sharp objects

Blisters

Burns

Insect bites

Pressure ulcers

Musculoskeletal

Fractures or other musculoskeletal trauma

Heterotopic ossification

Reproductive

Sexual intercourse or stimulation

Ejaculation

Electroejaculation or vibratory ejaculation

Scrotal compression

Epididymitis

Menstruation

Labor and delivery

(continued)

Other
Boosting (intentional inducement of AD to enhance athletic performance)
Functional electrical stimulus
Venous thrombo-embolism
Stimulants, excess caffeine, excess alcohol, substance abuse
Surgical procedures

Denervation hypersensitivity of peripheral adrenergic receptors below the level of injury may also contribute to the pathophysiology.

Course and Natural History

AD does not occur till after the phase of spinal shock when reflexes return, and it is unusual to see AD in the first month after SCI, although it has been reported within the first few days of injury.

CLINICAL CONSIDERATIONS

Assessment

History and Physical Examination
Signs and symptoms of AD are summarized in Table 33C.2.

The feature of most concern with AD is the significant and potentially life-threatening elevation in blood pressure.

Blood pressure can exceed 200 mmHg or higher for both systolic and diastolic readings during an episode of AD. However, even a blood pressure of

Table 33C.2

Symptoms and Signs of Autonomic Dysreflexia

Sudden, significant increase in blood pressure

Pounding headache

Flushing of the skin above the level of the SCI, or possibly below

Blurred vision, appearance of spots in the patient's visual fields

Nasal congestion

Profuse sweating above the level of the SCI, or possibly below the level

Piloerection or goose bumps above the level of SCI, or possibly below

Bradycardia (may be a relative slowing only and still within normal range)

Cardiac arrhythmias

Feelings of apprehension or anxiety

Minimal or no symptoms, despite a significantly elevated blood pressure

140/90 mmHg may represent AD in patients with tetraplegia who typically have a low baseline blood pressure. Blood pressure of 20 to 40 mmHg above baseline (15 mmHg for adolescents and children) may be a sign of AD. It is important to use appropriate sized cuff to measure blood pressure in children (width of cuff ~ 40% of arm circumference); too large cuffs tend to underestimate and small cuffs tend to overestimate blood pressure.

In addition to the rise in blood pressure, increased sympathetic outflow can also result in symptoms such as pallor and piloerection.

Compensatory parasympathetic response with vasodilation above the level of injury may cause pounding headache, nasal congestion, flushed skin above the level of injury, constricted pupils, and sometimes a relative bradycardia. Headache is the most common symptom and typically occurs in the frontal or occipital regions. AD should always be considered and blood pressure evaluated with any complaints of headache in this population. Young children may not be able to readily communicate symptoms of headache.

The severity of AD varies considerably, but serious and potentially life-threatening complications may occur with untreated AD in conjunction with the rapid rise in blood pressure. These include cardiac arrhythmias, seizures, or intracranial bleeding. Retinal hemorrhage and detachment may occur.

Diagnostic Tests
AD is primarily a clinical diagnosis. Lab or imaging studies are typically not needed, but may be indicated to look for potential precipitating factors, such as a urinary tract infection, depending on the clinical assessment. Similarly imaging studies may be indicated in some cases if limb fracture or intra-abdominal pathology is suspected as a cause of AD.

Management

The Consortium for Spinal Cord Medicine has published clinical practice guidelines for the acute management of AD. Summary of these treatment guidelines is as follows[1]:

- Check the individual's blood pressure.
- If the blood pressure is elevated and the individual is supine, immediately sit the person up. The rationale is that upright posture may reduce blood pressure through venous pooling in the lower extremities.
- Loosen any clothing or constrictive devices. This allows for further blood pooling below the level of injury and removes potential triggers for noxious sensory stimulation.

---

[1] From the Consortium for Spinal Cord Medicine Clinical Practice Guidelines on Acute Management of Autonomic Dysreflexia. 2001. Paralyzed Veterans of America.

▓ Monitor the blood pressure and pulse frequently.

▓ Quickly survey the individual for the instigating causes, beginning with the urinary system.

▓ If an indwelling urinary catheter is not in place, catheterize the individual.

▓ Prior to inserting the catheter, instill 2% lidocaine jelly (if readily available) into the urethra and wait several minutes.

▓ If the individual has an indwelling urinary catheter, check the system along its entire length for kinks, folds, constrictions, or obstructions and for correct placement of the indwelling catheter. If a problem is found, correct it immediately.

▓ If the catheter appears to be blocked, gently irrigate the bladder with a small amount of fluid, such as normal saline at body temperature. Avoid manually compressing or tapping on the bladder.

▓ If the catheter is not draining and the blood pressure remains elevated, remove and replace the catheter.

▓ Prior to replacing the catheter, instill 2% lidocaine jelly (if readily available) into the urethra and wait several minutes.

▓ If the catheter cannot be replaced, consider attempting to pass a coude catheter, or consult an urologist.

▓ Monitor the individual's blood pressure during bladder drainage.

▓ If acute symptoms of AD persist, including a sustained elevated blood pressure, suspect fecal impaction.

▓ If the elevated blood pressure is at or above 150 mmHg systolic, consider pharmacologic management to reduce the systolic blood pressure without causing hypotension prior to checking for fecal impaction.

▓ Use an antihypertensive agent with rapid onset and short duration while the causes of AD are being investigated (Table 33C.3). Typically used medications include:

  ● Two percent nitroglycerin ointment, 1 inch applied to the chest or back. This has the advantage of easy removal in case of precipitous or excessive fall in blood pressure. Nitrates in other forms (e.g., sodium nitroprusside drip for acute management in the hospital setting) can also be used. Nitrates in any form, including nitroglycerin ointment, are contraindicated in patients who may have taken phosphodiesterase type 5 inhibitors (PDE5I), such as sildenafil, within the past 24 to 48 hours.

Table 33C.3

Commonly Used Medications for Acute Management of Autonomic Dysreflexia

Nitroglycerin 2% ointment, 1 inch applied to the chest or back

Nifedipine, 10 mg, bite and swallow[a]

Captopril 25 mg, sublingual

[a]Should be used with great caution in elderly individuals and those with coronary artery disease (see text).

- Nifedipine, 10 mg, immediate release form, with the patient instructed to bite the capsule and swallow its contents. Sublingual administration (or swallow without bite) is not recommended due to delayed or erratic absorption. It can be repeated, if needed, after 10 to 15 minutes. While concerns about association of nifedipine-related cardiovascular problems (shunting of blood away from the heart and reflex tachycardia) have discouraged its use in the general population, those have not been reported in the context of AD treatment in SCI and it is still fairly commonly used for this purpose. It should be used with great caution in elderly individuals or those with coronary artery disease.
  - Captopril 25 mg, administered sublingually, has also been used with good effect.
- Monitor the individual for symptomatic hypotension.
- If fecal impaction is suspected, check the rectum for stool, using the following procedure: With a gloved hand, instill a topical anesthetic agent such as 2% lidocaine jelly generously into the rectum. Wait approximately 5 minutes for sensation in the area to decrease. Then, with a gloved hand, insert a lubricated finger into the rectum and check for the presence of stool. If present, gently remove, if possible. If AD becomes worse, stop the manual evacuation. Instill additional topical anesthetic and recheck the rectum for the presence of stool after approximately 20 minutes.
- If precipitating cause of AD is not yet determined, check for other less frequent causes.
- Monitor the individual's symptoms and blood pressure for a least 2 hours after resolution of the AD episode to make sure that it does not recur.
- If there is poor response to the treatment specified above and/or the cause of the dysreflexia has not been identified, strongly consider admitting the individual to the hospital to be monitored, to maintain pharmacologic control of the blood pressure, and to investigate other causes of the dysreflexia.
- Document the episode in the individual's medical record. This record should include the presenting signs and symptoms and their course, treatment instituted, recordings of blood pressure and pulse, and response to treatment. The effectiveness of the treatment may be evaluated according to the level of outcome criteria reached:
  - The cause of the AD episode has been identified.
  - The blood pressure has been restored to normal limits for the individual (usually 90 to 110 systolic mmHg for a person with tetraplegia in the sitting position).
  - The pulse rate has been restored to normal limits.
  - The individual is comfortable, with no signs or symptoms of AD, of increased intracranial pressure, or of heart failure.
- Once the individual with SCI has been stabilized, review the precipitating causes with the individual, members of the individual's

family, significant others, and caregivers and provide education as necessary. Individuals with SCI and their caregivers should be able to recognize and treat AD and seek emergency treatment if it is not promptly resolved. It is recommended that an individual with a SCI be given a written description of treatment for AD at the time of discharge that can be referred to in an emergency.

Pharmacological treatment is sometimes indicated on an ongoing basis for those with frequent recurrent AD, not amenable to other measures to reduce precipitating factors.

■ Prazosin, a selective alpha-1 adrenoreceptor blocker that lowers blood pressure by vasodilation, started at 0.5 to 1.0 mg twice daily, is an appropriate option in those instances.

Prevention and Education
Individuals with SCI and their caregivers should be well educated to recognize and treat AD and seek emergency treatment if it is not promptly resolved. They should be aware of common potential precipitating causes and the importance of preventive measures.

AD is often not recognized by non-SCI providers given its unique occurrence in people with SCI. Measures to increase level of awareness among providers including primary care physicians, and emergency department and emergency medical service personnel are needed. This further underscores the importance of educating and empowering people with SCI and their families so they can help direct their own treatment in such settings. Individuals at risk for AD should carry a medical emergency card that provides a brief description of AD including its recognition and management.

Education and regulations to eliminate the use of boosting, that is, intentional inducement of AD to enhance physical performance in athletic events, is important to discourage the use of this unsafe practice. The International Olympic Committee has explicitly banned the use of this practice.

AD During Labor and Delivery
Recognition and prevention of AD during labor and delivery in women with SCI is critical. Onset of AD usually occurs in conjunction with uterine contractions in this setting. Epidural anesthesia is recommended as a measure to prevent and control AD in that setting.

Practice Pearls

AD should always be considered and blood pressure evaluated with any complaints of headache in individuals with SCI above the T6 neurological level.

KNOWLEDGE GAPS AND EMERGING CONCEPTS

As additional research emerges to identify the precise mechanisms involved in the development of AD, it could lead to development of additional treatments to prevent and manage AD.

Currently used medications for AD are largely used on an empirical basis, and additional studies are needed to determine which treatments are most effective.

SUGGESTED READING

Consortium for Spinal Cord Medicine. *Acute Management of Autonomic Dysreflexia: Individuals with Spinal Cord Injury Presenting to Health Care Facilities.* 2nd ed. Washington, DC: Paralyzed Veterans of America; 2001.

Helkowski WM, Ditunno JF Jr, Boninger M. Autonomic dysreflexia: incidence in persons with neurologically complete and incomplete tetraplegia. *J Spinal Cord Med.* Fall 2003;26(3):244-247.

Krassioukov A, Warburton DE, Teasell R, Eng JJ; Spinal Cord Injury Rehabilitation Evidence Research Team. A systematic review of the management of autonomic dysreflexia after spinal cord injury. *Arch Phys Med Rehabil.* 2009;90(4):682-695.

Ischemic Heart Disease

GENERAL PRINCIPLES

Heart disease is now a major cause of mortality and morbidity in people with spinal cord injury (SCI), and with the aging of this population, ischemic heart disease (IHD)-related issues have become increasingly important in the care of these individuals. Several aspects of IHD can be influenced by the presence of SCI.

Etiology

Specific risk factors for IHD may be increased in SCI (Table 33D.1). These include—low levels of high density lipoprotiens (HDL), physical inactivity, increased proportion of body fat, and higher incidence of glucose intolerance.

The significance of additional emerging IHD risk factors in SCI still needs to be defined, as does the role of underlying inflammation and/or pro-thrombotic factors or platelet dysfunction, and the potential contribution of autonomic dysfunction.

Epidemiology

Cardiovascular diseases are among the top few leading causes of death in chronic SCI.

It has been suggested that the prevalence of IHD is increased after SCI compared to the general population. However, there is conflicting literature and evidence for this is not definitive. Small number of subjects, inadequate control for confounding variables and differences in patient populations and outcomes studied may account for the discrepancy in results among different studies.

Pathophysiology and Risk Factors

Smoking
The link between smoking and IHD is well established.

Table 33D.1

Potentially Increased Cardiovascular Risk Factors After SCI

Decreased physical activity

Low HDL cholesterol

Impaired glucose tolerance, insulin resistance

Increased proportion of body fat

Psychosocial factors (Depression, Social isolation)

Hypothesized effects of SCI on emerging risk factors

Hypertension
There is a consistent and continuous association of blood pressure levels with cardiovascular disease and excellent evidence that treatment of hypertension decreases morbidity and mortality from cardiac disease. In patients with SCI, a low rather than high baseline blood pressure is typical. However, hypertension is common when SCI results from aortic disease or complications of aortic repair. Autonomic dysreflexia in people with SCI above T6 is clinically distinguishable from essential hypertension by its presentation, context, course, and episodic nature. The association, if any, between autonomic dysreflexia and chronic heart disease has yet to be established.

Cholesterol
Elevated low density cholesterol (LDL-C) level is a proven risk factor for IHD. HDL cholesterol is a strong protective factor, and high HDL levels are inversely related to the risk of IHD. There is evidence to suggest that HDL levels are lower in the population with chronic SCI as compared to the general population. About 24% to 40% of people with SCI were reported to have HDL cholesterol of less than 35 mg/dl, compared to only 10% of the general population. Levels of LDL cholesterol in people with SCI are similar to those of the general population.

Sedentary Lifestyle
There is strong evidence that a sedentary lifestyle is an independent risk factor for IHD. Several possible mechanisms for the beneficial effects of physical activity have been suggested. These include an antiatherogenic effect through increased HDL cholesterol and decreased LDL cholesterol and triglycerides, favorable effects on platelet adhesiveness and blood viscosity, increased insulin sensitivity, more effective cardiac use of oxygen with conditioning, and reduction of blood pressure. People with SCI often lead a sedentary lifestyle as a result of their impaired mobility, lack of access, limited exercise options, and stress-related musculoskeletal injuries; additionally, they have an altered physiologic response to exercise due to loss of exercising muscle mass as well as altered autonomic function.

Obesity
Obesity adversely affects cardiac function, increases the risk factors for IHD, and is an independent risk factor for cardiovascular disease. Once the acute injury phase is over, persons with SCI generally have lower energy expenditure than

able-bodied people (See Chapter 39A). Rates for those with chronic tetraplegia are generally lower than in those with paraplegia. As a result, excessive weight gain is not uncommon.

Diabetes

The risk for IHD is especially high for individuals with diabetes. Much of this risk is caused by lipid abnormalities, but factors such as insulin levels and blood glucose also appear to have an independent role. A positive association between insulin levels and the subsequent risk for cardiovascular disease has been demonstrated. The constellation of risk factors constituting the metabolic syndrome includes abdominal obesity, atherogenic dyslipidemia, raised blood pressure, insulin resistance, and prothrombotic and proinflammatory states. The prevalence of impaired glucose tolerance, insulin resistance, and hyperinsulinemia in individuals with chronic SCI has been reported to be increased; however the data is weak and inconclusive. Prevalence is highly dependent on the demographics of the population studied.

Atypical and Emerging Risk Factors

In addition to the classically identifiable risk factors described, studies have identified a diverse group of additional possible risk factors for IHD, although at present there are no conclusive guidelines regarding the significance or intervention strategies for many of these. Some of these factors include oxidants, platelet activators, elevated plasma homocysteine, lipoprotein, and inflammatory markers such as C-reactive protein (CRP) and other prothrombotic and proinflammatory markers. Whereas most of the reported studies for these are in the general population, there are a few reports relating to the SCI population. Some reports have suggested platelet abnormalities in SCI, including abnormalities of aggregation, resistance to inhibition by prostacyclin, and the presence of a prostacyclin receptor antibody. The significance of these findings is not clear at present. Other studies have suggested elevated CRP levels in the SCI population.

Key prevention targets for the above risk factors for IHD as listed in Table 33D.2.

Table 33D.2

Key Prevention Targets for Ischemic Heart Disease (IHD)
Smoking cessation
Lipid management to goal
Blood pressure control
Weight management
Physical activity
Diabetic management to goal
Additional components of secondary prevention with known IHD
Antiplatelet agents (aspirin), anticoagulants
Renin-angiotensin aldosterone system blockers
Beta blockers

CLINICAL CONSIDERATIONS

Assessment

History and Physical Examination
There are unique issues that influence the diagnosis of IHD after SCI (Table 33D.3). Individuals with SCI above T5 may not perceive chest pain with angina since cardiac pain impulses traveling via the afferent sympathetic nerves enter the spinal cord between T1 and T5.

They may present atypically with episodic dyspnea, nausea, unexplained autonomic dysreflexia, syncope, or changes in spasticity. On the other hand, gastro-esophageal reflux, which is common in SCI, may be mistaken for angina.

There may also be confusion in the interpretation of physical signs in differentiating congestive heart failure from lung crackles caused by atelectasis or dependent edema, both of which are common in SCI.

Diagnostic Tests

Traditional treadmill exercise stress test can typically not be done. Arm ergometry can be done in those with paraplegia. But arm exercise typically produces lower heart rates than leg exercise, and may miss detection of heart disease.

Pharmacological stress testing is often the most practical option. It consists of administration of a pharmacological agent such as dipyridamole (Persantin), adenosine, or dobutamine to induce cardiac stress, in combination with a form of cardiac imaging (thallium 201 scanning or 2-D echocardiography).

Table 33D.3

Unique Issues in the Diagnosis of IHD After SCI

Atypical presentations, lack of chest pain

Under-diagnosis of ischemic heart disease (IHD)

Delayed treatment; Inadequate secondary prevention

Confusing physical signs

    Dependent edema versus heart failure

    Atelectasis versus left ventricular failure

Nonspecific ST-segment and T-wave changes in SCI

Cardiac stress testing

    Inability to perform traditional treadmill test

    Suboptimal sensitivity of arm versus leg exercise

    Difficulty in interpreting significance of exercise induced hypotension

    Indication for pharmacologic stress testing

Management

The principles of management of IHD in SCI are essentially the same as for those in the general population, as are those for secondary prevention in those with known cardiovascular disease.

The spectrum of interventions, including lifestyle changes, medications, angioplasty, and cardiac revascularization, should be available to people with SCI as appropriate.

Reduction of Cardiac Risk Factors
Key prevention targets for IHD are listed in Table 33D.2. Because of exercise limitations in SCI, reduction of other cardiac risk factors is even more important. These include:

- Smoking cessation (counseling, behavioral techniques, nicotine patches or gum).
- Detection and control of hypertension. SCI may influence choice of antihypertensive agents. For example, thiazide diuretics that are often used as first-line agents in able-bodied adults would not be the optimal choice for the person with SCI using intermittent catheterization for bladder management.
- Weight control, diabetic control, and lipid management as needed.
- Physical Activity/ Exercise in SCI. Exercise capacity in SCI is limited by two main factors: paralysis of the large lower extremity muscles, and the blunted sympathetic response to exercise. Activities of daily living alone typically do not result in cardiovascular conditioning. Even modest exercise can achieve health benefits, though may not be able to exercise enough to produce definite cardiovascular benefits with higher levels of injury. Depending on the level of injury, exercise options may include arm-crank ergometry, hand cycling, endurance sports, swimming, circuit resistance training and electrically induced exercise.

Medical Management
People with SCI may not be able to tolerate traditional anti-anginal medication doses because of low blood pressure, so the introduction of medications at lower doses with careful blood pressure monitoring may be needed.

Aspirin and beta-blockers are routinely recommended for patients with atherosclerotic cardiovascular disease and postmyocardial infarction unless contraindicated.

Because of the use of sildenafil and other phosphodiesterase-5 (PDE-5) inhibitors for SCI-related erectile dysfunction, patients should be specifically questioned about their use if considering nitrate therapy for angina to avoid potential life-threatening hypotension with concurrent use of these drugs.

Angiotensin-converting enzyme (ACE) inhibitors have been shown to reduce the risk of further coronary events after myocardial infarction. These drugs should be used cautiously, with careful monitoring of electrolytes, blood urea nitrogen, and creatinine if there is underlying renal insufficiency due to SCI-related urologic problems. Additionally, because of the potentially significant role of the renin-angiotensin system in maintaining blood pressure in people with tetraplegia, severe hypotension may occur with ACE inhibitors in these patients, so caution and low initial dose is prudent when starting these drugs.

Cardiac Rehabilitation
Cardiac rehabilitation programs follow the same principles as in able-bodied individuals, and patients with SCI can be easily integrated into cardiac rehabilitation group classes. Adaptations to address mobility limitations may be needed. For example, progressive wheelchair propulsion may be substituted for a traditional progressive walking program, although success may be limited by musculoskeletal complications in shoulders, elbows, and wrists.

The energy requirements for wheelchair propulsion on a level surface by paraplegic individuals have been shown to be equivalent to those needed for able-bodied ambulation. Patients may need retraining in the use of energy conservation techniques during activities of daily living.

KNOWLEDGE GAPS AND EMERGING CONCEPTS

More research is needed to establish the interaction of aging and SCI in the development, presentation, and management of cardiovascular disease. Studies to determine presenting symptoms, risk factors, and outcomes will be helpful in planning for appropriate interventions.

SUGGESTED READING

Bauman WA, Spungen AM. Coronary heart disease in individuals with spinal cord injury: assessment of risk factors. *Spinal Cord.* 2008;46(7):466-476.

Carlson KF, Wilt TJ, Taylor BC, et al. Effect of exercise on disorders of carbohydrate and lipid metabolism in adults with traumatic spinal cord injury: systematic review of the evidence. *J Spinal Cord Med.* 2009;32(4):361-378.

Sabharwal S. Cardiovascular dysfunction in spinal cord disorders. In: Lin V, ed. *Spinal Cord Medicine.* 2nd ed. New York, NY: Demos Publishing; 2010:241-255.

Peripheral Vascular Disease

GENERAL PRINCIPLES

With aging, there is increasing comorbidity from complications of peripheral vascular disease, especially in diabetics and smokers. The presence of SCI can influence the presentation and management of peripheral vascular disease.

Etiology

Factors that may increase the predisposition to arterial disease in these patients include those for atherosclerosis, such as lipid abnormalities, smoking, and glucose intolerance.

Epidemiology

The prevalence of this condition in the spinal cord injury (SCI) population is not well established. Some reports suggest a relatively high incidence of limb amputation because of vascular disease in patients with SCI, and reduced arterial circulation to the legs has been reported in SCI.

CLINICAL CONSIDERATIONS

Assessment

History and Physical Examination
A delay in diagnosis of peripheral arterial disease (PAD) may occur in patients with SCI because of the lack of the cardinal symptom of intermittent claudication.

Symptoms of more advanced limb ischemia, such as rest pain or numbness, may also be absent, and patients may first present with gangrenous changes or other signs of advanced disease.

Peripheral vascular disease may present with nonhealing skin ulcers in SCI.

Examination of peripheral pulses and foot examination for ischemic skin changes should be performed routinely as part of the periodic evaluation of patients with SCI.

However, skin discoloration and cool temperature in the feet may occur in SCI even without evidence of significant peripheral vascular disease, and the dependent leg edema that occurs in SCI may make the palpation of foot pulses difficult.

Diagnostic Testing
Because of the limitations of history and physical evaluation of arterial disease in these patients, vascular testing may be indicated for diagnosis, assessment of disease severity, and the monitoring of disease progression or regression. Specific arterial tests include continuous-wave Doppler, segmental pressures, transcutaneous oximetry, and imaging studies.

Continuous-wave Doppler or duplex scanning detects blood motion. In the normal artery, the pulsatile waveform is usually triphasic. With mild stenosis, there is dampening of the signal. As severity worsens, the signal becomes monophasic.

Segmental pressures can be measured by sequentially inflating and deflating pneumatic cuffs around the limb or digit and using the continuous-wave Doppler to determine the systolic pressure at which arterial flow resumes during cuff deflation. The most commonly reported segmental pressure is an ankle-brachial index (ABI). An ABI of greater than 1.0 is considered normal, 1.0 to 0.8 reflects mild disease, 0.8 to 0.5 moderate disease, and less than 0.5 severe disease. ABI may prove to be a useful screening tool for PAD in individuals with SCI. This measurement cannot be used when blood vessel walls are noncompressible due to calcification, as occurs commonly in diabetics.

Transcutaneous oximetry is used to evaluate skin blood flow by using oxygen-sensitive electrodes. This measurement is also useful in determining the adequacy of skin perfusion for healing at a given amputation site. Values above 40 mmHg are generally adequate, whereas those below 20 mmHg are not.

Imaging modalities such as 2-D real-time ultrasound, computed tomography (CT), and magnetic resonance angiography are being increasingly used instead of invasive angiography.

Management

Minimizing risk factors such as smoking, diabetes, and hyperlipedemia is a key component of management.

Because ischemic heart disease (IHD) is a common comorbidity in those with peripheral vascular disease and a frequent cause of death in these patients, primary and secondary prevention measures for IHD are indicated.

Limb revascularization for the relief of claudication may not be an issue because of the lack of this symptom in patients with SCI. Arterial reconstruction for occlusive disease may be difficult because of small and atrophic arteries in SCI.

Consideration of amputation for patients with advanced disease should be a team decision that should include the patient and SCI physician in addition to the surgeons. The effect of amputation on balance and transfers, weight redistribution with new pressure areas, and skin breakdown of the insensate stump are some factors that should be included in the deliberations. After amputation, patients should be evaluated by the rehabilitation team. They often need a new wheelchair and retraining for transfers and wheelchair mobility, in addition to education for stump and skin care.

SUGGESTED READING

Grew M, Kirshblum SC, Wood K, Millis SR, Ma R. The ankle brachial index in chronic spinal cord injury: a pilot study. *J Spinal Cord Med.* 2000;23(4):284-288.

Lee BY. Management of peripheral vascular disease in the spinal cord injured patient. In: *Comprehensive Management of the Spinal Cord Injured Patient.* Philadelphia: WB Saunders; 1991:1-11.

Impaired Thermoregulation

GENERAL PRINCIPLES

Etiology and Epidemiology

People with spinal cord injury (SCI) have an impaired ability to control temperature. The degree of impaired thermoregulation is related to the neurological impairment; the higher and more complete the SCI, the greater the abnormality with thermoregulation.

People with complete tetraplegia are especially prone to hyperthermia (defined as rectal temperature above 101°F/38.4°C due to impaired thermoregulation) and hypothermia (defined as rectal temperature below 95°F/35°C). They are often poikilothermic; i.e., because of inability to control body temperature within a narrow range, their temperature may vary considerably depending on the surrounding temperature.

Pathophysiology

The hypothalamus normally interprets afferent information about external and internal body temperature and integrates thermoregulatory responses to maintain body temperature within a narrow range. Noradrenergic and cholinergic efferents from the hypothalamus control vasomotor responses, sudomotor or sweating function, as well as shivering and piloerection. With decrease in core body temperature, sympathetic noradrenergic efferents induce shivering, piloerection, and vasoconstriction to produce heat. When core temperature rises, vasodilation and sweating occur to cause cooling.

After SCI, there is reduced afferent input to the thermoregulatory center in the hypothalamus due to interruption of afferent pathways, including the spinothalamic tract that carries temperature sensation. Efferent responses from the hypothalamus are also impaired due to loss of sympathetic connections resulting in impaired vasomotor control, impaired sweating below the level of injury, and loss of shivering. The higher the injury, the larger the body surface area impaired, and the greater the thermoregulatory dysfunction.

Extreme hypo- or hyperthermia can impair several body functions.

CLINICAL CONSIDERATIONS

Assessment

People with complete tetraplegia may have a normal body temperature that is 1°F to 2°F lower than neurologically intact individuals. Therefore, even a low grade fever may indicate a significant infection in these individuals. On the other hand, high body temperature may be a result of hot ambient temperature or excess blankets.

While impaired thermoregulation can be a cause of increased body temperature, it is imperative to consider infectious causes for sustained or significant increases in temperature.

Symptoms of heat stroke can include headache, dizziness, confusion, and loss of consciousness.

Management

After acute injury, prehospital and emergency room management requires special attention to body temperature since these individuals may be poikilothermic. Measures to prevent hypothermia, such as the use of Mylar or space blankets, may be needed in the field in case of acute SCI occurring in cold environments.

People with SCI, especially those with tetraplegia, should remain vigilant about avoiding extremes of temperature. If temperature is over 90° F, they should stay in an air conditioned environment if feasible, remain hydrated by drinking water, wear light clothing, limit time and intensity of outdoor activity, and try to stay in shady and cooler areas. Strenuous exercise in hot and humid weather should be avoided. Various cooling strategies have been shown to be effective to prevent exercise-related hyperthermia in wheelchair users, including the use of cooling devices, cooling sprays, and cooling vests.

Individuals with tetraplegia are especially vulnerable during heat or cold advisories involving and should have an emergency plan and contact information in case of problems.

KNOWLEDGE GAPS AND EMERGING CONCEPTS

Additional research is needed to evaluate the thermoregulatory response of wheelchair athletes at different levels of SCI, and to evaluate the effectiveness of available and emerging cooling strategies to prevent exercise-induced hyperthermia.

SUGGESTED READING

Karlsson AK, Krassioukov A, Alexander MS, Donovan W, Biering-Sørensen F. International spinal cord injury skin and thermoregulation function basic data set. *Spinal Cord*. 2012; 50(7):512-516.

Khan S, Plummer M, Martinez-Arizala A, Banovac K. Hypothermia in patients with chronic spinal cord injury. *J Spinal Cord Med*. 2007;30(1):27-30.

Price MJ. Thermoregulation during exercise in individuals with spinal cord injuries. *Sports Med*. 2006;36(10):863-879.

CHAPTER 34

Genitourinary Consequences: Overview

GENERAL PRINCIPLES

Genitourinary (GU) complications and voiding dysfunction are very significant effects of spinal cord injury (SCI). Awareness and management of urinary dysfunction in SCI has greatly reduced mortality from related complications and renal failure over the past several decades, but GU problems remain a major source of morbidity. Urinary tract infections (UTI) are the leading cause of hospitalization in people with SCI.

Ongoing surveillance and management of GU function is a crucial part of SCI care. Goals of neurogenic bladder management are to: minimize lower tract complications, preserve the upper urinary tract, avoid incontinence, and be compatible with the person's lifestyle.

CLINICAL CONSIDERATIONS

Neurogenic bladder dysfunction after SCI is covered in detail in Chapter 34A

Complications of voiding dysfunction in SCI include:

- *UTI*: See Chapter 34B
- *Kidney and bladder stones*: See Chapter 34C
- *Hydronephrosis*:
  Hydronephrosis can occur from several causes after SCI. Poor bladder wall compliance, detrusor-sphincter-dyssynergia (DSD), or bladder outlet obstruction can increase intravesical pressure and cause a functional obstruction to urinary flow. Intravesical pressure greater than 40 cm H_2O on urodynamic testing has been associated with a

significantly increased prevalence of upper tract changes in patients with SCI or meningomyelocele (Chapter 34A). Vesicoureteral reflux (VUR) may also increase hydrostatic pressure within the distal ureter that blocks urine flow and can lead to hydronephrosis. It has also been suggested that certain bacterial species can suppress ureteral peristalsis and cause dilation of the ureters. Mechanical obstruction from a stone or stricture can also lead to hydronephrosis. Ongoing surveillance to identify and address the underlying cause are needed for prevention and management of hydronephrosis.

- *VUR:*
  VUR can result in renal function deterioration through recurrent pyelonephritis with scarring and by causing back pressure-related hydronephrosis. VUR can occur as a result of high bladder pressure, changes in the submucosal course of the ureters with an abnormal, persistently open ureter orifice as a result bladder wall thickening, recurrent UTI, or because of congenital anomalies of the ureteral orifice. Management includes lowering of intravesical pressure and measures to prevent UTI. Indwelling catheterization may be indicated in some refractory cases to achieve sustained urine flow and reduce bladder pressure.
- *Autonomic dysreflexia* (AD): GU factors are the precipitating cause of more than 75% of instances of AD. See Chapter 33C
- *Catheter- and bladder management-related complications*: See Chapter 33A For example, bladder cancer risk may be increased with long-term use of indwelling catheters.

SUGGESTED READING

Cameron AP, Rodriguez GM, Schomer KG. Systematic review of urological followup after spinal cord injury. *J Urol.* 2012;187(2):391-397.

Consortium for Spinal Cord Medicine. *Bladder Management for Adults with Spinal Cord Injury. Clinical Practice Guidelines for Health Care Professionals.* Washington, DC: Paralyzed Veterans of America; 2006.

Neurogenic Bladder

GENERAL PRINCIPLES

Anatomy and Physiology of the Genitourinary Tract

Anatomy of the Urinary Tract
The upper urinary tract includes kidneys and ureters. The kidney consists of the renal parenchyma which secretes, concentrates, and excretes urine, and the collecting system which drains urine into the renal pelvis and down into the ureter. The renal parenchyma includes the external cortex and the internal medulla. The ureters extend from the ureteropelvic junction of the kidney to base of the bladder where they course submucosally in an oblique direction at the ureterovesical junction and open in the ureteral orifices. The ureterovesical junction is anatomically designed to allow urine to flow into the bladder but to prevent any reflux. Increase in vesical pressure simultaneously compresses the ureter and creates a one-way valve.

The lower urinary tract includes the bladder, urethra, and sphincters. The bladder is divided into the detrusor and trigone. Functionally urethral sphincters include the bladder neck (internal sphincter) that is under the control of the autonomic nervous system, and the external urethral sphincter that is has skeletal muscle fibers which are under the control of the somatic system.

Neuroanatomy of Voiding
The frontal lobe of the cerebral cortex functions as a control center that has a net inhibitory effect on the micturition center.

The pontine micturition center (PMC) is the major relay/excitatory center and coordinates urinary sphincter and bladder contraction. Disruption of this control leads to detrusor-sphincter dyssynergia (DSD).

The spinal cord connects the central and peripheral control and mediates a sacral reflex at the S2–S4 level.

Bladder Innervation (Table 34A.1)
Parasympathetic innervation is via the pelvic nerve (S2–S4). It is excitatory and causes detrusor contraction, mediated via muscarinic receptors (M3, M2). The neurotransmitter is acetylcholine.

Sympathetic innervation is via the hypogastric nerve (T10-L2). It acts on adrenergic receptors; the neurotransmitter is norepinephrine. It promotes storage, with relaxation of bladder muscle (β receptors) and excitation of the bladder base/urethra (α_1 receptors).

Somatic innervation is via the pudendal nerve (S2–S4). It originates from the motor neurons in the ventral horn of the spinal cord (nucleus of Onuf). It acts on nicotinic receptors; the neurotransmitter is acetylcholine. It is excitatory, and causes external sphincter contraction. Volitional voiding is achieved with voluntary relaxation of the external sphincter.

Bladder Function
Filling/storage: Afferent signals from bladder filling travel to the cortex. The cortex inhibits voiding reflex. The bladder fills without detrusor contraction (accommodation).

Table 34A.1
Bladder Innervation

Type of Innervation	Spinal Cord Nucleus	Nerve	Receptors/ Neurotransmitter	Action
Parasympathetic	S2–S4	Pelvic	Muscarinic (M3, M2)/ acetylcholine	Bladder (detrusor) contraction
Sympathetic	T10-L2	Hypogastric	Adrenergic/ norepinephrine	Promotes storage, with detrusor relaxation (β receptors) and bladder base/urethra contraction (α_1 receptors)
Somatic	S2–S4 (Nucleus of Onuf)	Pudendal	Nicotinic/ acetylcholine	External sphincter contraction; volitional voiding is achieved with voluntary relaxation of the external sphincter

Emptying: Voluntary voiding occurs at the appropriate time through a coordinated reflex beginning in pons with simultaneous detrusor contraction and sphincter relaxation.

Pathophysiology of Neurogenic Bladder in Spinal Cord Injury

Supra-Sacral Spinal Cord Lesion
The injury is above the sacral micturition center, which remains intact. It causes a pattern of dysfunction that depends on level and completeness of lesion. However, the characteristics of bladder dysfunction are not always predictable by neurological exam, and can evolve over several months before stabilizing.

Supra-sacral injury is characterized by detrusor hyperreflexia, that is, an upper motor neuron (UMN) bladder (after resolution of spinal shock, which is typically present in the first few weeks after injury during which time the bladder reflex activity is suppressed). This occurs with or without DSD. With DSD the detrusor contracts against a closed external sphincter, which can lead to high detrusor pressure, vesico-ureteral reflux (VUR), and autonomic dysreflexia (AD).

Sacral Cord (Conus) and Cauda Equina Injury (or Disease, e.g., Myelomeningocele)
In these cases the injury is at or below the sacral micturition center (S2–S4). It results in an areflexic or lower motor neuron (LMN) bladder.

Complications of Neurogenic Bladder (See Chapters 34, 34B, and 34C)

Although renal failure is no longer a major cause of death in spinal cord injury (SCI), genito-urinary complications continue to be significant problems, and can have a significant effect on participation and quality of life. These complications include: urinary tract infection (UTI), kidney and bladder stones, hydronephrosis, VUR, AD, and bladder cancer.

CLINICAL CONSIDERATIONS

Assessment

History and Physical Examination
Symptoms of urinary dysfunction include urinary retention and incontinence. Voiding frequency and volume should be assessed.

Evaluation of the neurogenic bladder requires a multidimensional assessment. Bowel and sexual function is typically impaired concomitantly and should be assessed. Hand function and dexterity, mobility, cognitive function, lifestyle, preferences, and available assistance all influence choice of management options.

The neurological examination characterizes the neurological lesion/injury. It should include evaluation of sacral sensation, reflexes, anal sphincter tone, and voluntary anal control. Persistent absence of bulbocavernosus reflex (S2–S4) and lower limb muscle stretch reflexes suggests LMN bladder impairment. However, neurological exam doesn't always predict the type of bladder dysfunction.

Other urological problems (e.g., benign prostatic hyperplasia, stress incontinence, or UTIs) may coexist and should be considered in the evaluation of urinary dysfunction. The clinical evaluation should also assess the presence and frequency of complications related to bladder dysfunction (e.g., UTI, stones, AD).

Diagnostic Testing
Evaluation of the genitourinary tract includes assessment of both the upper and lower urinary tracts.

Lower Tract Evaluation
Post-void residual volume (if no indwelling catheter) is measured to assess bladder emptying. It can be done using bladder ultrasound or catheterization after voiding.

Urodynamic evaluation: This involves filling of the bladder while monitoring bladder sensation, capacity, compliance, detrusor leak point pressure, maximum detrusor pressure, sphincter activity (typically with surface electromyography), urinary flow, and ability to empty/post-void residual volume. Blood pressure monitoring is important for those at risk of developing AD during the procedure. Video-urodynamics combines radiologic imaging with multi-channel urodynamics.

Cystoscopy is used to evaluate bladder anatomy and may identify stones, bladder tumor, or cystitis.

Voiding cystourethrogram can assess bladder neck and urethral function during filling and voiding phases. It may identify VUR or urethral obstruction.

Upper Tract Evaluation
This includes assessment of anatomy (through ultrasound, computed tomography scan, or intravenous pyelogram) as well as function (e.g., radionuclide renal scans).

Laboratory studies for renal function include blood urea nitrogen and creatinine. Since bacterial colonization is common, there is little role for routine urine cultures in the absence of specific indications or suspected infection.

Follow-up and ongoing assessment: Scheduled urological evaluation is conducted on a periodic, often annual, basis although consensus on the frequency and components of this maintenance evaluation is lacking. More frequent evaluations may be indicated, for example, for rapidly evolving status in the initial months after injury, or for those with urinary complications.

Management

Goals

Goals of neurogenic bladder management are to:

- Minimize lower tract complications
- Preserve the upper urinary tract
- Avoid incontinence
- Be compatible with the person's lifestyle, that is, address the whole person, convenience, and facilitate community integration and participation

Bladder management in SCI depends on the characteristics of the dysfunction, and needs to be individualized, along with provision of appropriate education and support to facilitate success.

Bladder Management Methods (Table 34A.2)

Intermittent Catheterization

Intermittent catheterization (IC) should be considered for individuals with sufficient hand function or willing caregiver to perform IC. It is usually the preferred option for bladder management if feasible.

IC should be avoided with: inability to IC/no willing caregiver for IC, abnormal urethral anatomy (stricture, false passage), low bladder capacity (<200 mL), unwillingness/inability to adhere to catheterization schedule (poor cognition, lack of motivation), high fluid intake, adverse reaction to passing catheter multiple times, or tendency to develop AD with bladder filling despite treatment.

Table 34A.2

Nonsurgical Options for Management of the Neurogenic Bladder in SCI	
Bladder Management	**Indications**
Intermittent catheterization	Often the first choice, if feasible. Need sufficient hand skills or willing caregiver. Must be willing and able to follow catheterization time schedule
Indwelling catheterization (urethral or suprapubic)	Consider for poor hand skills and lack of caregiver assistance. Not able or willing to follow intermittent catheterization schedule. High fluid intake. Lack of success with less invasive measures. Temporary management of vesicoureteral reflux. Choose suprapubic with epididymo-orchitis, prostatitis
Credé and Valsalva	Generally avoided in cervical SCI (unless the patient had sphincterotomy)
Reflex voiding	Hand skills or willing caregiver to put on condom catheter, empty leg bag. Confirmed small postvoid residual volumes, low voiding pressure. Able to maintain condom catheter in place. Need to also decrease detrusor-sphincter dyssynergia, if present (e.g., with a blocker, botulinum toxin injection, stent, sphincterotomy). Not an option for female patients

Table 34A.3

Antimuscarinic Agents for Overactive Bladder

Medication	Brand Name	Dosage	Comments
Oxybutinin	Ditropan	2.5–5.0 mg 2–4 times a day	Anticholinergic side effects include dry mouth, constipation, and blurred vision
Oxybutinin extended release	Ditropan XL	5–30 mg once daily	Dry mouth is less common with XL
Oxybutinin extended-release transdermal patch	Oxytrol	3.0 mg system applied every 3–4 days	Less frequent dosage and lower incidence of side effects
Tolterodine	Detrol	1–2 mg twice daily	Dry mouth, though may be less than oxybutinin
Tolterodine extended release	Detrol LA	2–4 mg twice daily	Preferred form of drug because of fewer side effects
Darifenacin	Enablex	7.5–15 mg once daily	Newer agents, more selective, with fewer side effects
Solifenacin	VESIcare	5–10 mg once daily	
Tropsium chloride	Sanctura	20 mg twice daily	
Tropsium chloride extended release	Sanctura XR	60 mg once daily	

Fluid intake and/or catheterization schedule should be adjusted if bladder volumes are consistently greater than 500 mL. Leakage of urine between catheterizations should be investigated and treated. Anticholinergic medications (Table 34A.3) should be considered.

Potential complications of IC include: UTIs, bladder over-distension, urinary incontinence, urethral trauma with hematuria, urethral false passages, strictures, AD (SCI above T6), and bladder stones.

Credé and Valsalva

Credé involves application of suprapubic pressure to express urine. Valsalva is a method in which an individual increases intra-abdominal pressure through use of abdominal muscles and diaphragm to express urine from the bladder.

These methods may be considered with LMN injury and low outlet resistance or those with sphincterotomy. These are not recommended as primary methods of bladder emptying since the bladder usually does not empty completely with the use of these techniques. These methods should be avoided with

DSD, bladder outlet obstruction, VUR, or hydronephrosis, since these can be worsened by the increased abdominal pressure.

Complications of these techniques include incomplete bladder emptying, high intravesical pressure, and development or worsening of VUR or hydronephrosis.

Indwelling Catheterization
Indwelling catheterization is considered in situations with: poor hand skills and limited available assistance, high fluid intake, cognitive impairment, elevated detrusor pressure, or lack of success with other methods.

Suprapubic (vs urethral) catheter should be considered with: urethral abnormalities or discomfort, difficulty with urethral catheter insertion, perineal skin break from urine leak, from urethral incompetence, desire for sexual genital function, and prostatitis, urethritis, or epidydymo-orchitis.

Long-term use of indwelling catheters is associated with several complications. These include: bladder and kidney stones, urethral erosions, epididymitis, recurrent UTI, pyelonephritis, hydronephrosis (from bladder wall thickening or fibrosis), and bladder cancer or metaplasia. Cystoscopic surveillance is appropriate for those with chronic indwelling catheters, especially in people who have been injured for over 10 years.

Reflex Voiding
This method is appropriate for males with adequate bladder contraction who have: sufficient hand skills or willing caregiver to put on condom catheter and empty leg bag, ability to maintain a condom catheter in place, small bladder capacity, small postvoid residue, and low pressure voiding.

Various options can be considered to ensure low-pressure voiding during reflex voiding. Nonsurgical options to consider include alpha-blockers or botulinum toxin to the sphincter to reduce DSD. Surgical options include sphincterotomy or endourethral stent to ensure low pressure.

Complications of reflex voiding include: condom catheter leakage and/or failure, penile skin breakdown, poor bladder emptying, UTI, upper tract damage if high intravesical pressure is untreated, and AD (with SCI at T6 or above).

Pharmacological Treatment
Antimuscarinic/anticholinergic agents (Table 34A.3) are used to decrease detrusor hyperreflexia and increase bladder capacity based on the fact that detrusor contractions are primarily mediated via muscarinic receptors. Oxybutynin and tolterodine are well established medications that have been used for many years. Newer antimuscarinic agents (trospium, darefenacin) are more selective and may have fewer anticholinergic side effects such as dry mouth.

Adrenergic alpha-blockers may be used to reduce DSD. Side effects include worsening of orthostatic hypotension, fatigue, and ejaculatory impairment.

Botulinum toxin: An injection in the detrusor has been used to treat overactive bladder, and injection into the sphincter may be used to reduce DSD. Further evaluation of its role in the management of neurogenic bladder is warranted.

Capsaicin and resiniferatoxin (1,000 times more potent than capsaicin) produce a neurotoxic effect on C-fibers (which mediate detrusor contraction in response to bladder irritation, versus A-delta afferent fibers that respond to bladder distension and are the ones primarily involved in normal voiding). Intravesicular instillation of these neurotoxic agents for local chemodenervation and have been reported to be effective in some studies but their role is still investigational.

Surgical Procedures
Transurethral Sphincterotomy
Transurethral resection of the sphincter (TURS) involves cutting the sphincter to allow free flow of urine from the bladder into a condom catheter. There should be preserved effective bladder contraction to allow adequate urine flow. Complications include late scar formation with restriction of urine flow, and worsening of erectile and ejaculatory function.

Urethral Stent
A stainless steel wire-mesh urethral stent is an alternative to manage urethral obstruction instead of TURS. Unlike TURS, it is potentially reversible since the sphincter is not cut. Stents have been used effectively in men who void reflexly and have DSD. In that situation, it can be considered for those who are unable or unwilling to perform IC or experience failure with intolerance to anticholinergic medication for IC, want to reflexly void but have recurrent AD, and/or experience failure or intolerance to alpha-blockers with reflex voiding. It is inappropriate for people who are unable to manage a condom catheter or have urethral abnormalities, and is not an option for females. Potential complications include stent migration, stone encrustation, and stricture formation.

Electrical Stimulation With Posterior Sacral Rhizotomy
In this technique, an implantable stimulator is used for electrical stimulation of the sacral parasympathetic nerves (S2–S4). It is done in conjunction with posterior sacral rhizotomy to increase bladder capacity and compliance and reduce reflex incontinence. While it has been used quite extensively in Europe, the product insert for the currently available sacral stimulator in the United States (approved for treatment of urinary retention and management of an overactive bladder) states that safety and effectiveness has not been demonstrated in neurological disease.

Bladder Augmentation
The bladder is surgically augmented using intestinal segments. This provides increased bladder capacity and bladder wall compliance for patients who are self-catheterizing.

It may be considered for those who have intractable involuntary bladder contractions causing incontinence, the ability and motivation to perform IC, the desire to convert from reflex voiding to an IC program, or are at high risk for upper tract deterioration secondary to hydronephrosis or VUR as a result of DSD. It may be an option to consider in female patients with paraplegia due to lack of an effective external collection device for that population.

It should be avoided in patients with compromised renal function since they are more prone to develop fluid and electrolyte imbalance. Severe abdominal adhesions or pelvic irradiation are also contraindications.

Continent Urinary Diversion
A continent catheterizable stoma is created on the abdominal wall which can be catheterized. For example, the Mitrofanoff appendicovesicostomy may be a surgical option in some children with SCI (Chapter 11) or myelomeningocele.

These may be considered when bladder augmentation is not feasible, those that cannot access the urethra due to congenital abnormalities or functional limitations, those with unsalvageable bladders due to urethral fistula and erosions, and those who require cystectomy for bladder cancer.

Urinary Diversion
Ureters are transected above the bladder and connected to an intestinal segment (usually an ileal conduit) which is brought to the skin of the lower abdominal wall and an external appliance is placed over the stoma to collect the urine.

It is an alternative to augmentation cystoplasty and continent diversion when hand function does not allow self-catheterization.

Cutaneous Ileovesicostomy
This is a variant of urinary diversion but, to preserve the ureterovesical junction, rather than dividing the ureters and connecting them to the ileal segment, the ileal segment is connected to the bladder and then brought to the lower abdominal wall.

Management of Complications

Management of individual complications of neurogenic bladder dysfunction is discussed further in Chapters 34, 34B, and 34C.

KNOWLEDGE GAPS AND EMERGING CONCEPTS

Additional prospective studies are needed to compare the benefits, risks, and complications of the currently used bladder management methods.

Off-label use of botulinum toxin injections and other chemical neurotoxins in the management of neurogenic bladder needs further evaluation.

SUGGESTED READING

Cameron AP. Pharmacologic therapy for the neurogenic bladder. *Urol Clin North Am.* 2010;37:495-506.

Consortium for Spinal Cord Medicine. *Bladder Management for Adults with Spinal Cord Injury. Clinical Practice Guidelines for Health Care Professionals.* Washington, DC: Paralyzed Veterans of America; 2006.

Groah SL, Weitzenkamp DA, Lammertse DP, Whiteneck GG, Lezotte DC, Hamman RF. Excess risk of bladder cancer in spinal cord injury: evidence for an association between indwelling catheter use and bladder cancer. *Arch Phys Med Rehabil.* 2002;83(3):346-351.

Samson G, Cardenas DD. Neurogenic bladder in spinal cord injury. *Phys Med Rehabil Clin N Am.* 2007;18(2):255-274.

Urinary Tract Infections

GENERAL PRINCIPLES

Urinary tract infections (UTI) are among the most important complications of neurogenic bladder dysfunction after spinal cord injury (SCI), and cause significant morbidity.

Clinical implications make it important to differentiate symptomatic UTI from asymptomatic bacteriuria (ABU).

Etiology

The majority of UTI in people with SCI is caused by bowel flora, most commonly gram-negative bacilli and enterococci.

The spectrum of pathogens causing catheter-associated UTI (CAUTI) is considerably broader than that causing uncomplicated UTI. In addition to *Escherichia coli*, which accounts for the vast majority of uncomplicated UTI in the general population, pathogens including *Klebsiella* species, *Pseudomonas* species, *Proteus* species, *Serratia* species, *Enterococcus* species, *Citrobacter* species, *Acetinobacter* species, and *Staphyloccus* species, are common and account for a much higher percentage of UTI in individuals with SCI.

Epidemiology and Pathophysiology

UTI is the most common infection in people with SCI, occurring at an estimated rate of between 1.5 to 2.5 episodes per patient per year. It has been determined to be a leading cause of rehospitalizations in individuals with SCI.

Risk factors for UTI in SCI have been categorized into structural/physiological, behavioral, and demographic. Structural/physiological factors include over-distension of the bladder, large postvoid residuals, vesicoureteral reflux, high pressure voiding, urinary stones, and functional (e.g., detrusor sphincter dyssynergia) or structural (e.g., stricture) outlet obstruction.

The association between type of bladder management and incidence of symptomatic UTI is not clearly established. Risk of UTI is probably higher in those with indwelling catheters than those who manage their bladder with intermittent catheterization (IC), but there is conflicting data about that in the literature (although there is consensus that those with chronic indwelling catheters have higher, almost universal, prevalence of bacteriuria). Those who use an external condom catheter with reflex voiding also have been shown to have at least similar rates of UTI as those who perform IC.

Behavioral and demographic influences on UTI after SCI have not been well studied. Poor personal hygiene is cited as a risk factor, as is lower functional independence. Wheelchair athletes have been shown to have significantly lower rate of UTI than nonathletes at the same neurological level.

CLINICAL CONSIDERATIONS

Assessment

History and Physical Examination
Patients with SCI who develop UTI often present with atypical or nonspecific symptoms. Because of impaired sensation, dysuria may be absent. Patients may only report generalized malaise. There may be new onset of urinary incontinence, cloudy or strong-smelling urine, or hematuria. Occasionally urinary retention develops. Increased spasticity may occur in the lower abdomen or legs. Those with SCI above the T6 neurological level may present with symptoms of autonomic dysreflexia (AD) such as headache, sweating, and flushing. Sometimes, especially in older patients or those with previous cognitive impairment, increased confusion may be the primary presenting feature.

Features of Upper Versus Lower Tract Infection
In addition to the above symptoms and signs, those with upper tract infection often have fever and chills. Discomfort and tenderness in the costovertebral area may be present if sensation in that area is preserved.

Differential Diagnosis
When patients present with some of the nonspecific symptoms listed above, UTI is high on the list of differentials but there are several other conditions that could present with similar features in people with SCI. Other infectious processes, respiratory problems, fecal impaction, bowel obstruction, or several other medical problems may present with similar nonspecific symptoms. Localizing symptoms, such as new incontinence between catheterizations, may provide a clue to the condition but are not always present.

Diagnostic Tests
Urine analysis and culture are performed. It is important to obtain the culture before starting antibiotics whenever feasible. Blood cultures are drawn when systemic infection is a consideration. Other laboratory tests include complete blood count with differential, blood urea nitrogen, and serum creatinine.

UTI Versus ABU

The distinction between UTI and ABU is crucial, but often not straightforward. ABU is common in people with SCI. There are clinical and microbiological criteria to distinguish ABU from UTI. The traditionally cited microbiologic criterion is usually greater than or equal to 10^5 bacterial colony forming units (cfu)/mL without a catheter and greater than or equal to 10^2 cfu/ml in CAUTI, but many clinicians consider the presence of symptoms essential to the diagnosis of UTI in SCI regardless of the bacterial count in the urine.

Pyuria, that is, the presence of leukocytes in the urine, is a good indicator of UTI in the non-SCI population. However, in people with SCI the significance of pyuria (e.g., determined by the leukocyte esterase test) is sometimes difficult to interpret and may not necessarily be helpful in distinguishing between UTI and ABU. The irritating effect of a urinary catheter, especially indwelling catheter, on the bladder wall or routine change of catheter causes a significant increase in urinary white cell count without altering the bacterial colony count. While infection with gram negative organisms is typically associated with significant pyuria, gram positive bacteria such as *Staphylococcus epidermidis* and *Streptococcus fecalis* may elicit minimal pyuria, even with high colony counts. Thus while the presence of significant pyuria may be indicative of UTI with bacterial tissue invasion, that is not always the case. And while the absence of pyuria makes a UTI less likely, it does not rule it out.

Management

Symptomatic UTI should always be treated. Unexplained signs and symptoms consistent with UTI may also warrant empiric treatment.

ABU should not be treated in most cases, except before urologic instrumentation. Attempted treatment of ABU in individuals with high-grade reflux, the presence of hydronephrosis, or with urea-splitting organisms has been recommended by some, but that is not uniform practice and other considerations may play a role in deciding whether or not to treat with antibiotics in those situations.

Antibiotic Treatment

Urine culture should be obtained prior to starting antibiotic treatment. Empiric antibiotic treatment could be started pending results of the culture, and adjusted as needed based on results of the culture and sensitivity.

Those with mild symptoms can be started on oral antibiotics, often a fluoroquinolone. Duration of treatment is typically 7 to 10 days.

Hospitalization should be considered in those with high fever, chills, or dehydration, and broad spectrum antibiotics started pending culture results. Antibiotic treatment for at least 14 days is recommended in such cases where the clinical picture is consistent with pyelonephritis. Bladder distension should be avoided and an indwelling catheter may need to be placed during fluid hydration. Lack of response within 48 to 72 hours merits repeat cultures and consideration of imaging studies to rule out urinary tract pathology.

Not uncommonly, growth of more than one organism is seen in urine cultures obtained from people with SCI being treated for UTI. Since it is difficult to accurately differentiate which of the organisms is contributing to the clinical infection, treatment to cover all potentially pathogenic organisms grown from urine cultures is reasonable.

Follow-Up Management
Once the infection is treated and has responded clinically, routine follow-up urine cultures are typically not recommended, since the urinary tract often becomes colonized with other organisms.

In patients with persistent or recurrent UTI, testing to evaluate the urinary tract is indicated to look for presence of an anatomical nidus or cause (e.g., stone, abscess, or stricture) or a functional abnormality (e.g., high postvoid urinary residual volumes or vesicoureteral reflux).

Prophylaxis of UTI
Consistently following good hygiene practices and correct technique of catheter insertion are important elements of UTI prevention, as is proper bladder management and avoidance of large-postvoid residual urinary volumes.

Prophylactic antibiotics don't have a long-term effect and often facilitate growth of resistant organisms so they are not indicated in most cases, except prior to urological testing that requires instrumentation.

The role of cranberry supplements and of methenamine hippurate in reducing UTI in people with SCI has conflicting literature, with more recent studies reporting no significant benefit. Routine bladder irrigation with antimicrobial agents has not been shown to be effective.

There are some reports suggesting that the use of hydrophilic-coated catheters for IC may be associated with less frequent UTI than nonhydrophilic catheters. This merits further study.

Practice Pearl

The often nonspecific and atypical presentation of UTI in people with SCI should be recognized so that the diagnosis is not missed. At the same time, it is important to consider and adequately evaluate other causes of such nonspecific symptoms and avoid overtreatment of bacteriuria with antibiotics.

KNOWLEDGE GAPS AND EMERGING CONCEPTS

Colonization of the bladder with nonpathogenic organisms (e.g., certain nonpathogenic strains of *Escherichia coli*), with the goal of causing bacterial interference to reduce the presence of pathogenic urinary organisms, has shown promising results in initial studies.

The role of prophylactic antibiotics in the presence of high-grade reflux, the presence of hydronephrosis, or with urea-splitting organisms is not well-defined and needs further study.

SUGGESTED READING

Darouiche RO, Hull RA. Bacterial interference for prevention of urinary tract infection. *Clin Infect Dis.* 2012;55(10):1400-1407.

D'Hondt F, Everaert K. Urinary tract infections in patients with spinal cord injuries. *Curr Infect Dis Rep.* 2011;13(6):544-551.

Edokpolo LU, Stavris KB, Foster HE Jr. Intermittent catheterization and recurrent urinary tract infection in spinal cord injury. *Top Spinal Cord Inj Rehabil.* 2012;18(2):187-192.

Li L, Ye W, Ruan H, Yang B, Zhang S, Li L. Impact of hydrophilic catheters on urinary tract infections in people with spinal cord injury: systematic review and meta-analysis of randomized controlled trials. *Arch Phys Med Rehabil.* 2013;94(4):782-787.

Opperman EA. Cranberry is not effective for the prevention or treatment of urinary tract infections in individuals with spinal cord injury. *Spinal Cord.* 2010;48(6):451-456.

Urinary Stones

GENERAL PRINCIPLES

Etiology and Epidemiology

The risk of developing bladder stones after spinal cord injury (SCI) is reported to be around 35% and the risk of renal calculi around 8% to 10%. Those with upper tract stone formers are more likely to have had previous bladder stones.

The risk of renal stones in the first few months after SCI is thought to be associated with the hypercalciuria that occurs during this period, although its role in pathogenesis is unclear. Some studies show similar rates of hypercalciuria between stone formers and nonstone formers, and other factors such as urinary stasis likely play an important part even with early stones.

After the first 2 years of injury, one study found that 98% of renal stones were either magnesium ammonium phosphate (struvite) or calcium phosphate (apitate). Recurrent or chronic urinary infections are important factors in the formation of these stones. Renal stones are likely associated with the choice of bladder drainage, although reports comparing indwelling vs. intermittent catheterization in this regard are conflicting. The presence of vesico-ureteral reflux has been shown to be associated with higher risk of renal stones. While some studies have demonstrated a higher incidence in patients with complete tetraplegia compared to lower or incomplete injuries, that association may be largely explained by differences in bladder drainage options for that group.

Bladder stones are more likely to occur in those with indwelling catheters. Bladder infections and urinary stasis are also important factors. Bladder stones may also originate from stones in the upper urinary tract.

Pathophysiology

Struvite stones are associated with urinary tract infections (UTI). Irritation and inflammation of the urinary endothelium facilitates bacterial adherence to the urinary endothelium. Struvite and apitate crystals get incorporated in the bacterial biofilm. The risk is higher with urease-producing bacteria. These include *Proteus mirabilis*, although several other bacterial species also produce

300

urease. Urease catalyzes a reaction that produces ammonium and bicarbonate from breakdown of urea and water. The resulting alkaline urine promotes crystallization of struvite and apitate.

Staghorn calculi are stones that occupy the renal pelvis and extend into two or more of the renal infundibula; these are most commonly composed of struvite.

In case of bladder stones, an indwelling catheter acts as a foreign body and bacteria attach to it, forming a biofilm. The above described process involving bacterial adherence to urinary endothelium and crystallization of struvite and apitate promotes bladder stones.

Natural History

Renal calculi have been demonstrated to be among the most important factors associated with permanent deterioration in renal function in people with SCI (along with vesico-ureteral reflux and recurrent pyelonephritis). Stone size and location are also important in that regard. Staghorn calculi left untreated can severely compromise renal function on the involved side. Bladder calculi by themselves are not associated with renal failure in the absence of other urinary problems, but can serve as a nidus for infections.

CLINICAL CONSIDERATIONS

Assessment

History and Physical Examination
Classic symptoms of colic are often absent in people with SCI. One of the commonest presentations of urinary stones is recurrent or intractable UTI.

Autonomic dysreflexia (AD) may occur in those with injury above T6. Nonspecific symptoms may be the only presentation and include increased spasticity, sweating, fatigue, anorexia, or poorly localized abdominal discomfort. Nausea and vomiting may occur.

Hematuria may be present. Encrustation of an indwelling bladder catheter has been shown to be strongly suggestive of the possibility of bladder stones. Repeated catheter blockage may occur in those cases.

Diagnostic Tests
Imaging
Imaging studies identify the presence of stones, and can indicate their location, size, and presence of associated complications.

Plain radiographs can identify calcified renal stones, although less dense stones or small stones may be difficult to visualize, and may be concealed by stool in the gastrointestinal tract. Bladder stones are often not seen on plain radiographs. *Helical computed tomography* (CT) is becoming one of the imaging method of choice for urinary stones, especially in acute situations. It identifies both radiolucent and radiopaque stones, shows other abdominal pathology, has high sensitivity and specificity, and is relatively noninvasive. *Abdominal ultrasound* can demonstrate renal and bladder stones but is less specific and can miss ureteral stones. It can also identify associated renal complications such as abscess or hydronephrosis. It is an often used screening tool for urological surveillance as part of a scheduled periodic evaluation. *Intravenous pyelogram* is much less frequently used now than it was in the past. It requires potentially nephrotoxic intravenous contrast injection. *Retrograde pyelogram* can be done while performing a cystoscopy, and can potentially be used to identify stones for removal during the procedure.

Laboratory testing is done to determine renal function and to identify coexisting urinary infection.

Cystoscopy can confirm bladder stones, and potentially treat them at the same time.

Practice Pearl

Symptoms of urinary stones can be quite nonspecific in people with SCI, and overlap with presentation of other complications. It is important to consider urinary stones in the differential diagnosis of such nonspecific presentations (e.g., increasing spasticity, sweating, episodes of AD), especially in people with history of recurrent UTI.

Management

Management includes stone removal and treatment of associated complications.

Surgical Indications
Small stones that are not enlarging or associated with infection, obstruction, or impaired renal function can be observed without surgical intervention. Stones not meeting those criteria should be removed.

Preprocedure Management
Any identified urinary infection should be treated with antibiotics. While sterilization of the urine may not be possible, preprocedure antibiotic prophylaxis is usually recommended. Adequate hydration, and control of nausea, vomiting, or associated discomfort is initiated. Assessment of contractures and available range of motion may be important to plan for positioning for proper access.

If there is acute obstruction by the stone, it should be treated emergently especially in the presence of associated infection. Retrograde drainage using a ureteral catheter or stent, or antegrade drainage with a percutaneous nephrostomy tube, is done to relieve the obstruction and divert the urine.

Surgical Options for Stone Removal
Options for renal stones include percutaneous nephrolithotomy (PCNL), extracorporeal short wave lithotripsy (ESWL), or a combination of both. ESWL alone may be effective for small stones, but PCNL is indicated for stones greater than 2 cm in diameter. Large stones may require fragmentation with lithotripsy or laser prior to extraction by PCNL, and sometimes multiple procedures are needed. Complications include AD and urosepsis.

Ureteral stones may be treated ureteroscopy and lithotripsy or by ESWL.

Bladder stones are treated with cystoscopy or cystolitholapaxy (i.e., stone fragmentation prior to removal).

Open surgery is rarely performed now with the advent of less invasive surgical procedures for stone removal.

Prevention and Monitoring
Lifelong upper tract surveillance is important, especially given the often nonspecific or silent presentation of urolithiasis after SCI and the risk of significant complications including recurrent infections and renal impairment. Uniform consensus about the frequency and specifics of assessment is lacking, although most agree that periodic surveillance should include evaluation of upper tract structure and function.

KNOWLEDGE GAPS AND EMERGING CONCEPTS

Specific literature on management of urinary stones in people with SCI is quite limited, and larger studies will be helpful.

While renal failure as a cause of death after SCI has decreased dramatically with modern management and surveillance, morbidity from complications such as urolithiasis remains high and additional research is needed to further enhance preventive measures.

SUGGESTED READING

Linsenmeyer MA, Linsenmeyer TA. Accuracy of bladder stone detection using abdominal x-ray after spinal cord injury. *J Spinal Cord Med*. 2004;27(5):438-442.

Linsenmeyer MA, Linsenmeyer TA. Accuracy of predicting bladder stones based on catheter encrustation in individuals with spinal cord injury. *J Spinal Cord Med*. 2006;29(4):402-405.

Ost MC, Lee BR. Urolithiasis in patients with spinal cord injuries: risk factors, management, and outcomes. *Curr Opin Urol*. 2006;16(2):93-99.

Ramsey S, McIlhenny C. Evidence-based management of upper tract urolithiasis in the spinal cord-injured patient. *Spinal Cord*. 2011;49(9):948-954.

Welk B, Fuller A, Razvi H, Denstedt J. Renal stone disease in spinal-cord-injured patients. *J Endourol*. 2012;26(8):954-959.

CHAPTER 35

Sexual Function and Reproductive Health After SCI

GENERAL PRINCIPLES

Related Anatomy and Physiology

Neurologic Pathways (Table 35.1)
Parasympathetic Innervation
Parasympathetic innervation of the genitalia is via the pelvic nerve. The parasympathetic neurons are located in the intermediolateral column of the sacral spinal cord (S2-S4). Parasympathetic stimulation causes erection in men and genital engorgement in women.

Sympathetic Innervation
Sympathetic innervation of the genitalia is via the hypogastric nerve. Sympathetic neurons are located in the intermediolateral column of the thoracolumbar spinal cord (T10-L2). Sympathetic stimulation is primarily responsible for ejaculation in men and rhythmic contractions of the smooth muscles in the fallopian tubes and uterus with orgasm in women.

Neurophysiology of Arousal
Erections can be psychogenic or reflexogenic. Normally these two mechanisms act in synergy. Sensory stimulation of the genitals causes reflexogenic erection in men. This reflex occurs at the S2-S4 level of the spinal cord. Afferents are the pudendal nerve which carries sensory afferents from the genitals, and the efferent pathway is through the pelvic nerve as mentioned above. Psychogenic erection involves more complex pathways. In psychogenic erection, various visual, auditory, tactile, and/or imaginative afferent stimuli are processed through central pathways. After passing via different pathways, these fibers travel in the hypogastric nerve to reach the pelvic plexus, where the effect is integrated with parasympathetic function. The sympathetic nervous system, working in conjunction with the parasympathetic system, thus plays an important role in the occurrence of psychogenic erection.

In women, these pathways are similarly involved in reflex and psychogenic genital vasocongestion and lubrication.

Table 35.1

Autonomic Control of Sexual Function				
Type of Innervation	Spinal Cord Nucleus	Nerve	Physiological Effect in Men	Physiological Effect in Women
Parasympathetic	S2-S4	Pelvic	Erections (reflexogenic and psychogenic)	Genital arousal and engorgement
Sympathetic	T10-L2	Hypogastric	Involved in psychogenic erection (in conjunction with parasympathetic); and in ejaculation	Role in psychogenic arousal and lubrication

Ejaculation

Ejaculation is a neurologically more complicated phenomenon and relies on the coordination of the sympathetic (T11-L2) and parasympathetic nervous systems (S2-4) in addition to the somatic nervous system through the pudendal nerve (S2-5). Semen expulsion is produced by rhythmic contraction of the urethral smooth muscle (via sympathetic innervation) and ischiocavernosus and bulbocavernosus muscles (somatic innervation).

Biochemical Pathway for Erection

The primary neurotransmitter involved in parasympathetic-mediated erection is nitric oxide (NO). NO is released following parasympathetic stimulation, and crosses into the arteriolar smooth muscle cell. NO activates guanyl cyclase, which converts guanosine monophosphate (GMP) to cyclic GMP (cGMP), a potent vasodilator. Smooth muscle relaxation of the arterioles allows the rapid filling of the cavernous sinusoidal space. As erectile tissue of the corpora cavernosa fills with blood, the veins that drain the erectile tissue are compressed and venous outflow decreases, contributing further to the erection. Reversal of this process involves conversion of cGMP into GMP by the enzyme phosphodiesterase 5. This is the basis of using phosphodiesterase inhibitors (PDE5I) in the management of erectile dysfunction (ED).

Pathophysiology and Epidemiology

Effect of SCI on Sexual Response (Table 35.2)

Over 80% of men regain some erectile function after SCI within 2 years of injury, although the quality or sustainability of erections frequently remains impaired. The effect of spinal cord injury (SCI) on sexual function can be understood based on the above physiology (summarized in Table 35.2). Complete SCI involving the sacral S2-S4 level is expected to result in loss of reflex erection in men. Reflex erection is spared in SCI above the sacral level. Psychogenic erections are generally absent in SCI at or above T10, but often preserved with injury below T10-L2. In women, similar generalizations apply to the effect of SCI on reflex and psychogenic lubrication.

Table 35.2
Predicting Sexual Dysfunction Based on SCI Level and Completeness[a]

With complete supra-sacral (UMN) injury, reflex erections are preserved in 90% of men

With complete SCI above T10, psychogenic erections are typically absent; with supra-sacral injury, but below T10-L2 (i.e., exam findings of preserved sensation in T10-L2 dermatomes), psychogenic erections are often preserved

With complete sacral (LMN) SCI (absent bulbocavernosus reflex and anal wink response on exam) reflex erections are absent; psychogenic erections may be present in about 25%

With incomplete SCI, the more incomplete the injury is, the greater the likelihood of preserved reflex and psychogenic erections

Similar generalizations likely apply to the effect of SCI on reflex and psychogenic genital engorgement and lubrication in women, although have been less extensively studied

Spontaneous ejaculation in men with complete SCI above T11 is rare. Ejaculation can occur in about 20% of men with complete SCI below that level, generally in those with retained psychogenic erections

[a]Even in those with some preserved erectile function after SCI, impairment in the quality or sustainability of erections is common.

Preservation of sensation in T10-L2 dermatomes has been associated with preservation of psychogenic arousal as indicated by genital engorgement in women and erections in men. Reflex genital arousal has been associated preservation of intact reflex function (bulbocavernosus reflex, anal wink) in the S2-S4 dermatomes. In those with incomplete SCI, the more incomplete the injury is, the greater the likelihood of reflex and psychogenic erections and ejaculation in men and genital lubrication and orgasm in women.

Overall, after SCI the ability to ejaculate spontaneously is present in less than 10% of men with complete SCI. Ejaculation in men with complete SCI above T10 is rare. Ejaculation can occur in about 20% of men with complete SCI below that level, generally in those with retained psychogenic erections. Positive indications about ability to ejaculate after SCI either with self or partner stimulation include incomplete injury, degree of genital sensation and voluntary anal control, and presence of a strong bulbocavernosus reflex.

Other Factors Affecting Sexual Function in SCI
In addition to the direct effect of SCI on sexual response, other factors can significantly affect sexual function. These include pain, spasticity, difficulty positioning, impaired hand function, neurogenic bowel and bladder-related issues, and psychological/emotional issues related to depression, self-esteem, or relationships.

Semen Abnormalities and Male Fertility
Impaired sperm motility is common after SCI, even though sperm concentration is less affected. The causes are likely multifactorial and not fully understood.

Stasis of the semen associated with seminal vesicle dysfunction has been documented. Elevated cytokine and leukocyte levels in semen have been reported, suggesting an inflammatory component. Other factors such as scrotal hyperthermia have been suggested, but their significance is unclear. The method of obtaining semen may itself contribute to some semen abnormalities. Only a small percent of men with SCI are able to father children without medical intervention.

Menstruation and Female Fertility
Temporary cessation of menses is typical after SCI, but normal menstruation is restored within 6 to 12 months in most women. While not well studied, fertility after that period is assumed to be normal. There are several SCI-related factors that impact pregnancy and labor, which are discussed later in this chapter.

CLINICAL CONSIDERATIONS

The clinical practice guideline on *Sexuality and Reproductive Health in Adults with Spinal Cord Injury* developed by the Consortium for Spinal Cord Medicine provides excellent guidance on this topic.

Based on consideration of individual readiness to discuss such information, the subject should be approached in a straightforward and nonjudgmental manner during the course of rehabilitation, with open-ended questions that encourage ongoing dialogue. Referral to professionals with additional expertise in this area should be made at the appropriate time. A suggested framework for intervention related to sexuality is the PLISSIT model. PLISSIT is an acronym for four levels of intervention: Permission, Limited Information, Specific Suggestions, and Intensive Therapy (Table 35.3).

Due attention to privacy and respect for professional boundaries is especially important at all times when addressing a sensitive topic like sexual function.

Assessment

History and Physical Examination
Assessment of neurological factors and medical conditions that can impact sexual function is an important aspect of evaluation. A detailed neurological, musculoskeletal, and functional assessment should be conducted. Examination using the International Standards for Neurological Classification of Spinal Cord Injury (ISNCSCI), should include special attention to the preservation of sensation from T10-L2 and S2-5 along with determination of the presence of voluntary anal contraction and reflexes to assess sexual function.

Medical comorbidities such as diabetes, cardiovascular disease, chronic pain, and drug or alcohol use, should be evaluated. Current medications are also important to consider since several, including drugs for depression or spasticity, can affect sexual function.

Table 35.3

The PLISSIT Model as a Framework for Intervention Related to Sexuality

Level of Intervention	Description
Permission	Creating an atmosphere in which it is clear to individuals that discussion about sex will be well received
Limited Information	This relates to an individual's readiness to receive information regarding the impact of his or her specific condition on sexual expression; it will vary from one individual to another. Some may want health care providers to do nothing more than clear up misconceptions; others may be ready for more detailed information about their sexual function
Specific Suggestions	Refers to suggestions aimed at specific sexual difficulties. This level may require advanced knowledge and clinical skill on the part of the provider because it involves obtaining a detailed sexual history, identifying specific problems, and setting goals for specific interventions, education, or compensatory strategies
Intensive therapy	Requires referral to a specialist with formal training and documented competence in sex therapy, sexuality counseling, or psychotherapy

Referral to the psychologist or appropriate provider with expertise should be considered, for assessment of relevant emotional and psychological factors, including depression, previous experiences and relationships, and current relationships.

International Standards to document remaining Autonomic Function after Spinal Cord Injury (ISAFSCI), published by the American Spinal Injuries Association, include guidance about specific documentation of sexual function. For sexual function it is recommended that the presence of psychogenic genital arousal (penile erection or vaginal lubrication) is recorded as well as documentation of reflex genital arousal. Ability to achieve orgasm is recorded.

The presence of antegrade ejaculation is documented for males. The ability to sense menses (cramping, pain, etc.) relative to before injury is documented for females.

Management

It is important to address the issue of sexual function in the context of the whole person, rather than as an isolated physiological phenomenon. As appropriate, opportunities should be provided to include the individual's partner in discussions and education. Promotion of healthy relationships, self-esteem, and intimacy, are an integral part of the overall management.

Practical Consideration Regarding Sexual Activity After SCI
Several factors related to SCI can pose practical challenges for sexual activity, and should be addressed with education, advice, and assistance as appropriate.

These include issues with positioning, bladder and bowel function, risk of autonomic dysreflexia (AD), and skin breakdown (Table 35.4).

Treatment of ED

ED in men with SCI should be treated with the least invasive methods before prescribing interventions that may produce an adverse reaction. The full range of options should be discussed, with development of an individualized treatment plan.

Phosphodiesterase Type 5 Inhibitors

PDE5I are highly effective in the SCI population, except for those individuals with cauda equina and conus medullaris injuries. They are generally safe and well tolerated by men with SCI, and are often the first choice option. Absolute contraindications include the concomitant use of nitrates (e.g., nitropaste to treat AD), certain alpha blockers, or the presence of retinitis pigmentosa. Sildenafil was the initially approved medication, and subsequently vardenafil and tadalafil have been approved for ED.

Intra-Cavernosal Injections

Intracavernosal injections are commonly used when oral medications are ineffective. An injection of alprostadil (prostaglandin E1 or alprostadil with various combinations of papaverine and phentolamine) is injected by the person with SCI or his partner. Dose is titrated to the level to allow for an erection to occur within 5 to 10 minutes and last approximately 1 hour. Maintaining pressure on the site for several minutes reduces penile scarring at the injection site. Priapism is a potential complication.

Table 35.4
Practical Advice Regarding Sexual Activity in People With SCI

Complete bladder and bowel care prior to sexual activity and explore contingency plans, as necessary, if incontinence should occur. Special measures may be needed if using indwelling catheter or condom for bladder drainage.

Inspect insensate skin surfaces, particularly around the genitalia and buttocks, immediately after sexual activity as these areas may have received excessive friction, pressure, or tears.

People with SCI at T6 or above have the potential to experience autonomic dysreflexia (AD) with sexual activity. If AD is experienced, the sexual activity should stop and the person should sit up immediately, and seek treatment. The use of prophylactic medications for AD prior to activity may be considered.

May need to experiment with/learn about optimal positioning during sexual activity and/or about obtaining assistance from caregivers in preparation. Safety issues to prevent injury during sexual activity should be reinforced, as appropriate.

Understand risk for acquiring or transmitting sexually transmitted diseases, and take appropriate preventive measures

Vacuum Device
With this device, a vacuum is created in a tube placed over the penis that causes blood to fill the corporal chambers of the penis. When the penis achieves a satisfactory degree of rigidity, an elastic penile ring is slipped off the tube and placed over the base of the penis to maintain the erection. The constriction ring should never be left in place for more than 30 minutes. The device requires some degree of manual dexterity or partner assistance. Complaints include unnatural erections and lack of spontaneity. Use of anticoagulant medication is a contraindication.

Intra-Urethral Medications
Intra-urethral vasodilators, most often alprostadil, have been used, but are relatively ineffective in SCI and are now seldom prescribed.

Penile Implants
These can be very effective, but are typically the last resort since they cause irreversible damage to penile tissue. There are two types of implants: a silicone malleable prosthesis and an inflatable hydraulic prosthesis.

Evaluation and Treatment of Testosterone Deficiency
Testosterone deficiency occurs in a higher rate in men with SCI; evaluation should be considered in men presenting with suppressed libido, reduced strength, fatigue, or poor response to PDE5I for erection enhancement, to determine if testosterone replacement is indicated.

However, it is important to be aware that exogenous testosterone replacement will suppress spermatogenesis and therefore should not be the treatment of choice in hypogonadal men with SCI who wish to pursue biological fatherhood.

Options for Assisted Fertility and Fatherhood
Assistance with fertility for biological fatherhood is often necessary in men with SCI. Semen analysis should be performed in such cases. For men with incomplete lesions, natural ejaculation and insemination with vaginal intercourse may be possible. For couples considering pregnancy, factors such as semen retrieval, quality of semen, partner fertility, and availability and affordability of assisted reproductive techniques (ART) need to be considered.

Options for semen retrieval (in order of least invasiveness and preference as initial options) include natural ejaculation with self or partner masturbation, vibratory stimulation, electroejaculation, and surgical sperm retrieval. AD can occur with both vibratory stimulation and electroejaculation with SCI above T6. Surgical sperm retrieval can be used if less invasive procedures are not possible or are ineffective. ARTs involve processing the retrieved sperm for placement in the uterus or extracting individual sperm to combine with extracted eggs for in vitro fertilization (IVF) and/or intracytoplasmic sperm injection.

Reproductive Health in Women With SCI
Preventive Health
Women with SCI should have full access to recommended preventive health care services and routine gynecological procedures and screenings; barriers should be identified and addressed as feasible.

Birth Control
Options should be discussed to identify the safest feasible birth control method for women with SCI. One of the preferred options for birth control in women with SCI is condom use by the partner. Other options include permanent sterilization and oral contraceptive pills. Hormonal birth control must be prescribed with caution and avoided altogether in women within 1 year of injury. Barrier methods, such as intrauterine devices, are associated with higher risk of pelvic inflammatory disease, which is increased in women with SCI due to frequent urinary tract infections and the inability to detect pain. Diaphragms and cervical caps require hand dexterity, and may create vaginal wall breakdown.

Pregnancy
Information should be provided about fertility and pregnancy. In some cases, adoption may be a preferred option to complete a family. Issues of child-rearing should be considered before proceeding with pregnancy. Prenatal care should begin early. Extra assistance may be needed during pregnancy for transfers, dressing, monitoring skin surfaces, and bowel and bladder care. Weight gain, skin breakdown, immobility, incontinence, digestion issues, and respiratory difficulties may be problems during pregnancy. Proper adjustment of wheelchair seating throughout pregnancy is crucial, with the need to progressively increase the seat-to-back angle to allow for the increasing abdominal mass.

Labor and Delivery
Premature delivery is relatively common. Frequent checks for effacement and dilation of the cervix should begin at 28 weeks of gestation. Diminished sensation and absence of pain may result in unrecognized conventional labor symptoms, especially in women with SCI at T10 and above. One of the most critical complications of labor and delivery is AD in women with SCI above T6. AD must be differentiated from preeclampsia (where blood pressure elevation is persistent, rather than episodic as in AD). Epidural anesthesia is usually the recommended method to prevent and reduce AD risk during labor and delivery.

KNOWLEDGE GAPS AND EMERGING CONCEPTS

Research is being done on new drugs to treat ED, including new PGE5I that may be more selective than the currently available agents and cause less hypotension and cardiovascular side effects. There is a need for better outcome measures to assess the efficacy of interventions for sexual dysfunction. Additional areas of investigation include further study of mechanisms and potential treatments for sperm abnormalities in men with SCI.

SUGGESTED READING

American Spinal Injury Association. International standards to document remaining autonomic function after spinal cord injury (ISAFSCI). *Spinal Cord.* 2012; Atlanta, GA.

Brackett NL, Lynne CM, Ibrahim E, Ohl DA, Sønksen J. Treatment of infertility in men with spinal cord injury. *Nat Rev Urol.* 2010;7(3):162-172.

Brown DJ, Hill ST, Baker HW. Male fertility and sexual function after spinal cord injury. *Prog Brain Res.* 2006;152:427-439.

Consortium for Spinal Cord Medicine. Sexuality and reproductive health in adults with spinal cord injury: a clinical practice guideline for health-care professionals. *J Spinal Cord Med.* 2010;33(3):281-336.

Dimitriadis F, Karakitsios K, Tsounapi P, et al. Erectile function and male reproduction in men with spinal cord injury: a review. *Andrologia.* 2010;42(3):139-165.

Elliott SL. Problems of sexual function after spinal cord injury. *Prog Brain Res.* 2006;152: 387-399.

Everaert K, de Waard WI, Van Hoof T, Kiekens C, Mulliez T, D'herde C. Neuroanatomy and neurophysiology related to sexual dysfunction in male neurogenic patients with lesions to the spinal cord or peripheral nerves. *Spinal Cord.* 2010;48(3):182-191.

Rizio N, Tran C, Sorenson M. Efficacy and satisfaction rates of oral PDE5 is in the treatment of erectile dysfunction secondary to spinal cord injury: a review of literature. *J Spinal Cord Med.* 2012;35(4):219-228.

CHAPTER 36

Gastrointestinal Consequences: Overview

GENERAL PRINCIPLES

Gastrointestinal (GI) problems are common after spinal cord injury (SCI), and an important cause of morbidity and mortality. The neurogenic bowel, one of the most significant GI consequences of SCI, is discussed in Chapter 36A along with its related complications.

In addition there are several GI issues that involve the upper gastrointestinal tract as a direct or indirect result of SCI. These are summarized in Table 36.1.

CLINICAL CONSIDERATIONS

SCI also has an effect on presentation, diagnosis, and management of abdominal emergencies and acute abdomen (Table 36.2). Mortality after an acute abdominal emergency is reported to be higher than average and high index of suspicion is necessary to avoid missed or delayed diagnosis.

SCI can affect colon cancer screening. False positive results may occur with blood testing in the presence of hemorrhoids which are more prevalent in people with SCI (Chapter 36A). While bowel preparation for colonoscopy is more difficult than usual, it is important to comply with guidelines for colon cancer screening as in the general population.

Table 36.1

Upper Gastrointestinal Tract-Related Problems in SCI	
Condition	Considerations
Poor dental hygiene	- Individuals with tetraplegia have difficulty performing dental hygiene due to impaired upper extremity function, contributing to an increased prevalence of dental and gum disease
	(continued)

313

Table 36.1
Upper Gastrointestinal Tract-Related Problems in SCI (*continued*)

Condition	Considerations
	- An additional contributing factor to potential for dental problems is reduced access to dental care, since only some dental offices are able to accommodate power wheelchairs
Dysphagia	- Dysphagia is common during the acute and initial rehabilitation phase in people with tetraplegia - Risk factors include the presence of a tracheostomy, mechanical ventilation, spinal surgery via an anterior approach, and increased age - Swallowing evaluation, and appropriate swallowing precautions, are indicated in these circumstances
GERD	- Reduced gastroesophageal sphincter tone, increased acid secretion, medications, recumbency, and immobilization may contribute to a higher incidence of GERD in people with tetraplegia - Characteristic symptoms of heartburn may be absent
Erosive gastritis and ulcers	- Increased risk, especially with higher level and completeness of injury, during the acute phase - Intact gastric vagal innervation with loss of sympathetic innervation may contribute by increasing gastric acid secretion - Stress ulcer prophylaxis is indicated for the first 4 weeks after SCI, with PPIs or histamine H2-receptor antagonists, but should not be continued indiscriminately since the risk greatly diminishes. Prolonged PPI use has been associated with increased *Clostridium difficile* infection
Impaired gastric motility	- May lead to early satiety and epigastric bloating
SMA syndrome	- SMA syndrome is a rare condition in which the third portion of the duodenum is intermittently compressed by the overlying SMA - Predisposing factors include: rapid weight loss (loss of mesenteric fat that separates the duodenum from the SMA), use of a constricting body jacket/orthosis, and prolonged supine positioning - Symptoms include epigastric pain, fullness, and vomiting, especially when supine - Barium study shows a cutoff between the third and fourth portions of the duodenum in the supine position - Management includes: upright positioning for meals, assuming the side-lying position (vs. supine) after eating, and restoration of lost weight. Surgery is rarely indicated
Pancreatitis	- Acute pancreatitis risk may be increased in acute injury possibly due to parasympathetic predominance and sphincter of Oddi dysfunction. High dose steroids, if given after acute SCI, may increase risk

(continued)

Condition	Considerations
	- Symptoms may be absent in tetraplegia. Diagnosis is supported by lab testing (amylase, lipase)
Gall bladder disease	- Prevalence may be increased though is not established
	- Bile stasis due to impaired sympathetic innervation, impaired enterohepatic circulation, and altered biliary lipid excretion are proposed theoretical reasons
	- May not present with classic symptoms due to sensory loss

Abbreviations: SCI, spinal cord injury; GERD, gastro-esophageal reflux disease; PPI, proton pump inhibitors; SMA, superior mesenteric artery.

Table 36.2
Acute Abdomen After SCI: Special Considerations

Pain and tenderness may be absent or atypical (e.g., only referred to shoulder) in patients with cervical or high thoracic injury

Loss of motor and reflex function may mask rigidity and guarding

Rigidity may also be difficult to evaluate in the presence of abdominal spasticity

High index of suspicion is warranted to avoid missed or delayed diagnosis

The presence of nausea, vomiting, or nonspecific malaise may be the only clinical symptoms

Low grade fever or tachycardia may be the only clinical findings

Bowel sounds may be increased, decreased, or absent depending on the pathology

May present with increased spasticity

The presentation may include autonomic dysreflexia in people with injury above T6

A low threshold for lab testing and imaging (abdominal ultrasound, computed tomography) is warranted for nonspecific findings that are not readily explained

SUGGESTED READING

Chen D, Nussbaum SB. The gastrointestinal system and bowel management following spinal cord injury. *Phys Med Rehabil Clin N Am.* 2000;11(1):45-56.

Ebert E. Gastrointestinal involvement in spinal cord injury: a clinical perspective. *J Gastrointestin Liver Dis.* 2012;21(1):75-82.

Enck P, Greving I, Klosterhalfen S, Wietek B. Upper and lower gastrointestinal motor and sensory dysfunction after human spinal cord injury. *Prog Brain Res.* 2006;152:373-384.

Gondim FA, de Oliveira GR, Thomas FP. Upper gastrointestinal motility changes following spinal cord injury. *Neurogastroenterol Motil.* 2010;22(1):2-6.

Kirshblum S, Johnston MV, Brown J, O'Connor KC, Jarosz P. Predictors of dysphagia after spinal cord injury. *Arch Phys Med Rehabil.* 1999;80(9):1101-1105.

Shem K, Castillo K, Wong S, Chang J. Dysphagia in individuals with tetraplegia: incidence and risk factors. *J Spinal Cord Med.* 2011;34(1):85-92.

Neurogenic Bowel

GENERAL PRINCIPLES

Anatomy and Physiology of the Bowel

Colon Anatomy
The colon extends from the ileocaecal sphincter to the anal sphincter. The internal anal sphincter (IAS) consists of smooth muscle. The external anal sphincter (EAS) is composed of striated muscle, and contracts with the pelvic floor. Puborectalis muscle loops around the proximal rectum and maintains the nearly 90° anorectal angle.

Innervation of the Colon (Table 36A.1)
The innervation of the colon is both extrinsic (parasympathetic, sympathetic, and somatic) and intrinsic (myenteric and submucosal plexus). The specifics of these different innervations are summarized in Table 36A.1.

Colonic Reflexes (Table 36A.2)
Colonic reflexes play an important role in the pathophysiology and are the basis of several aspects of bowel management after spinal cord injury (SCI), so it is important to understand their underlying mechanisms and relevance in SCI.

Important colon reflexes are summarized in Table 36A.2. The gastrocolic, colocolonic, and rectocolic reflexes stimulate colon mobility. The recto-anal inhibitory reflex (RAIR) and anorectal excitatory reflex are involved in defecation. EAS and puborectalis muscle (voluntary) contraction prevents defecation and maintains continence in the presence of rectal contraction; this is also known as the holding reflex.

Colon Physiology
The functions of the colon include:

Storage: The colon forms and contains stool, supports symbiotic bacteria, and secretes mucus for fecal lubrication.
Propulsion: This is under chemical control (neurotransmitters, hormones), local neurogenic control (enteric nervous system), and facilitated

Table 36A.1

Innervation of the Colon

Type of Innervation	Nerve Supply	Effect on the Bowel
Parasympathetic	Vagus nerve (Cranial X) up to splenic flexure; Pelvic nerve (S2-S4) from splenic flexure to anal sphincter	Increased peristalsis and gut motility;Increased secretions;Relaxation of smooth muscle sphincters
Sympathetic	Hypogastric nerve (T10-L2)	Decreased peristalsis and gut motility;Decreased secretions;Contraction of smooth muscle sphincters
Somatic	Pudendal nerve (S2-S5)	Contraction of external anal sphincter (EAS) and pelvic floor
Intrinsic	Myenteric (Auerbach) plexus between inner circular and outer longitudinal layers of the colon wall;	Control of tone and rhythmic contractility, assisting in stool propulsion throughout the colon
	Submucosal (Meissner) plexus	Controls intestinal secretion and absorption

Table 36A.2

Colon Reflexes

Reflex	Mediation	Effect	Relevance in SCI
Gastrocolic reflex	Cholinergic	Increased colonic activity after a meal	Reported to be present, exaggerated, or decreased after SCI; provides the basis for performing bowel program after a meal
Colocolonic reflex	Mediated by the myenteric plexus	Causes colonic smooth muscle above the dilation to constrict and below the dilation to relax, thus facilitating caudal stool propulsion	Preserved in neurogenic bowel

(continued)

Table 36A.2

Colon Reflexes (*continued*)			
Reflex	Mediation	Effect	Relevance in SCI
Rectocolic reflex	Mediated by the pelvic nerve	Causes colonic peristalsis in response to mechanical or chemical stimulation of the rectum or anus	Preserved in UMN neurogenic bowel. provides the basis for use of digital stimulation or suppositories for bowel program
Recto-anal inhibitory reflex (RAIR)	Is an entero-enteric response, mediated by the myenteric plexus	Rectal distension with stool causes relaxation of internal anal sphincter, initiates defecation through rectal contraction	Preserved in SCI since it is independent of spinal control
Anorectal excitatory reflex		Maintains rectal contraction (and defection) as stool passes through the anal canal	

by extrinsic reflex pathways (facilitatory via parasympathetic, rectocolic reflex).

Continence: The closed IAS and acute angle of the anorectal canal in resting helps in maintaining continence. Sympathetic (L1-L2) discharges increase IAS tone. *Defecation:* Begins with involuntary advancement of stool into rectum. The RAIR causes decreased IAS tone with rectal dilation. There is an urge to defecate from rectal and puborectalis stretch. Willful defecation occurs with voluntary EAS and puborectalis relaxation. Stool passage is driven by peristalsis and increased abdominal pressure (Valsalva).

Pathophysiology of Neurogenic Bowel

SCI impacts bowel activity through multiple mechanisms that include: temporary loss/depression of reflex activity (e.g., spinal shock), effect on colo-rectal compliance and mobility, increased colonic transit times, and alterations in anal sphincter control.

There are similarities between the genitourinary and gastrointestinal (GI) tracts in terms of smooth internal and striated external sphincters, innervation, blood supply, and response to cholinergic and adrenergic stimuli. So it follows that those with difficulty in micturition associated with neurogenic bladder are also likely to experience problems with defecation.

Upper Motor Neuron and Lower Motor Neuron Bowel (Table 36A.3)

Depending on the level of SCI and the related impairments, neurogenic bowel may be reflexic or areflexic.

Reflexic or Upper Motor Neuron (UMN) Bowel
Characteristics include:

- Injury above sacral segments (S2-S4) of the spinal cord
- People with SCI above T5 lack functioning abdominal muscles and generate abdominal pressure by intercostals and diaphragmatic contraction; those with cervical SCI rely solely on diaphragmatic contraction
- Reflex coordination of stool propulsions is preserved with intact nerve connections between spinal cord and colon. Rectal distension causes brief EAS contraction, which prevents leakage
- Bowel is hyperreflexic and there is reduced rectal compliance
- Stool retention occurs due to inability to voluntarily initiate defecation with EAS relaxation, pelvic spasticity
- Transit time is prolonged
- Typically results in constipation and mild incontinence

Areflexic or Lower Motor Neuron (LMN) Bowel
Characteristics include:

- Injury at sacral segments (conus medullaris) or cauda equina (or pelvic nerves)
- Loss of spinal cord mediated reflex peristalsis
- Myenteric plexus coordinates slow stool propulsion
- Sluggish stool movement; dryer, rounder shape (scybalous)

Table 36A.3

Upper Motor Neuron (UMN) vs. Lower Motor Neuron (LMN) Bowel		
Characteristic	UMN Bowel	LMN Bowel
Level of injury	Above sacral segments of the spinal cord	Sacral spinal cord (conus medullaris), cauda equina, or pelvic nerve
Pathophysiology	Reflex bowel contractions present, hyperreflexic, dysrhythmic contractions	Loss of spinal cord mediated reflex peristalsis, sluggish stool movement
Primary symptoms	Constipation, fecal incontinence is typically mild	Constipation, fecal incontinence, increased stool frequency, dry round (scybalous) stool

(continued)

Table 36A.3

Upper Motor Neuron (UMN) vs. Lower Motor Neuron (LMN) Bowel (continued)

Characteristic	UMN Bowel	LMN Bowel
Examination findings	Pelvic and external anal sphincter spasticity	Hypotonic, patulous anal sphincter
Management:		
Desired stool consistency	Soft formed stool	Firm (though not hard) stool
Bowel program frequency	Every 1–3 days	Daily (sometimes more often)
Rectal stimulation	Rectal suppository and/ or digital stimulation to initiate defecation	Rectal suppository and digital stimulation are often not effective
Manual evacuation of stool	Typically not routinely needed (though may be done prior to suppository insertion to facilitate contact with rectal mucosa or in case of complications such as fecal impaction)	Often needed as part of the bowel program. Involves insertion of lubricated gloved fingers to hook or break up stool in rectum and pull it out
Valsalva maneuver	Less often used than with LMN bowel	Gentle Valsalva maneuver, with bladder emptied prior to avoid vescico-ureteral reflux may be used to assist elimination by increasing intra-abdominal pressure

- Hypotonic anal sphincter and levator ani muscles with risk of fecal incontinence
- Typically results in constipation, incontinence, and increased frequency of defecation

Differences between UMN and LMN bowel are summarized in Table 36A.3.

Complications of Neurogenic Bowel

Complications of the neurogenic bowel include constipation, fecal impaction, diarrhea, rectal bleeding, and hemorrhoids. Assessment and management of these complications are discussed later in this chapter.

Autonomic dysreflexia (AD) may result from constipation or other complications of neurogenic bowel in people with SCI above the T6 neurological level.

Decreased respiratory excursion may occur with abdominal distension.

Table 36A.4

Elements of a Typical Bowel Program for an UMN Bowel (Goals: Predictable and Effective Elimination; Minimize Complications, Compatible With the Individual's Lifestyle)

Individualize for each person, while following the general principles below

Consistent schedule established, performed at around the same time each day (to develop a habitual, predictable response)

Frequency: daily or every other day (depending on amount and type of diet and fluid intake, type of bowel impairment, individual variations, and preinjury patterns of elimination)

Food or liquid taken about 30 min prior (to make use of gastrocolic reflex)

Seated position preferred when feasible (vs in bed) to utilize gravity (faster, more effective), otherwise side-lying

Digital stimulation and/or rectal suppository to initiate defecation using the least noxious stimulation that is effective; digital stimulation (lubricated finger moved slowly in a clockwise manner) usually performed for 15–20 secs, repeated every 5–10 mins if needed

Use appropriate adaptive equipment needed for bowel care (e.g., padded commode or shower chair based on level of injury, digital bowel stimulator or suppository inserter for those with impaired hand function)

Individualized assistive techniques may be used in some instances to aid bowel emptying (e.g., abdominal massage, deep breathing, or ingestion of warm fluids)

Medications (not always needed): stool softener (e.g., docusate sodium 100 mg three times a day), peristaltic stimulant (e.g., senna), and docusate suppository (see Table 36A.5)

Maintain skin and fall precautions during bowel care

Ensure adequate education and training

Monitor effectiveness and adherence

Modify as/if needed to simplify or to increase effectiveness; maintain 3–5 cycles (in the absence of adverse reactions and complications) before making changes; change one element at a time

CLINICAL CONSIDERATIONS

Assessment

History

Key elements of patient history include premorbid gastro-intestinal function and medical conditions, current bowel program (including satisfaction), current bowel related symptoms, defecation frequency and duration, stool character, and medication use. Fluid intake, diet, and activity level should be assessed.

There should be a systemic assessment of bowel function, including: time of day, frequency, assistance required, and duration, facilitative techniques, type of rectal stimulation, medications for bowel function, characteristics of stool (amount, consistency, color, mucus, presence of blood), and presence or absence of desire to have a bowel movement. Signals of upcoming defecation may include abdominal pressure, prickling sensation, increased spasticity, goose bumps, or sweating.

Difficulties with evacuation should be evaluated, including inquiry about delayed or painful evacuations, constipation, diarrhea, and unplanned evacuations or fecal incontinence.

Symptoms of AD may sometimes result from constipation or other complications of neurogenic bowel.

Fecal impaction or other abdominal pathology may present with atypical or nonspecific symptoms such as anorexia and nausea.

Physical Examination
Abdomen examination includes inspection for distension, hernia, or other abnormalities; palpation for any hard stool, tenderness, or masses; percussion; and auscultation of bowel sounds.

The anal orifice should be examined. It may be patulous or gaping (e.g., due to trauma or distension). The anocutaneous reflex (mediated by the pudendal nerve, S2-S4) is checked by tugging perianal hair or stroking with a broken swab stick. It should be checked bilaterally.

Perianal pin-prick sensation should be checked.

Digital rectal exam should be done to check for deep anal pressure, presence of the palpable ridge of the puborectalis muscular sling, voluntary anal contraction, bulbocavernosus reflex, and the presence of stool, hemorrhoids, or masses.

International Standards to document remaining Autonomic Function after SCI (ISAFSCI) specify the following as recommended surrogate measures of autonomic control of the distal bowel: sensation of the need for bowel movement, continence of stool, and presence of voluntary sphincter contraction during anorectal examination.

Functional assessment is important in determination of the most appropriate bowel program. It should include evaluation of the ability to learn, ability to direct others, sitting tolerance, sitting balance, upper extremity strength, sensation, function, transfer skills, presence and risk of skin breakdown. Home accessibility and equipment needs should be assessed.

Diagnostic Tests
A flat plate abdominal radiograph can show feces and abnormal gas patterns in case of fecal impaction.

Stool testing for occult blood should be done age 50 and above as part of colon cancer screening, although false positive results can occur due to hemorrhoids. Colonoscopy is another option for cancer screening but requires good preprocedure bowel preparation for proper visualization of the colon mucosa.

Other tests may be indicated in special circumstances, for example, in investigating obscure cause of symptoms, or when contemplating bowel surgery. Stool examination for leukocytes, pathogens, and clostridium difficile toxin may be indicated when investigating unexplained diarrhea.

Management

Bowel program in people with SCI should be comprehensive, individualized (based on neurological impairment, needs, availability of caregiver assistance, use of adaptive equipment, activity level, and lifestyle), and patient-centered.

Goals of a scheduled bowel program are: to achieve effective, predictable, and efficient elimination, prevent fecal incontinence, and minimize complications.

Components of a Bowel Program (See Table 36A.4)
Diet
The diet should have adequate fiber content but should be individualized. It is not recommended that patients automatically be placed on high fiber diets. Diet having greater than 15 gm fiber may be started initially, and then titrated. Effect of high fiber diet in SCI is debated with conflicting results in different studies. Some reports suggest that higher levels of fiber increased rather than decreased gastro-intestinal transit time in people with SCI. Foods that cause flatulence or adversely affect stool consistency should be identified and avoided if possible.

Fluids
Fluid needs for stool consistency have to be balanced with fluid intake parameters for bladder management. Increased fluid intake helps prevent hard, impacted stool. However, the frequency of intermitted catheterization may need to be increased to avoid bladder over-distension from the increased fluid intake.

Physical Activity
Movement causes mechanical stimulation and may increase intestinal peristalsis, so regular physical activity is helpful.

Scheduled Bowel Care
A consistent schedule for elimination should be established based on factors that influence elimination, preinjury patterns of elimination, attendant care, personal goals, and lifestyle considerations. Bowel care should be scheduled at the same time of the day. A frequency of at least once every 2 days is recommended to avoid chronic colorectal distension. As much as feasible, the goal should be to keep the time to complete an established bowel program less than 45 to 60 minutes.

Triggering of defecation is done with digital stimulation, glycerin suppository, or if needed, bisacodyl suppository. These are often administered 20 to 30 minutes after a meal (to utilize the gastro-colic reflex) and having the patient attempt defecation after 10 minutes. Individualized assistive techniques may be helpful in facilitating defecation. Seating for upright bowel care should be done when feasible to make use of gravity and the mechanical advantage for abdominal muscles to facilitate defecation in the seated position.

The program should be initiated in acute care and continued throughout life. Simplification of the program can be considered if elimination occurs consistently with no unplanned evacuations in between. Monitoring program effectiveness and assessment of adherence to treatment is important, with revisions to the program as/if needed. Typically at least 3 to 5 cycles of bowel care are needed to assess adequacy after each revision, before making additional changes.

Manual Evacuation of Stool (for LMN Bowel)
The recto-colic reflex is impaired in patients with LMN injury who typically have an areflexic bowel, so triggering of bowel care by digital stimulation or suppository is often not effective. Manual evacuation of the stool done daily or more frequently is often required in these cases for adequate elimination and to reduce incontinence between scheduled evacuations (Table 36A.3).

Patient and Caregiver Education
Education of both patients and caregivers is crucial. The educational program should encompass, anatomy, process of defecation, the effect of SCI on bowel function, goals and rationale of the bowel program, measures to facilitate regular and effective elimination, the involved techniques, and prevention, recognition, and managements of related complications.

Medications to Aid Bowel Function (Table 36A.5)
Oral medications may help to facilitate bowel care, though are not always required. Medications include stool softeners (e.g., docusate), bulk forming agents that can stimulate peristalsis through increased stool bulk, peristaltic

Table 36A.5

Bowel Medications			
Medication Class	Drug Examples/ Dosage	Mechanism of Action	Side Effects/ Considerations
Stool softeners	Docusate sodium (Colace); docusate calcium (Surfak)	Emulsify fat and decrease water absorption in colon, so increase water content of stool to make it soft	Adequate fluid intake is necessary, have to balance intake with bladder management considerations

(continued)

Medication Class	Drug Examples/ Dosage	Mechanism of Action	Side Effects/ Considerations
Bulk forming agents	Psyllium (Fibercon, Metamucil, Naturacil), calcium polycarbophil (Fibercon), methylcellulose (Citrucel)	Increase stool bulk by absorbing water	Diarrhea with excess use; risk of bowel obstruction if fluid intake not adequate
Peristaltic stimulants and prokinetic agents	Senna (Senokot)	Directly stimulates Auerbach plexus to induce colonic peristalsis	Melanosis coli (staining of colonic mucosa seen on colonoscopy), decreased responsiveness over time may lead to atonic bowel;Prokinetic agent, cisapride was taken off the market due to serious cardiac arrhythmias
Contact irritants	Bisacodyl (Dulcolax) oral tablet, suppository, and enema	Increase colonic peristalsis by direct irritation or stimulation of the colonic mucosa	Oral form is not recommended for regular use and reserved for occasional use only when there are problems with the bowel program. Suppository: Polyethylene glycol (PGB) based bisacocodyl suppository or in a combination small-volume mini-enema have been shown to be more effective than hydrogenated vegetable oil-based bisacodyl suppositories in some studies.

stimulants (e.g., senna), and contact irritants (e.g., bisacodyl). Information about these medications, including mechanism of action, side effects, and other considerations are summarized in Table 36A.5.

Other Interventions
Biofeedback has been tried but is of questionable effectiveness. Pulsed irrigation evacuation (with warm tap water pulses administered rectally) has been used in children and more recently, in adults. While there are some reports of effectiveness, it needs to be further evaluated before routine use can be recommended.

Surgical Options
Surgical options in intractable cases include colostomy, or appendicocecostomy to create an antegrade continence enema (ACE) (Malone procedure). Surgical decision-making and planning involves interdisciplinary evaluation and input, ensuring that suitable nonsurgical options have given adequate trial, and the individual's expectations, goals, and limitations.

ACE or the Malone procedure involves bringing the appendix to the abdominal wall after mobilizing the colon, and amputating its tip to create a catheterizable stoma on the abdominal wall through which an enema can be administered. This method has primarily been used in children (Chapter 11), but there are reports of its increasing and effective use in adults with SCI.

Colostomy may be an appropriate option to consider in individuals for whom there has been a failure to establish an adequate and acceptable bowel program despite sustained efforts. Careful patient selection is crucial; for the appropriate candidate who has had severe problems or difficulty with conservative management, understands limitations and side effects of surgery, and demonstrates capacity to manage the colostomy, the procedure can significantly reduce burden of care and improve quality of life. Appropriate placement of the stoma is important to allow for access and visualization. It may occasionally also be performed as a temporary or permanent measure to divert feces away from pelvic pressure ulcers.

Management of Complications
Constipation
Balanced diet, adequate fluid and fiber intake are important components in management and prevention of constipation. Increased activity is helpful through mechanical stimulation of peristalsis. Reduction or elimination of constipating medications should be attempted as/if feasible. Bulk forming agents and laxatives given at least 8 hours before planned bowel care may be helpful if the other measures alone are not effective.

Fecal Impaction
Fecal impaction is confirmed with colonic palpation, rectal exam, and/or abdominal radiograph.

Manual evacuation should be attempted if feces is palpable in rectum. Anesthetic ointment or jelly should be used to reduce noxious stimulus and occurrence of AD in at-risk individuals (SCI above T6), and it is important to monitor and treat AD if it occurs in these individuals. For more proximal impaction, one may need to use oral stimulants, for example, magnesium citrate or bisacodyl tablets. Caution is needed in case of suspected bowel obstruction, since intestinal perforation could result. Oil retention enemas may be helpful in combination with oral agents to loosen stool.

Hemorrhoids

Development of hemorrhoids is minimized by maintain soft stools and minimizing trauma during anal stimulation. Symptoms may include pain, bleeding, mucus incontinence (due to prolapsed mucosa), or symptoms of AD. Management of clinically significant and/or symptomatic hemorrhoids includes: discouragement of straining and minimizing digital stimulation during bowel care, and increased stool softeners to avoid hard stool, use of topical anti-inflammatory creams or suppositories. Hemorrhoidectomy may be considered for persistent bleeding or AD that are unresponsive to conservative treatment.

Practice Pearls

It is important to recognize that fecal impaction may present only with nausea and loss of appetite. Anti-nausea medications, which have anticholinergic and constipating properties, will worsen the problem if given mistakenly.

Liquid stool may pass around the blockage in fecal impaction, and should not be mistakenly diagnosed or treated as diarrhea.

KNOWLEDGE GAPS AND EMERGING CONCEPTS

Effect of dietary fiber intake on the neurogenic bowel needs additional evaluation. Results of currently available studies are conflicting. Long term effects of bowel medications needs further study.

SUGGESTED READING

Chen D, Nussbaum SB. The gastrointestinal system and bowel management following spinal cord injury. *Phys Med Rehabil Clin N Am.* 2000;11(1):45-56.

Consortium for Spinal Cord Medicine. *Neurogenic Bowel Management in Adults with Spinal Cord Injury. Clinical Practice Guidelines for Health Care Professionals.* Washington, DC: Paralyzed Veterans of America; 1998.

Ebert E. Gastrointestinal involvement in spinal cord injury: a clinical perspective. *J Gastrointestin Liver Dis.* 2012;21(1):75-82.

Steins SA, Bergman SB, Goetz LL. Neurogenic bowel dysfunction after spinal cord injury: clinical evaluation and rehabilitative management. *Arch Phys Med Rehabil.* 1997;78: S86-S100.

CHAPTER 37

Pressure Ulcers

Pressure ulcers are a major cause of morbidity, reduced participation and quality of life, hospitalization, and cost of care for people with spinal cord injury (SCI) throughout their lifetime.

GENERAL PRINCIPLES

The National Pressure Ulcer Advisory Panel (NPUAP) definition of a pressure ulcer is: a localized injury to the skin and/or underlying tissue usually over a bony prominence, as a result of pressure, or pressure in combination with shear.

Etiology

The etiology of pressure ulcers is multidimensional. Following SCI, the neurologically impaired skin undergoes significant alterations that make it more susceptible to breakdown. These include autonomic changes, biochemical factors, and mechanical factors.

Loss of mobility and impaired sensation limit ability to perform pressure relief. Pressure, friction, and shear are the primary factors associated with development of pressure ulcers. Moisture associated with bladder or bowel incontinence can be an important contributor, as can systemic factors including impaired medical status or nutrition.

Epidemiology

Lifetime risk of pressure ulcer is estimated to be over 50% in people with SCI although precise estimates are not available. Older age is associated with increased risk. SCI-related risk factors for pressure ulcers include completeness of injury, longer duration of SCI, and lesser functional independence. Diabetes or vascular disease adds to risk.

Previous history of pressure ulcer is a strong predictor of future pressure ulcer risk. Recurrence rates are high, although there is significant variation in the reported rate depending on the population being studied.

In the early postinjury stage, the most common sites of pressure ulcers are the sacrum, followed by heels and ischium. After 2 years postinjury, most common sites are ischium, sacrum, and trochanter.

Pathophysiology

The precise mechanisms of pressure ulcer formation are still not fully understood. Pressure, shear, and the resulting deformation of tissue are primary factors leading to formation of pressure ulcers. Muscle is more sensitive to ischemia than is skin. Pressure ulcers usually develop over bony prominences; prolonged pressure on these areas compresses skin and muscle, occluding vascular supply.

CLINICAL CONSIDERATIONS

Assessment

Multidimensional assessment is essential in the context of pressure ulcer prevention and treatment. Aspects of assessment include: evaluating the whole person, assessing risk, assessing the skin/wound, assessing complications, and assessing healing or deterioration.

Risk Assessment
Comprehensive risk assessment for pressure ulcers includes evaluation of:

▦ Demographic factors: Age, duration of injury, ethnicity, marital status, education
▦ Physical and medical factors: Level and completeness of injury, activity and mobility, bowel and bladder status including continence, and medical comorbidities
▦ Nutritional status: Dietary intake, anthropometric measurements, biochemical parameters including prealbumin, albumin, and hemoglobin. A short half-life of 2 to 3 days makes prealbumin the most sensitive indicator for monitoring adequacy of nutrition
▦ Psychological and social factors: Cognitive status, psychological distress, substance abuse, and behavioral issues including adherence to recommended preventive measures

Existing risk assessment tools are imprecise for use in the SCI population, and their predictive value requires additional investigation. In the absence of an optimal risk assessment tool, a commonly used scale is the Braden scale (Table 37.1) although most individuals with SCI would be classified at risk with use of this scale. The Salzberg scale and Norton scale are other risk assessment tools. Several other scales have been developed but most have been used on a limited basis with inadequate demonstration of validity.

Table 37.1

Braden Scale Criteria and Scoring

Criteria/Subscales

Sensory perception

Moisture

Activity

Mobility

Nutrition

Friction and shear

Scoring

Each subscale is scored from 1 (highest risk) to 4 (lowest risk) except "friction and shear" which scores from 1 to 3, for a total score range of 6 to 23

The lower the score the greater the risk for pressure ulcer

Risk categories range from no risk (total score 19–23) to very high risk (score less than 9)

Cut-off point ranging from 11–19 are cited for establishing at-risk status, but are not well established for individuals with SCI

Assessment Following Development of a Pressure Ulcer
Systemic Assessment
Comprehensive systemic assessment is important. Contributing factors and circumstances that led to the development of the pressure ulcer should be identified if possible. Evaluation should include: complete history and examination to evaluate for above-mentioned systemic risk factors; psychological and behavioral health, social and financial resources; availability and utilizations of care assistance; positioning, posture, and related equipment; and systemic complications such as sepsis, pain, and worsening of spasticity.

Assessment and documentation of the pressure ulcer should include:

- Location
- General appearance of wound base
- Size (length, width, depth, wound area)
- Stage
- Exudate
- Odor
- Necrosis
- Undermining
- Margins
- Surrounding tissue
- Sinus tracts
- Evidence of infection (Table 37.2)
- Healing (i.e., granulation, epithelialization)

Staging of pressure ulcers (Table 37.3): NPUAP redefined the stages of pressure ulcers in 2007, including the original four stages and adding two stages on deep tissue injury and unstageable pressure ulcers (Table 37.3).

Table 37.2
Indicators of Wound Infection

Local

Erythema

Edema

Warmth

Induration

Pain

Purulent drainage

Systemic

Fever

Chills

Leukocytosis

Altered mental status

Tachycardia

Autonomic dysreflexia

Increased spasticity

Table 37.3
Staging of Pressure Ulcers (NPUAP)

Stage	Definition	Additional Description
Stage I: Nonblanchable erythema	Intact skin with nonblanchable redness of a localized area usually over a bony prominence.	The area may be painful, firm, soft, warmer, or cooler as compared to adjacent tissue. Stage I may be difficult to detect in individuals with dark skin tones. Darkly pigmented skin may not have visible blanching; its color may differ from the surrounding area.
Stage II: Partial thickness	Partial thickness loss of dermis presenting as a shallow open ulcer with a red pink wound bed, without slough. May also present as an intact or open/ruptured serum-filled blister.	This stage should not be used to describe skin tears, tape burns, perineal dermatitis, maceration, or excoriation.

(continued)

Table 37.3
Staging of Pressure Ulcers (NPUAP) (*continued*)

Stage	Definition	Additional Description
Stage III: Full thickness skin loss	Full thickness tissue loss. Subcutaneous fat may be visible but bone, tendon, or muscle are not exposed. Slough may be present but does not obscure the depth of tissue loss. May include undermining and tunneling.	The depth of a stage III pressure ulcer varies by anatomical location. The bridge of the nose, ear, occiput, and malleolus do not have subcutaneous tissue and stage III ulcers can be shallow. In contrast, areas of significant adiposity can develop extremely deep stage III pressure ulcers. Bone/tendon is not visible or directly palpable.
Stage IV: Full thickness tissue loss	Full thickness tissue loss with exposed bone, tendon or muscle. Slough or eschar may be present on some parts of the wound bed. Often include undermining and tunneling.	The depth of a stage IV pressure ulcer also varies by anatomical location. Stage IV ulcers can extend into muscle and/or supporting structures (e.g., fascia, tendon, or joint capsule) making osteomyelitis possible. Exposed bone/tendon is visible or directly palpable.
Unstageable: Full thickness skin or tissue loss—depth unknown	Full thickness tissue loss in which the base of the ulcer is covered by slough (yellow, tan, gray, green, or brown) and/or eschar (tan, brown, or black) in the wound bed.	Until enough slough and/or eschar is removed to expose the base of the wound, the true depth, and therefore stage, cannot be determined. Stable (dry, adherent, intact without erythema, or fluctuance) eschar on the heels serves as the body's biological cover and should not be removed.
Suspected Deep Tissue Injury	Purple or maroon localized area of discolored intact skin or blood-filled blister due to damage of underlying soft tissue from pressure and/or shear. The area may be preceded by tissue that is painful, firm, mushy, boggy, warmer, or cooler as compared to adjacent tissue.	Deep tissue injury may be difficult to detect in individuals with dark skin tones. Evolution may include a thin blister over a dark wound bed. The wound may further evolve and become covered by thin eschar. Evolution may be rapid, exposing additional layers of tissue even with optimal treatment.

Abbreviation: NPUAP, National Pressure Ulcer Advisory Panel.

Reassessment and monitoring of the pressure ulcer is needed on a consistent and ongoing basis to determine adequacy of the treatment plan. Measurement of wound surface area, including wound depth and undermining is a reliable and valid method of assessing wound healing. A photographic record of the wound can be helpful in documenting progress.

The Pressure Ulcer Scale for Healing (PUSH) is a simple scale for evaluating healing of pressure ulcers based on size (length, width), exudate amount, and tissue type.

Investigation for Possible Osteomyelitis and Other Complications

Suspected osteomyelitis may be evaluated with imaging studies. Bone scan is more sensitive than plain film but specificity in differentiating from soft tissue infection is limited. Indium white cell scans are more specific. Magnetic resonance imaging (MRI) may show anatomical detail. Bone biopsy is the most definitive form of diagnosis but there may be reluctance to perform it unless surgery is otherwise indicated.

Long-standing ulcers of 20 years or longer duration may occasionally develop squamous cell carcinoma (Marjolins ulcers). Clinically, these may present with increased discharge, wart-like growths and/or bleeding from the wound. If clinically suspected, biopsy of suspicious areas is performed to identify the lesion.

Management

The Consortium for Spinal Cord Medicine has developed practitioner as well as consumer guidelines for pressure ulcer prevention and treatment following SCI. Clinical practice guidelines for pressure ulcer management have also been developed by NPUAP.

Comprehensive Treatment Plan

Elements of a comprehensive treatment plan include cleansing, debridement, dressings, surgery as indicated, support surfaces and positioning to manage tissue loads, attention to general health, nutrition, and other systemic factors. The treatment plan should be reevaluated and modified if the ulcer shows no evidence of healing within 2 to 4 weeks. Education and reinforcement of preventive measures are critical for minimizing recurrence.

Attention to General Health and Systemic Complications

Management of underlying contributing factors is critical. Aggressive nutritional support and hydration is important for healing. Supplemental intake to ensure adequate protein and caloric intake should be provided as needed. Identified nutritional deficiencies should be corrected. However, routine use of supplemental micronutrients has not been proven to enhance healing.

A large randomized controlled trial did not demonstrate any improvement in healing of stage III or IV pressure ulcers with addition of an anabolic steroid (oxandrolone).

Comorbid conditions that interfere with wound healing should be treated. Bladder and bowel incontinence needs to be appropriately managed. Smoking cessation is important to emphasize.

Systemic antibiotics may be needed to treat infected wounds. Osteomyelitis treatment includes antibiotic treatment for 6 to 12 weeks.

Cleansing the Wound
Cleansing is done to remove visible debris and aid assessment after a wound has initially occurred, to remove excess slough and exudate, and to remove remaining dressing material.

Wounds should be cleansed at each dressing change. Normal saline is a good cleansing agent. Irrigation is the method of choice for cleansing wounds. This may be carried out utilizing a syringe in order to produce gentle pressure without causing trauma to the wound. Antiseptic agents (e.g., povidone-iodine or hydrogen peroxide) can be cytotoxic and should be avoided.

Pulsatile lavage therapy is a form of hydrotherapy that may be a preferred alternative to whirlpool for patients with large amounts of exudate and necrotic tissue.

Debridement
Method of wound debridement depends on the clinical situation. Eschar and devitalized tissue should be removed. Debridement methods include autolytic, enzymatic, mechanical, sharp (using sterile instruments that only remove necrotic tissue without anesthesia or significant bleeding in viable tissue), or surgical debridement.

Dressings (Table 37.4)
Dressings should be used with the goal of keeping the ulcer bed continuously moist and the surrounding skin dry. Functions of a dressing are to protect the wound from contamination or trauma, provide compression if swelling or bleeding are anticipated, apply medications, absorb drainage, and/or debride necrotic tissue.

The condition of the wound and desired function determine the choice of dressing. Each product has advantages and disadvantages and no single dressing is suitable for all wounds. See Table 37.4 for categories and indications of available dressings.

Table 37.4

Dressing Categories for Skin Wounds

Dressing Type	Examples	Advantages	Disadvantages	Indications	Contraindications
Transparent film	Opsite, Tegaderm	Barrier to external contamination, comfortable, allows inspection, minimizes friction	Nonabsorptive so exudate may pool, may be traumatic to remove, especially for fragile skin, application may be difficult	Superficial wounds (Stage I–II), as a secondary dressing, cover for hydrophilic powder or paste	Highly exudative wounds, infected wounds
Hydrocolloid dressing	Duoderm	Retains moisture, painless removal, facilitates autolytic debridement, nonadhesive, water-proof	Opaque, edges may roll up, odor on removal so can confuse with infection	Partial thickness wounds, as preventive dressing for high-risk friction areas	Heavy exudate, sinus tracts
Hydrogel	Curasol SoloSite	Nonadherent, trauma-free removal, comfortable rehydrates dry wound bed, promotes autolysis	Some require secondary dressing to secure, may macerate surrounding skin	Partial and full-thickness wounds, wounds with necrosis or slough	Heavily exudative wounds
Foams	Lyofoam, Polymem	Moist, absorbent and protective	Set size of foam may be limited by wound size	Wounds with mild to moderate exudate	Dry wounds, dry eschar, wounds that need frequent review
Alginate	Sorbsan, Seasorb	Highly absorbent, fills dead space, can pack cavities, promotes hemostasis	May require secondary dressing, gel can be confused with slough or pus	Moderately or highly exudative infected or noninfected wounds, wounds that require packing and absorption	Dry wounds or hard eschar

(continued)

Table 37.4

Dressing Categories for Skin Wounds (*continued*)

Dressing Type	Examples	Advantages	Disadvantages	Indications	Contraindications
Composites	Covaderm plus, Alldress	Combination of two or more physically distinct products manufactured as a single dressing that can serve multiple purposes	Varies with product	Adhesive border may limit use on fragile skin	Some products are contraindicated for Stage IV ulcers
Collagens	Fibracol	Absorbant, nonadherent, conforms well	Requires secondary dressing to secure	Partial and full thickness wounds, surgical wounds	Necrotic wounds
Enzymatic debriders	Accuzyme, Santyl	Nonsurgical method of debridement	Inactivated by soaps and detergents, some enzymatics can damage healthy tissue	To debride wounds	Healing wounds that don't require debridement
Gauze dressings	Kendall Curity	Readily available, effective as packing agent, can be used with infected wounds, can be used for mechanical debridement (wet to dry)	Can delay healing with inappropriate use, pain on removal, labor intensive	Vary with product and method of use, draining wounds, necrotic wounds	Clean wounds with healthy granulation tissue

Practice Pearl

It is important to address specific wound characteristics and needed functions of dressing treatment at various points, and change dressing progression accordingly. For example an infected Stage IV sacral ulcer with yellow necrotic slough and exudate may be treated with calcium alginate rope to absorb wound exudate and to promote autolytic debridement. As the wound heals and develops a red, granulating base the dressing choice may change to hydrocolloid paste and dressing to fill the dead space in the wound cavity and to provide a moisture-retaining occlusive healing environment. With further healing, as the wound becomes pink and is re-epithelializing, hydrocolloid dressing may be used by itself to protect the new epithelium.

Adjunctive Therapies
Adjunctive therapies that have been used to promote healing include electrical stimulation, hyperbaric oxygen, and use of negative pressure wound therapy (NPWT).

NPWT devices include a suction pump with foam and occlusive dressing to create negative pressure on the treated wound. This therapy is proposed to facilitate wound healing through multiple mechanisms including decreased bacterial load and edema while promoting granulation and improving local circulation. A tight seal and conformance to the anatomical surface is required for effective use.

Positioning
Proper positioning to reduce tissue load is needed since SCI significantly restricts the individual's ability to move and change positions. Periodic repositioning is needed to relieve pressure over bony prominences. An optimal turning schedule in bed should be established.

Positioning patients directly on a pressure ulcer should be avoided. Closed cutouts or donut-type cushions should be avoided.

The time the head of the bed is elevated should be limited, and the lowest degree of elevation consistent with medical considerations and other indications is recommended since elevating the head of the bed can increase shear and friction forces between the skin and bed surface.

Bed Support Surfaces
Appropriate bed support surfaces should be used to reduce tissue load in prevention and treatment of pressure ulcers. Specialized support surfaces redistribute an individual's weight over skin and subcutaneous tissues as it presses against the bed (or chair, in the case of cushions).

Bed support surfaces can be classified as dynamic or static.

■ Dynamic surfaces include: air fluidized, low air loss, and alternating air mattresses
■ Static surfaces include static flotation, foam, and standard mattress

Static support surface can be used for individuals who can be positioned without weight-bearing on an ulcer without bottoming out on the support surface. A dynamic support surface is indicated if the person can't be positioned without putting pressure on an ulcer, when a static support surface bottoms out, in case of a nonhealing ulcer or development of a new ulcer while on a static support surface. Low air-loss and air-fluidized beds are used for pressure ulcers on multiple turning surfaces or to manage moisture and heat in the presence of Stage III or IV ulcers. Air-fluid beds are expensive, heavy, and noisy, make transfers difficult, limit the ability to elevate the head of the bed, require increased attention to pulmonary toileting, and increase vulnerability to dehydration.

Wheelchair Positioning, Weight Shifting, and Cushions
Wheelchairs should be prescribed and fitted to promote proper postural alignment and to allow for changes in body pressure distribution based on the functional abilities of the individual (Chapter 29).

Weight shifts are a critical element of pressure reduction. A power weight-shifting wheelchair system should be prescribed for individuals who are unable to perform manual weight shifts independently. A push-up pressure relief while seated in a manual wheelchair can off-load the buttocks but requires sufficient arm strength and can contribute to upper extremity overuse problems over time. A forward lean will unweight ischial tuberosities, and a side-lean can be done to unweight the contralateral side while seated.

A proper sitting schedule needs to be established. As much as possible, positioning the wheelchair-seated individual directly on a pressure ulcer should be avoided.

Pressure mapping may be used as an adjunctive measure to identify areas of high pressure and evaluate effectiveness of different seating surfaces and alignments. The device consists of arrays of sensors on a flexible mat that measures pressure between the user and the support surface, and the information is displayed as a color-coded image to illustrate pressure magnitudes.

Wheelchair cushions include: foam, gel, air, and alternating air cushions. Proper cushion maintenance and inspection is important. Seating cushions should be examined to make sure they are not "bottoming out." Ring (donut) cushions increase venous congestion and edema and should not be used.

Surgery

Surgery may be indicated for complex full thickness pressure ulcers. Surgical procedures include those that prepare the wound for successful healing (e.g., surgical debridement, or un-roofing of sinuses or cavities), or those that provide definitive closure.

In addition to local wound considerations, general evaluation is important for proper patient selection including medical status, ability to tolerate surgery, and ability and motivation to comply with needed postoperative and ongoing care (which is, however, often difficult to quantify objectively).

Local and systemic factors should be optimized preoperatively as much as possible including smoking cessation, spasticity management, treatment of infection, and optimization of nutrition.

Muco-cutaneous or fascio-cutaneous flaps are the procedures of choice for definitive surgical closure. Elements of surgical treatment include: excision of ulcer, surrounding scar, and underlying necrotic or infected bone, filling dead space, enhancing vascularity of the healing wound, distributing pressure off bone, and preserving options in case of future breakdown. Prophylactic ischiectomy is not recommended since it does not prevent recurrence, but can cause secondary problems including increased weight bearing in other at-risk areas.

Postoperatively patients are put on bed-rest on a low air loss or air fluidized mattress, typically for 3 to 6 weeks after which a progressive mobilization protocol is initiated. Once patients are able to tolerate passive range of motion of the hips to 90° flexion without stressing the surgical site, sitting for short intervals (10–15 minutes) is initiated and gradually progressed with careful attention to ensure no deterioration in surgical site healing. Special attention to smoking cessation, nutrition, and spasticity management is important in the postoperative period.

Ongoing Preventive Measures

Prevention of pressure ulcers is an important aspect of SCI care throughout the care continuum.

Prolonged immobilization should be avoided whenever feasible. Pressure relief measures should be instituted as soon as possible and continued throughout the care continuum.

Patient education is critical. Education should emphasize the need for meticulous skin care, avoidance of skin dryness or excess moisture, regular skin inspection (including use of a long-handled mirror to visualize hard-to-see bony prominences), importance, frequency, and techniques for regular pressure relief, proper nutrition, avoidance of tobacco, and maintenance of support surfaces and cushions.

KNOWLEDGE GAPS AND EMERGING CONCEPTS

SCI-specific risk assessment tools for pressure ulcers still need to be developed and studied.

Studies are also needed to develop standard methods for measuring wounds and reporting healing rates.

The precise role and indications of NPWT need to be further delineated to facilitate optimal use in people with SCI.

There are new and promising adjuvant therapies being developed and used in treating pressure ulcers including growth factors (e.g., recombinant platelet-derived growth factor and nerve growth factor) and cellular therapies, but more information is needed to determine effectiveness and define their role in managing pressure ulcers.

SUGGESTED READING

Bauman WA, Spungen AM, Collins JF, et al. The effect of oxandrolone on the healing of chronic pressure ulcers in persons with spinal cord injury: a randomized trial. *Ann Intern Med.* 2013;158(10):718-726.

Consortium for Spinal Cord Medicine. *Pressure Ulcer Prevention and Treatment Following Spinal Cord Injury. Clinical Practice Guidelines for Health Care Professionals.* Washington, DC: Paralyzed Veterans of America; 2000.

European Pressure Ulcer Advisory Panel and National Pressure Ulcer Advisory Panel. *Prevention and Treatment of Pressure Ulcers: Quick Reference Guide.* Washington, DC: National Pressure Ulcer Advisory Panel; 2009.

Henzel MK, Bogie KM, Guihan M, Ho CH. Pressure ulcer management and research priorities for patients with spinal cord injury: consensus opinion from SCI QUERI Expert Panel on Pressure Ulcer Research Implementation. *J Rehabil Res Dev.* 2011;48(3):xi-xxxii.

Reddy M, Gill SS, Kalkar SR, Wu W, Anderson PJ, Rochon PA. Treatment of pressure ulcers: a systematic review. *JAMA.* 2008;300(22):2647-2662.

Regan MA, Teasell RW, Wolfe DL, Keast D, Mortenson WB, Aubut JA. Spinal Cord Injury Rehabilitation Evidence Research Team. A systematic review of therapeutic interventions for pressure ulcers after spinal cord injury. *Arch Phys Med Rehabil.* 2009;90(2): 213-231.

CHAPTER 38

Neurological and Musculoskeletal Consequences: Overview

GENERAL PRINCIPLES

Spinal cord injury (SCI) can be associated with several neurological and musculoskeletal complications. These include conditions that involve the spine/spinal cord, one or more of the extremities, or are generalized and involve multiple regions such as spasticity (Chapter 38A) or below-level neuropathic pain (Chapter 38C).

Neurological and musculoskeletal conditions involving the spine and/or spinal cord are summarized in Table 38.1, and those involving the extremities are summarized in Table 38.2.

Table 38.1

Neurological and Musculoskeletal Complications Involving the Spine/Spinal Cord After SCI

Condition	Considerations
Posttraumatic syringomyelia	- See Chapter 38B
Scoliosis	- Most prevalent in pediatric SCI prior to attainment of skeletal maturity; rare in adult-onset SCI (see Chapter 11)
Tethered cord syndrome	- Spinal arachnoiditis after SCI can lead to scarring and tethering of the nerve roots or cauda equina
Vertebral pain and degeneration around injury site (with spinal cord or nerve root compression)	- Progressive degenerative changes can occur in proximity to the deformed or immobile vertebral segments at the injury site. These include: degenerative disk disease, spinal stenosis, kyphosis, nonunion of previous surgical fixation, and segmental instability. There may also be loosening, or breakage of surgical hardware, or infection - Neurological worsening due to spinal cord or nerve root compression, or localized pain can develop - Imaging of the spine is needed to establish a diagnosis - Management may include symptomatic treatment of pain, immobilization, and/or surgical revision
Charcot spine/neuropathic arthropathy	- Motion above and below the vertebral level of spinal fusion or instrumentation can lead to erosive destruction of cartilage and bone over time, and development of a spinal pseudarthrosis; proprioceptive deficits with loss of protective mechanisms contribute to pathogenesis - Presenting symptoms and signs include: back pain, audible crepitus or clunking on spinal motion, new neurological deficits due to cord compression resulting from spinal instability, loss of sitting balance, conversion from upper to lower motor neuron bowel/bladder or loss of reflexogenic erections (due to lumbosacral root involvement) - Diagnosis confirmed by imaging; differentiate from infection or malignancy - Treatment is primarily surgical. However, there is risk of recurrence of pathology below the surgical revision

Table 38.2
Neurological and Musculoskeletal Complications of the Extremities After SCI

Condition	Considerations
Fractures sustained during acute injury	- Traumatic fractures may be sustained concomitantly with acute SCI, and are usually treated surgically (unlike pathological fractures in chronic SCI) - Surgical fixation is performed as appropriate without consideration of completeness of SCI - Temporary weight-bearing restrictions may require modification of SCI rehabilitation
Fractures in chronic SCI (osteoporotic fractures)	- See Chapter 39B
Heterotopic ossification	- See Chapter 38D
Musculoskeletal overuse syndromes	- See Chapter 27 and Table 27.3 for joint protection techniques to reduce upper limb overuse injury - Shoulder pain is most common. See Chapter 38C for additional discussion - Other soft tissue disorders of the upper limb include lateral epicondylitis (extensor tendinosis) or medial epicondylitis (flexor tendinosis), olecranon bursitis, DeQuervain's tenosynovitis (involving the abductor pollicis longus and extensor pollicis brevis) - Lower limb overuse injuries may occur in ambulatory individuals
Entrapment neuropathies	- The most common entrapment neuropathies after SCI are median nerve compression at the wrist (carpal tunnel syndrome) and ulnar nerve compression at the elbow (Table 38B.2)
Spasticity and Contractures	- See Chapter 38A

SUGGESTED READING

Biering-Sørensen F, Burns AS, Curt A, et al. International spinal cord injury musculoskeletal basic data set. *Spinal Cord.* 2012;50(11):797-802.

Goldstein B. Musculoskeletal conditions after spinal cord injury. *Phys Med Rehabil Clin N Am.* 2000;11(1):91-108.

Paralyzed Veterans of America Consortium for Spinal Cord Medicine. Preservation of upper limb function following spinal cord injury: a clinical practice guideline for health-care professionals. *J Spinal Cord Med.* 2005;28(5):434-470.

Widerström-Noga E, Biering-Sørensen F, Bryce T, et al. The international spinal cord injury pain basic data set. *Spinal Cord.* 2008;46(12):818-823.

Spasticity

GENERAL PRINCIPLES

Spasticity has been defined as a motor disorder characterized by a velocity-dependent increase in tonic stretch reflexes or muscle tone with exaggerated tendon jerks, resulting from hyper-excitability of the stretch reflex as one component of the upper motor neuron (UMN) syndrome.

Spasticity involves a constellation of tonic and phasic features that include increased muscle tone, exaggerated muscle stretch reflexes, involuntary muscle spasms, and clonus.

Etiology/Pathophysiology

The mechanisms underlying spasticity are complex and not fully understood. The primary mechanism is believed to be due to the loss of descending inhibitory modulating signals as a result of the spinal cord injury (SCI). Loss of descending inhibition results in hyperactivity of segmental reflexes.

Another contributing mechanism is thought to be denervation hypersensitivity that occurs at the receptor level over time, resulting in decreased threshold for motor unit activation and a heightened response to stimuli.

Abnormal branching and communication of intact spinal interneurons may also be a contributing factor.

Epidemiology

Spasticity is common after SCI, reportedly affecting 50% to 75% of individuals following injury. Higher incidence is reported in persons with cervical and upper thoracic injury in comparison with those with lower levels of injury.

Natural History

During the period of spinal shock, muscle tone is often reduced. Spasticity appears over time; time of onset and progression as well as severity is quite variable even between those with similar level and completeness of injury.

344

CLINICAL CONSIDERATIONS

Assessment

History and Physical Examination
Evaluation should include assessment of severity and localization of spasticity, identification of triggering factors that could precipitate or worsen spasticity, and effect on function, comfort, and sleep.

Triggering Factors
Any noxious stimulus can worsen spasticity. Causes include conditions such as urinary tract infections, bladder stones, bowel impaction, hemorrhoids, ingrown toe nail, pressure ulcers, fractures, menstruation, posttraumatic syringomyelia, or intra-abdominal pathology.

Consequences of Spasticity
Spasticity is a frequent source of complaints and complications, causing pain, discomfort, reduced mobility, and range of motion. It can disrupt seating stability and sleep. It can interfere with the individual's ability to perform activities of daily living and make it difficult for caregivers to optimally assist with dressing, grooming, and hygiene. Complications of severe and chronic spasticity include joint contractures, joint subluxation, and pressure ulcers.

Self-rating scales have been used to quantify the effect of spasticity on daily life of the individual. An example is the SCI Spasticity Evaluation Tool (SCI-SET).

Physical Examination

Clinical examination demonstrates resistance to passive stretch that is velocity dependent. Weakness, hyperactive muscle stretch reflexes, and abnormal primitive reflexes (i.e., Babinski response), which are part of the UMN syndrome, are often present.

Clinical Scales to Assess Spasticity
Although these scales are convenient and easy to learn and use, the accuracy and consistency of the measurement can be variable depending on the interpretation of the examiner and patient self-report. The most common clinically administered scale to quantify spasticity is the Modified Ashworth Scale.

The *Modified Ashworth Scale* (Table 38A.1) is ideally determined with the patient in the supine position and instructed to relax. If testing a muscle that primarily flexes a joint, the joint is placed in a maximally flexed position and moved to a position of maximal extension over one second (count of "one-one-thousand") by the examiner. If testing a muscle that primarily extends a joint, the joint is placed in a maximally extended position and moved to a position of maximal flexion over one second. It is graded from 0 to 4 with 0 denoting no increase in muscle tone (there is no designation for reduced tone in this scale) and 4 indicating that the affected part is rigid in flexion or extension.

Table 38A.1

Modified Ashworth Scale[a]

Score	Description
0	No increase in muscle tone
1	Slight increase in muscle tone, manifested by a catch and release or by minimal resistance at the end of the range of motion when the affected part(s) is moved in flexion or extension
1+	Slight increase in muscle tone, manifested by a catch, followed by minimal resistance throughout the remainder (less than half) of the range of motion
2	More marked increase in muscle tone through most of the range of motion, but affected part(s) easily moved
3	Considerable increase in muscle tone, passive movement difficult
4	Affected part(s) rigid in flexion or extension

[a]If testing a muscle that primarily flexes a joint, the joint is placed in a maximally flexed position and moved to a position of maximal extension over one second (count of "one-one-thousand"). If testing a muscle that primarily extends a joint, the joint is placed in a maximally extended position and moved to a position of maximal flexion over one second.

The *Penn Spasm Frequency Scale* is a 5 point self report scale ranging from 0 (no spasms) to 4 (spasms occurring more than 10 times per hour).

Diagnostic Tests

Biomechanical assessment can be done with techniques such as the pendulum test, biomechanical gait analysis, and isokinetic dynamometry. The pendulum test is done in a seated position with the leg hanging over the edge of the testing surface. Motion around the knee is assessed with a goniometer, and the degree of reduced swing can be quantified as a measure of spasticity. This test has limited clinical value, but has been shown to have good reliability and has been used as a quantifiable outcome measure in research settings.

Electrophysiological assessment utilizes surface EMG to measure threshold of activation for motor unit activity, and measures include the Hoffmann reflex (H reflex) and the H/M ratio (amplitude of H reflex to that of the compound motor action potential). The H/M ratio is increased in people with spasticity and has been found to correlate well with the Ashworth Scale.

These tests have limited clinical value, but have been shown to have good reliability and have been used as quantifiable outcome measures in research settings.

Management

Approach to Treatment
Considerations for treatment take into account not only the presence or sever-ity of the symptoms but also on the impact on the daily activities and life of the individual with SCI. Decisions to treat should be based on factors such as interference of spasticity with function, presence of pain related to spasms or tone, interference with sleep, the risk of developing the previously described complications.

Not all spasticity needs to be treated. Some people may use spasticity to their benefit, for example, to assist with transfers and bed positioning. Persons with incomplete SCI may depend on lower extremity extensor tone to assist with knee stability in standing and walking activities. Some degree of spasticity has been suggested to be beneficial in maintenance of bone or muscle mass and for prevention of deep venous thrombosis.

The usual approach to spasticity management is stepwise. It begins with identification and removal of noxious triggers in conjunction with position-ing, stretching, and, as needed, orthoses. Oral medications are then added and titrated for optimal management. Chemodenervation is considered, espe-cially in where the management of localized spasticity is the goal. Intrathecal baclofen is considered for those instances when oral medications are not ade-quately effective or not well tolerated.

Addressing Triggering Factors
Identification and management of other underlying pathophysiological pro-cesses is important. Increased spasticity may be secondary to urinary tract infections, bladder calculi, ingrown toenails, hemorrhoids, constipation, or bowel impaction. Irritation from urethral catheters, fractures and menstrua-tion, deep venous thrombosis, pressure ulcers, appendicitis, cholecystitis, or other abdominal process may also worsen spasticity.

Physical Treatments
Slow, sustained stretching may reduce motor neuron excitability and prevent contractures. There may be a carry-over of reduced spasticity for several hours after treatment. Weight bearing on a tilt table or standing frame or other stand-ing activities may provide prolonged stretch.

Posture and positioning can play an important role. Adequate lumbar support in wheelchairs and avoidance of sacral sitting can reduce symptom triggers. Sling style sitting surface may cause excessive internal femoral rotation and should be avoided.

Tone reducing orthotics such as ankle-foot orthoses (AFOs) may improve gait patterns. Serial casting has been utilized as a key component for treatment for joint contracture. Casts can be bivalved for skin inspection. Casting is sometimes preceded by chemodenervation to improve the stretch.

Cold application (e.g., with a cold pack or a cooling spray) to lower intramuscular temperature may help reduce clonus and spasticity. Electrical stimulation of the symptomatic muscles has been reported to have a short term effects.

*Oral Medications (*Table 38A.2*)*
Selection of medication should include consideration for the person's age, co-morbidities, and cognitive status.

Baclofen is an analog of gamma amino butyric acid (GABA) which is an inhibitory neurotransmitter that binds presynaptically at the GABA-B receptors. It exerts its effect by reducing flexor spasms, increasing range of motion, and decreasing spastic hypertonia. It is often used as the first-line drug in management of SCI-related spasticity. Dose ranges from 15 to 80 mg per day, though some patients require higher doses. It has a short half-life of 3.5 hours and may require frequent dosing to sustain therapeutic effect throughout the day and night. It may have anxiolytic and analgesic properties. Side effects include sedation, fatigue, weakness, nausea, dizziness, paresthesias, and hallucinations. Discontinuation must be tapered to prevent withdrawal symptoms that may include seizures, visual disturbances, and hallucinations. It is excreted by the kidneys and may need adjustment for people with impaired renal function.

Benzodiazepines include diazepam and clonazepam. These drugs act through the GABA system though don't directly bind to the GABA receptor. Diazepam binds at a site near the GABA-A receptor on presynaptic neuron and enhances GABA-mediated chloride conductance into nerve terminals and thereby increases inhibitory activity of the neurons. It also facilitates postsynaptic effects of GABA. The use of this class of drugs is limited by the known and prevalent side effects that include sedation, depression, cognitive impairment, and tolerance.

Alpha 2 agonists (clonidine and tizanidine) bind to presynaptic alpha 2 receptors on interneurons in the dorsal horn of the spinal cord, and are believed to depress polysynaptic reflexes by decreasing the release of excitatory amino acids such as glutamate and aspartate and facilitating the action of glycine, an inhibitory amino acid neurotransmitter. Clonidine can be delivered orally, transdermally, and intrathecally. The transdermal patch is available in two strengths, is designed to deliver the designated dose over 7 days, and has fewer side effects than the oral form. Known side effects include sedation, hypotension, and dry mouth. It should be initiated at a low dose and titrated cautiously to minimize side effects.

Tizanidine has shorter half-life and a much lower incidence of hypotension than clonidine. Hallucinations have been reported in a small percentage in the initial weeks of starting treatment. It can cause elevated liver enzymes in 5% of cases, and liver function tests are recommended at baseline, and periodically at 1, 3, and 6 months.

Table 38A.2

Oral Medications for Spasticity

Medication	Mechanism of Action	Starting Dose	Recommended Maximum Dose	Side Effects/ Precautions
Baclofen	Presynaptic inhibition of GABA B receptors	2–5 mg	40–80 mg in divided doses	Sedation, cognitive impairment, seizures with abrupt withdrawal
Gabapentin	Unknown (may involve binding to a calcium channel receptor in neurons)	100–300 mg	3600 mg/day in divided doses	Off-label use, dizziness, drowsiness
Tizanidine	α_2 adrenergic agonist	2–4 mg	36 mg/day in divided doses	Dry mouth, elevated liver enzymes, periodic liver testing
Clonidine	α_2 adrenergic agonist	0.1 mg	0.4 mg in divided doses	Dry mouth, hypotension, drowsiness, constipation
Diazepam	GABA-A receptor agonist, facilitates post-synaptic effects of GABA	2 mg	40 mg in divided doses	Sedation, cognitive impairment, impaired motor coordination, tolerance
Dantrolene	Calcium release inhibitor, interferes with excitation contraction coupling needed for muscle contraction	25 mg	400 mg in divided doses	Hepatotoxicity (to monitor liver enzymes), muscle weakness, diarrhea
Cyproheptadine	Antiseratogernic	4 mg	36 mg in divided doses	Sedation, dry mouth

Gabapentin is structurally related to neurotransmitter GABA but does not interact with GABA receptors. Its activity may involve voltage-gated calcium channels, but its exact mechanism of action in reducing spasticity is not known. It is exclusively excreted via the kidney. Blood levels and liver enzymes do not require monitoring.

Dantrolene acts directly on muscle tissue, exerting its effect by preventing neutrally induced release of calcium ions from the sarcoplasmic reticulum along muscle fibers, thereby decreasing calcium dependent excitation–contraction coupling. The drug is nonselective and may act on normal and spastic tissues to cause weakness, which may be a concern for those with marginal strength. It may cause hepatotoxicity and, rarely, fulminant hepatic failure so baseline and periodic liver function testing is indicated.

Cyproheptadine is a nonselective serotonergic antagonist that also has antihistamine activity. Side effects include dry mouth, sedation, fatigue, and weight gain.

Cannabis: Patients report significant benefit in spasticity from marijuana. Although prohibited by federal law, it may be a therapeutic option in the states where its prescription and use is allowed for medicinal purposes.

Intrathecal Medications
Intrathecal delivery of medication such as baclofen is an option for people who either failed oral regimen of antispasticity medication or could not tolerate side-effects. The treatment entails the use of an implanted device to deliver the medication continuously into the intrathecal space to bypass the blood brain barrier. It is generally preferred in persons with diffuse symptoms of spasticity and is more effective in treating spasticity in the lower extremities than in the trunk and upper extremities. However, placement of the catheter and manipulation of the delivery mode have been proposed to improve coverage of upper extremity symptoms.

Screening includes a trial of intrathecal injection of baclofen via lumbar puncture followed by objective and subjective monitoring for effectiveness. Fifty microgram of baclofen is administered. Onset of effect is within 45 to 60 minutes, peak effect is usually noted at around 4 hours, and is lost by 8 hours.

Pump placement: The pump is implanted subcutaneously in the anterior abdominal wall with the catheter tunneled subcutaneously and inserted in to the spinal canal at the L1 vertebral level and threaded into the subarachnoid space to the desired level.

Pump management includes refilling at scheduled intervals in conjunction with pump interrogation. For refills, the pump reservoir is accessed through a central access port, remaining medication in the reservoir removed, and the new medication refilled then injected into the reservoir. Pump programming is done to update information about reservoir volume, drug concentration, dosing regimen, and alarm dates.

Complications include catheter disconnection, kinking, or blockage, pump failure, infection, and baclofen over-dosage.

Baclofen withdrawal: Table 38A.3 summarizes causes of delivery failure of intrathecal medications. Early signs of under-dosing include increased spasticity, pruritis, hypotension, and paresthesias. Abrupt withdrawal can lead to fever or hyperthermia, altered mental status, exaggerated spasticity, and muscle rigidity. If not treated promptly, it can sometimes progress to rhabdomyolysis, multiple organ system failure, and death, so it requires immediate attention. Baclofen is either restored intrathecally or, if not feasible to do right away, high oral baclofen is given though improvement may take several hours with oral treatment. Intravenous benzodiazepines have also been given. In the presence of severe hyperthermia, dantrolene administration is indicated.

Baclofen over-dosage: Symptoms of intrathecal baclofen over-dosage include drowsiness, light-headedness, dizziness, and somnolence. Respiratory depression, seizures, progressive hypotonia, and impaired consciousness can occur.

Chemoneurolysis
Chemical neurolysis can be done with various agents including motor point blocks with phenol or alcohol, and botulinum toxin injection.

Phenol neurolysis and motor point blocks can be used to treat focal spasticity by targeting motor nerve branches or motor points of affected muscles. Electrical stimulation guidance is used to localize the greatest concentration of motor end plates within the target muscle. It is more economical than botulinum toxin but requires more precise injection of the drug to avoid painful dysesthesia. Effect can last for several months to over a year. Often a relatively intense stretching program or serial casting is done following the block for additive benefit.

Table 38A.3

Potential Causes of Delivery Failure of Intrathecal Medication

Pump	No or low drug in reservoir
	Low battery
	Pump failure
Catheter	Kink or blockage
	Disconnection from pump
	Leakage or tears
	Migration
Human factors	Programming error
	Incorrect concentration or drug
	Incorrect refill technique

Botulinum toxin injections block the release of acetylcholine at the neuromuscular junction and interfere with muscle activation. It is injected directly into the muscle. The effect is dose dependent and is decided based on muscle bulk and severity of symptoms. There are various subtypes of botulinum toxin. Only botulinum toxin type A and B have been developed for clinical use. Onabotulinum toxin A has received Food and Drug Administration (FDA)-approved indication for spasticity management, though that is limited to upper extremity spasticity of the flexor muscles of the elbow, wrist, and fingers in adult patients. The most common side effect is excessive weakness of the injected muscle, with occasional spread to nontarget muscles. In 2009, FDA mandated a new label warning and risk mitigation strategy for botulinum toxin products sold in the United States, in view of potential spread from the injection area to other areas of the body causing symptoms due to muscle weakness. The smallest effective dose should be injected, and the interval between treatments should be 3 months or longer.

KNOWLEDGE GAPS AND EMERGING CONCEPTS

Emerging knowledge about the precise mechanisms of spasticity at the cellular level is likely to lead to development of newer therapeutic options.

SUGGESTED READING

Adams MM, Hicks AL. Spasticity after spinal cord injury. *Spinal Cord*. 2005;43:577-586.

Dietz V, Sinkjaer T. Spasticity. *Handb Clin Neurol*. 2012;109:197-211.

Francisco GE. The role of intrathecal baclofen therapy in the upper motor neuron syndrome. *Eur Med Phys*. 2004;40:131-143.

Rekand T. Clinical assessment and management of spasticity: a review. *Acta Neurol Scand Suppl*. 2010;(190):62-66.

Neurological Decline After SCI

GENERAL PRINCIPLES

Neurological decline after the initial spinal cord injury (SCI) is estimated to occur in about 15% of patients, and can be due to several potential causes (Table 38B.1). The additional neurological deterioration can occur in the initial weeks or months following SCI, but often occurs after several years. It can have significant negative effect on functional abilities and create anxiety about further loss in independence and worsening function following adjustment to SCI.

Entrapment neuropathies of the upper limb that may occur after SCI (most commonly the median nerve at the wrist followed by ulnar nerve at the elbow) are summarized in Table 38B.2. Tethering of the spinal cord and nerve roots/cauda equina due to spinal arachnoiditis may be a cause of late neurological decline after SCI. Manifestations are similar to spinal arachnoiditis from other causes as discussed in Chapter 19. Conditions involving spinal compression of nerve roots and/or spinal cord, such as vertebral pseudoarthrosis or deformity are summarized in Chapter 38, Table 38.1.

The focus of the remaining chapter is on posttraumatic syringomyelia (PTS), which is among the commonest causes of late neurological decline after SCI (also see Chapter 23 for discussion about developmental syringomyelia).

Etiology and Epidemiology of PTS

PTS is a condition in which an expanding cyst develops within the spinal cord at some point after an injury. PTS has been reported as early as 1 month after SCI to as late as several decades later.

Following SCI many patients show fluid filled cysts on magnetic resonance imaging (MRI) that represent myelomalacia rather than PTS. Expanding PTS is reported in about 15% to 20% of patients after SCI; symptomatic PTS with neurological decline is much less common, occurring in 3% to 8%.

PTS is more common with complete than incomplete injuries.

Table 38B.1
Causes of Additional Neurological Decline After SCI

- Posttraumatic syringomyelia
- Entrapment neuropathies (see Table 38B.2)
- Tethered cord syndrome (often involving cauda equina)
- Nerve root and/or spinal cord compression from spinal:
  - Instability
  - Deformity
  - Pseudarthrosis, Charcot's arthropathy
  - Degeneration, stenosis

Abbreviation: SCI, spinal cord injury.

Table 38B.2
Upper Extremity Entrapment Neuropathies in People With SCI

Median Nerve at the Wrist (Carpal Tunnel Syndrome)

- Most common entrapment neuropathy after SCI
- Estimated prevalence 40%–60%; causes significant neurological decline in ~3%–5%
- Caused by repetitive forces during wheelchair propulsion, transfers, and weight shifts
- For preventive measures during activities and wheelchair set-up see Chapter 27, Table 27.3 and Chapter 29, Table 29.3 respectively
- Clinical findings: numbness/tingling and decreased sensation in median nerve territory (lateral 3½ digits); nocturnal discomfort, weakness/clumsiness of hand, positive Phalen sign (wrist held at 90° flexion for 30–60 s); positive Tinel sign (tapping over wrist); loss of two-point discrimination (filament testing)
- Confirmed by electrodiagnostic testing (prolonged motor and sensory distal latency of median nerve, focal slowing or conduction block in carpal tunnel)
- Management: modifying activities as feasible to comply with preventive measures referenced above is most important, night splint, anti-inflammatory medications, steroid injection into carpal tunnel, surgical release (with planning for restrictions and temporary increased dependence for 6–8 weeks in postoperative period)

Median Nerve Compression in Forearm

- Anterior interosseous nerve syndrome: may occur with repetitive elbow flexion and pronation of forearm, purely motor branch, weakness of pinch, unable to make "Ok" sign with thumb and second digit
- Pronator syndrome: compression of median nerve between two heads of pronator teres muscle in forearm, may occur with repetitive pronation/supination, presents with forearms pain, hand weakness and numbness over thumb/index finger (and thenar eminence, which distinguishes it from carpal tunnel syndrome)

Ulnar Nerve Compression at Elbow (Cubital Tunnel Syndrome)

- Second most common entrapment neuropathy in SCI
- Compression may occur with repetitive flexion and contraction of elbow during wheelchair propulsion or due to direct pressure from habitually resting elbow on hard surface

(continued)

Ulnar Nerve Compression at Elbow (Cubital Tunnel Syndrome)
■ Clinical findings: numbness of little and ring fingers, hand intrinsic muscle weakness, ulnar claw hand (benediction posture), Froment sign (inability to hold piece of paper between thumb and index finger using thumb adductor, so substitute with thumb inter-phalangeal flexion), Wartenberg sign (passively abducted fifth digit due to palmer interosseous weakness) ■ Electrodiagnostic testing shows decreased conduction velocity across the elbow ■ Management: Avoid pressure on medial elbow or prolonged elbow flexion, anti-inflammatory medications, surgical release

Ulnar Nerve Compression at Wrist (Guyon's Canal)
■ Can occur during repeated pressure over hypothenar eminence during wheelchair propulsion or crutch walking, differentiated from compression at elbow by sensory loss limited to volar aspect of lateral 1½ fingers with spared sensation over dorsal surface of digits (due to sparing of proximally originating dorsal ulnar cutaneous nerve), +ve Tinel sign over hypothenar eminence, treated with activity modification, anti-inflammatory medications, surgical release

Radial Nerve Compression
■ Not as common but can occur in SCI at the axilla (crutch palsy), spiral grove, forearm/supinator (posterior interosseous syndrome, purely motor), and at the wrist (dorsal hand sensory loss); principles of management are similar to other entrapment neuropathies in SCI

Abbreviation: SCI, spinal cord injury.

Pathophysiology of PTS

The pathophysiology of PTS is currently not well understood and may involve different mechanisms for initiation and for continued expansion of the syrinx. Hemodynamic changes due to impaired cerebrospinal fluid (CSF) circulation, possibly due to obstruction or narrowing of the subarachnoid space, are likely involved in many cases. This can lead to PTS either by high pressure or by creating a suction effect that draws CSF into the syrinx. Another suggested factor is the possibility of bioactive molecules that change water and solute transport and may cause CSF to enter the syrinx. Local ischemia of the cord may also be involved in the initiation.

Natural History

The natural history of PTS is quite variable. A significant number remain stable without any significant clinical change. Typically there is slow progression of symptoms over many years; in a smaller percent the decline can be quite rapid. Early-onset PTS often progresses rapidly.

CLINICAL CONSIDERATIONS

Assessment

History
Patients with PTS may present with subtle symptoms and high degree of vigilance is indicated.

Pain is common at or above the site of injury in individuals with post-traumatic PTS and may be referred to the neck and upper arms, sometimes in a cape-like distribution. Pain is dull, aching, or burning in character and may be inter-mittent or constant. It may be worsened by coughing, sneezing, straining, or postural changes.

Progression of previously stable neurological deficits after SCI should prompt consideration of PTS. Patients may notice new or ascending sensory loss. Occasionally the sensory loss may be noted after inadvertent burns or injury to the insensate area. Weakness or clumsiness of hands may be reported, although motor symptoms usually occur later in the course.

Symptoms are often asymmetrical or unilateral at the onset.

Less common presentations include new or worsening orthostatic hypoten-sion, hyperhidrosis, worsening autonomic dysreflexia, increased or decreased muscle spasticity, loss of reflex bladder emptying, or scoliosis.

Physical Examination
Typical exam findings in PTS include a dissociated sensory loss, with loss of pain and temperature sensation (due to involvement of crossing spinothalamic fibers by the syrinx) and preservation of tactile sensation, vibration, and posi-tion (posterior columns) until later stages. Loss of reflexes in the upper extrem-ity may be noted. Muscle atrophy is less common and occurs later. Scoliosis may occasionally be present due to asymmetrical involvement of trunk muscles.

Horner's syndrome may occur due to involvement of autonomic pathways descending in the lateral columns.

Sensory loss over the nose and mouth (extending outward over the face as the syrinx expands) occurs in case of spread of the syrinx to the brainstem.

Serial neurological examination is important for detection and monitoring of the syrinx. Quantitative measurements, such as grip and pinch strength, or hand-held myometry are helpful for monitoring weakness progression.

Diagnostic Tests
Imaging
MRI is the modality of choice for diagnosis, and can also provide useful infor-mation about the anatomical extent and lobulation of the syrinx. Sometimes the PTS image is obscured by metallic instrumentation from spine surgery. In case of poor visualization computed tomography (CT) or CT myelogram may be done.

Electrodiagnosis
Electrodiagnostic tests may show abnormalities, but have limited utility for mak-ing the diagnosis of PTS. These are primarily useful for identifying other causes of neurological decline such as entrapment neuropathies, and are occasionally

used as a supplemental monitoring tool. Early changes on electrodiagnostic testing of PTS include prolonged F-waves; later changes include reduced compound muscle action potential (CMAP), large motor units consistent with a denervation process, and reduced maximal firing rate during voluntary effort.

Differential Diagnosis
Other central and peripheral conditions can cause neurological decline after SCI (Table 38B.1). However, it is important to consider the possibility of PTS regardless of finding the presence of another considerably prevalent condition such as carpal tunnel syndrome on electrodiagnostic testing that may be co-existing. Of course, non-SCI related causes of new neurological deficits, such as stroke or central nervous system neoplasms, can occur in people with SCI as well.

Management

Conservative Treatment
Patients should be monitored with serial neurological examination, quantitative testing, and serial imaging. Serial electrophysiological testing may have a supplemental role.

Maneuvers that create Valsalva-like effects should be avoided, given the possibility that increased pressures generated may contribute to the pathogenesis of the syrinx, although the utility of this measure is not definite. It may include avoidance of straining for bowel movement or Valsalva maneuver to aid in emptying the bladder, straining during transfers, and other activities.

Symptomatic management of pain, and rehabilitation interventions to compensate for lost function, can be helpful. Vigilance about avoidance of burns or injuries on new areas of reduced temperature and pain sensation is important to stress.

Surgical
Indications for surgery include rapid deterioration of neurological function or intractable pain. The role of surgical intervention in early or very slowly progressive PTS is less clear. Surgery can prevent progression and improve function but outcomes are quite variable. There is often improvement in pain and sensory function; motor, bladder, or bowel improvement is considerably less common, although progression may be slowed or stopped.

Several surgical procedures have been used. If PTS is associated with spinal canal narrowing and significant arachnoiditis, untethering the cord and nerve roots, combined with duraplasty may be indicated, with the premise that improved CSF flow will ameliorate the condition. Shunting of the syrinx is another surgical option, with the shunt draining the cyst into a low pressure area with high absorptive capacity. Shunt options include syringopleural, syringoperitoneal, or syringosubarachnoid shunt. Complications include shunt malfunction, shunt failure, and infection. Some investigators have also reported good results with selective spinal cordectomy as a method to drain CSF.

KNOWLEDGE GAPS AND EMERGING CONCEPTS

Cellular therapies, with cell transplants to fill the cyst are being investigated as a potential strategy. As understanding of the pathophysiology of PTS improves, more therapies will hopefully emerge.

SUGGESTED READING

Bursell JP, Little JW, Stiens SA. Electrodiagnosis in spinal cord injured persons with new weakness or sensory loss: central and peripheral etiologies. *Arch Phys Med Rehabil.* 1999;80(8):904-909.

Falci SP, Indeck C, Lammertse DP. Posttraumatic spinal cord tethering and syringomyelia: surgical treatment and long-term outcome. *J Neurosurg Spine.* 2009;11(4):445-460.

Paralyzed Veterans of America Consortium for Spinal Cord Medicine. Preservation of upper limb function following spinal cord injury: a clinical practice guideline for health-care professionals. *J Spinal Cord Med.* 2005;28(5):434-470.

Shields CB, Zhang YP, Shields LB. Post-traumatic syringomyelia: CSF hydrodynamic changes following spinal cord injury are the driving force in the development of PTSM. *Handb Clin Neurol.* 2012;109:355-367.

Spinal Cord Injury-Related Pain

GENERAL PRINCIPLES

Persistent or chronic pain is a significant problem for people with spinal cord injury (SCI) and one of the most frequently reported reasons for reduced quality of life after SCI.

Etiology

Pain after SCI can be due to numerous causes and is often multifactorial. Various classifications for pain after SCI have been used. A currently accepted classification, based on expert consensus, is the International SCI Pain Classification (ISCIP). The ISCIP classification organizes SCI pain into three tiers: Tier 1 categorizes pain type as nociceptive, neuropathic, other, and unknown; Tier 2 includes various subtypes for neuropathic and nociceptive pain; and Tier 3 is used to specify the primary pain source and/or pathology (Table 38C.1).

Nociceptive Musculoskeletal Pain
Musculoskeletal pain is most often due to overuse in people with SCI. It can sometimes be aggravated or precipitated by an acute injury. Overuse injuries commonly occur at the muscle-tendon junction, but can also involve cartilage, bursa, or bone. In people with paraplegia, shoulder pain is usually due to overuse. In those with tetraplegia, shoulder pain is more often related to shoulder instability (due to weakness of shoulder stabilizers) and/or contractures or capsulitis resulting from spasticity or lack of range of motion. Elbow pain from medial or lateral epicondylitis may occur from excessive forces or poor technique during wheelchair propulsion, and elbow or wrist pain may arise from weight bearing during repeated transfers or crutch use.

Nociceptive Visceral Pain
Visceral pain can be caused by any visceral pathology. Examples include fecal impaction, bowel obstruction, cholecystitis, gall stones or biliary duct stones, appendicitis, or pyelonephritis.

Table 38C.1

International Spinal Cord Injury Pain (ISCIP) Classification

Tier 1: Pain Type	Tier 2: Pain Subtype	Tier 3: Primary Pain Source and/or Pathology
Nociceptive pain	Musculoskeletal pain	E.g., glenohumeral arthritis, lateral epicondylitis, femur fracture
	Visceral pain	E.g., myocardial infarction, abdominal pain due to bowel impaction, cholecystitis, renal stone
	Other nociceptive pain	E.g., autonomic dysreflexia headache, migraine headache, surgical skin incision
Neuropathic pain	At level SCI pain	E.g., spinal cord compression, nerve root compression, syringomyelia
	Below level SCI pain	E.g., spinal cord ischemia, spinal cord compression
	Other neuropathic pain	E.g., carpal tunnel syndrome, trigeminal neuralgia, diabetic polyneuropathy
Other pain		E.g., fibromyalgia, Complex Regional Pain Syndrome type I, irritable bowel syndrome
Unknown pain		

Neuropathic Pain

At-level neuropathic pain can be caused by focal damage or lesion involving the spinal cord or nerve roots in the vicinity of the level of injury. Examples include nerve root compression due to vertebral deformity or instability around the level of injury. Below-level pain occurs as a result of the SCI itself. Other neuropathic pain includes that resulting from compressive or entrapment neuropathies.

Epidemiology

Significant pain is estimated to occur in approximately two-thirds of people with SCI, though the incidence varies considerably between reports based on the population studied and the criteria used to define and diagnose chronic pain.

Incidence of chronic neuropathic pain is reported to be higher in those with violence-associated SCI, especially if related to gunshot wound.

Shoulder pain is present in 30% to 70% of people with SCI. It is more common in older age, and increases with severity of injury, manual wheelchair use, reduced flexibility or stability of the shoulder joint, and increased body mass index.

Pathophysiology

Pathophysiology of pain depends on the type. Nociceptive musculoskeletal pain after SCI arises from activation of sensory nociceptive receptors in musculoskeletal tissues. It is most often the result of overuse injury because of repetitive forces on the upper extremity during activities such as wheelchair propulsion, overhead reaching, and transfers.

Neuropathic pain pathophysiology is not fully understood, but likely includes both central and peripheral mechanisms. Mechanisms may include cortical reorganization, neuronal hypersensitivity due to changes in receptors and ion channels, abnormal sprouting and connections, ectopic impulse generation, loss of inhibitory interneurons, and altered function of descending inhibitory and facilitatory pathways.

In addition to pathophysiological mechanisms, psychosocial mechanisms are important in pain generation and pain maintenance, and in pain-related suffering.

Complications and Associated Conditions

Chronic pain is associated with several comorbidities including depression, sleep disturbance, and functional limitations.

CLINICAL CONSIDERATIONS

Assessment

History
The international SCI pain basic data set provides guidance about a standardized way to collect and report data regarding pain in people with SCI. Assessment should include information to help distinguish between the different types of pain (Table 38C.2).

Pain intensity can be quantified using a standardized scale such as visual analogue scale (VAS) or the numerical rating scale (NRS, rating pain from 0 to 10). In addition evaluation of pain characteristics/descriptors, location, time course, radiation, associated features, and aggravating and relieving factors should be completed.

Pain interference with daily activities, mood, and sleep, should be assessed. Assessment of comorbidities such as depression is important. Responsiveness to previous and current treatments should be evaluated.

Table 38C.2

Distinguishing Features of Various Pain Types

Musculoskeletal Pain	Visceral Pain	Neuropathic Pain
Described as "dull" or "aching"	Described as "cramping," "dull," or "tender." Often poorly localized	Described as "hot-burning," "tingling," "pricking," "pins and needles," "sharp," "shooting," "squeezing," "painful cold" and "electric shock-like"
Affected by movement or a change in position	Affected by food intake or other visceral functions; associated nausea, loss of appetite, sweating	Sensory deficits present within the pain distribution area
Tenderness of musculoskeletal structures on palpation	Tenderness on palpation of the abdomen	Allodynia or hyperalgesia within the pain distribution
Evidence of consistent skeletal pathology on imaging	Evidence of visceral pathology on imaging or other testing	
Responsive to anti-inflammatory medication		

Pre-existing musculoskeletal or neuromuscular conditions that could be contributing to the pain should be noted.

Physical Examination

In addition to a focused examination of the region where the pain is localized, it is important to include a careful general physical, neurological, and musculoskeletal examination given the often multifocal nature of the pain and the high prevalence of atypical or overlapping presentations.

For example, in evaluating shoulder pain a thorough musculoskeletal examination of the shoulder region is needed, including special provocative tests for impingement or rotator cuff injury. In addition, however, neck or abdomen examination may identify possible sources of referred pain to the shoulder. Increase in pain with movement and localized tenderness to palpation suggest a musculoskeletal origin of the pain, whereas evidence of allodynia (pain evoked by normally nonpainful stimuli such as light touch) or hyperpathia (an exaggerated level of pain in response to nociceptive stimuli) suggest a neuropathic origin. New sensory or motor deficits found on examination may provide a clue to the possibility of a cervical syringomyelia as the cause of shoulder pain. Abdominal distension or tenderness may suggest a visceral source of referred pain (Table 38C.3).

Table 38C.3

Differential Diagnosis of Shoulder Pain After SCI

Etiology of Shoulder Pain	Suggestive Features
Musculoskeletal	
■ Rotator cuff/subacromial pain syndrome	Affected by movement or positioning
	Local tenderness
• Rotator cuff tendinitis	Limited range of motion
• Supraspinatus tendinitis	Positive provocative maneuvers
• Biceps tendinitis	Responsive to anti-inflammatory drugs
• Sub-acromial bursitis	
• Impingement syndrome	
■ Muscle strain	
■ Myofascial pain	
■ Acromioclavicular joint arthritis/strain	
■ Glenohumeral arthritis	
■ Frozen shoulder/capsulitis	
■ Osteolysis of distal clavicle	
■ Osteonecrosis of humeral head	
■ Musculoskeletal pathology of the cervical spine	
• Degenerative disease	
• Mechanical instability	
Visceral	
■ Acute abdomen	Fever, chills
• Cholecystitis	Nausea, loss of appetite
• Appendicitis	New or worsening autonomic dysreflexia
• Perforated peptic ulcer	or sweating
■ Renal stone	Abdominal tenderness, distension
■ Gallstone	
■ Ileus, bowel impaction	
■ Myocardial ischemia	
■ Other abdominal, pelvic pathology	
Neuropathic	
■ Syringomyelia	New sensory or motor impairment
■ Cervical radiculopathy	Burning, tingling pain/discomfort
■ Transitional zone pain	
Other	
■ Complex regional pain syndrome	Allodynia, hyperpathia
	Vasomotor changes

Abbreviation: SCI, spinal cord injury.

Diagnostic Tests

Imaging

Depending on the clinical presentation, imaging and other diagnostic tests are done to identify underlying pathology. For example, imaging of the shoulder may be indicated to evaluate persisting shoulder pain in a person with chronic SCI;

cervical spine imaging may also be indicated to assess for possible referred pain. Magnetic resonance imaging (MRI) of the cervical spine may be done to look for a syringomyelia if the characteristics of the pain and associated symptoms and signs suggest that possibility.

Similarly, abdominal imaging (ultrasound, MRI) may be needed to evaluate poorly localized abdominal discomfort that could be visceral in origin.

Laboratory Studies
These may be indicated, based on clinical assessment, to evaluate a potential visceral source of pain or systemic problems such as inflammatory arthritis.

Other Testing
Electromyography and nerve conduction testing may be helpful to evaluate possible nerve compression (e.g., carpal tunnel syndrome).

Differential Diagnosis
It is important to have an expanded differential diagnosis when evaluating pain in a person with SCI, given the often multifocal nature of the discomfort and the high prevalence of atypical or overlapping presentations (Table 38C.3).

Management

Management of Nociceptive Musculoskeletal Pain
Joint protection techniques are crucial both in prevention of overuse injuries and in their management (Chapter 27, Table 27.3). Flexibility exercise programs to maintain normal glenohumeral motion and pectoral muscle mobility should be incorporated into an overall fitness program for wheelchair users, as well as individualized and progressive resistance training.

Acute or subacute injuries are treated using the same principles as in the able-bodied population. However, relative rest may be difficult to achieve because of functional demands on the upper limb. Resting night splints may be helpful in carpal tunnel syndrome. Home modifications or additional assistance may allow for relative rest. Alternative techniques for activities, for joint protection, are even more important to consider when upper limb pain or injury is present.

If surgical intervention is considered for musculoskeletal pain in people with SCI, it is important to be aware of and plan for the postoperative recovery time of weeks to months when a period of increased functional restriction and dependence is to be anticipated. Temporary use of a power wheelchair, home modifications, and/or additional assistance may be considered during this time.

Pharmacological Management of Neuropathic Pain
Pharmacological management of neuropathic pain is quite suboptimal at this time, and not always effective. Recommended first line treatment includes tricyclic antidepressants (e.g., amitriptyline), calcium channel α_2-δ ligands

gabapentin and pregabalin, and mixed serotonin-noradrenaline reuptake inhibitors (Table 38C.4). Tricyclic antidepressants or mixed serotonin-noradrenaline reuptake inhibitors have the advantage of treating co-existing depression, if that is a prominent feature.

Pregabalin, a calcium channel α_2-δ ligand, was approved by the Food and Drug Administration (FDA) for SCI-related pain in 2012 based on results of supporting randomized controlled trials. It can be started at 150 mg/day in two to three divided doses and titrated up to 300 to 450 mg/day based on response. Gabapentin is administered three times daily, starting with a low initial dose and titrating up till pain relief, dose-limiting side-effects, or dosage of 3600 mg is achieved.

Second line agents include opioids, and tramadol (an analgesic that has low-affinity binding for the mu opioid receptors and inhibits reuptake of serotonin and norepinephrine). With opioids, major side effects include constipation, nausea, and sedation. Another important concern is that of abuse, misuse, or addiction. Risk factors include previous substance abuse and family history of substance abuse. An opioid drug agreement should be considered. Cannabinoids have had mixed efficacy in clinical trials. Intrathecal treatment

Table 38C.4

Medications Used for Pain Management in SCI	
Nonopioid analgesic	Acetaminophen
	Nonsteroidal anti-inflammatory drugs, salicylates
	Tramadol
Anticonvulsant— calcium channel α_2-δ ligands	Gabapentin
	Pregabalin
Other anticonvulsants	Carbamazepine
	Other (phenytoin, valproic acid, lamotrigine)
Tricyclic antidepressant	Amitriptyline
	Nortriptyline
SNRI	Duloxetine
	Venlafaxine
Opioid	Morphine sulfate
	Oxycodone
	Hydrocodone
	Fentanyl (transdermal)
Local anesthetic	Lidocaine patch
Neuroblocking cream	Capsaicin

Abbreviations: SCI, spinal cord injury; SNRI, serotonin-noradrenergic reuptake inhibitor.

with clonidine and morphine, or with neurotoxins such as ziconotide, has been used for severe refractory neuropathic pain.

Surgical Procedures
For intractable neuropathic pain following SCI, invasive treatments including deep brain stimulation, dorsal column stimulation, cordotomy, and dorsal root entry zone lesions have been tried, but without substantial evidence of success.

Multimodal Management of Pain, Emotional Distress, and Reduced Functioning
A multidisciplinary approach, using a biopsychosocial model, is recommended for chronic pain management. Due attention needs to be paid to the often accompanying emotional distress, reduced functioning, and impaired sleep patterns. Use of alcohol and illicit substances and misuse of prescription medications should be assessed and addressed as appropriate. Nonpharmacological measures including biofeedback or acupuncture may be helpful and cognitive behavioral therapy (CBT) may improve coping and functioning with pain and reduce pain-related depressive symptoms.

KNOWLEDGE GAPS AND EMERGING CONCEPTS

Emerging knowledge about the cellular and molecular changes that are involved in of neuronal hyper-excitability and other mechanisms in the pathogenesis of pain offers potential targets for new mechanism-based treatments.

SUGGESTED READING

Bryce TN, Biering-Sørensen F, Finnerup NB, et al. International spinal cord injury pain classification: part I. Background and description. *Spinal Cord.* 2012;50(6):413-417.

Cardenas DD, Felix ER. Pain after spinal cord injury: a review of classification, treatment approaches, and treatment assessment. *PM R.* 2009;1(12):1077-1090.

Cardenas DD, Nieshoff EC, Suda K, et al. A randomized trial of pregabalin in patients with neuropathic pain due to spinal cord injury. *Neurology.* 2013;80(6):533-539.

Dijkers M, Bryce T, Zanca J. Prevalence of chronic pain after traumatic spinal cord injury: a systematic review. *J Rehabil Res Dev.* 2009;46(1):13-29.

Dyson-Hudson TA, Kirshblum SC. Shoulder pain in chronic spinal cord injury, Part I: Epidemiology, etiology, and pathomechanics. *J Spinal Cord Med.* 2004;27(1):4-17.

Finnerup NB, Baastrup C. Spinal cord injury pain: mechanisms and management. *Curr Pain Headache Rep.* 2012;16(3):207-216.

Mehta S, Orenczuk K, McIntyre A, et al. Neuropathic pain post spinal cord injury part 1: systematic review of physical and behavioral treatment. *Top Spinal Cord Inj Rehabil.* 2013;19(1):61-77

Michailidou C, Marston L, De Souza LH, Sutherland I. A systematic review of the prevalence of musculoskeletal pain, back and low back pain in people with spinal cord injury. *Disabil Rehabil.* In press.

Teasell RW, Mehta S, Aubut JA, et al. A systematic review of pharmacologic treatments of pain after spinal cord injury. *Arch Phys Med Rehabil.* 2010;91(5):816-831.

Widerström-Noga E, Biering-Sørensen F, Bryce T, et al. The international spinal cord injury pain basic data set. *Spinal Cord.* 2008;46(12):818-823.

Heterotopic Ossification

GENERAL PRINCIPLES

Heterotopic ossification (HO) is characterized by formation of lamellar bone in soft tissues, usually around joints.

Etiology and Epidemiology

The estimated incidence after spinal cord injury (SCI) is around 25% to 30%, though only half of those cases are clinically or functionally significant. Progression to bony ankylosis occurs in a less than 5% of patients with SCI.

In people with SCI, risk factors for HO include: complete injury, prolonged immobility, spasticity and, in some but not all reports, thoracic level of injury and associated pressure ulcers.

HO occurs below the level of SCI. The most commonly involved joint is the hip (involved in 80%–90%, usually on the anterior or antero-medial aspect), followed by the knee (medial aspect), elbow, and shoulder.

Pathophysiology

The pathophysiology of HO is not well understood. It likely involves abnormal activation of mesenchymal cells to differentiate into bone-forming cells under the influence of bone morphogenic protein (BMP). The triggers for this process are not known, but may involve a combination of factors including inflammation, proprioceptive dysfunction, local trauma, tissue hypoxia, abnormal sympathetic activity, and/or immobilization hypercalcemia.

The bone formation in HO occurs primarily in the connective tissue between muscle planes, rather than within the muscle itself. Lamellar bone formation starts peripherally and progresses centrally, and is surrounded by a capsule of compressed muscle fibers and connective tissue.

Complications and Associated Conditions

Loss of joint mobility due to HO can interfere with mobility, positioning, hygiene, and activities of daily living. HO can also lead to breakdown of overlying skin, and increased spasticity. Autonomic dysreflexia can occur in people with SCI above T6. In rare instances, nerve compression or vascular occlusion may occur.

Natural History

Clinically detectable HO most commonly begins 1 to 4 months after SCI, sometimes later. Progression to mature bone often takes 12 to 24 months.

CLINICAL CONSIDERATIONS

Assessment

History and Physical Examination
Loss of range of motion (ROM) of the involved region is a common presenting feature. There may be associated pain or tenderness in case of preserved sensation, as well as local swelling or redness. It may be preceded or accompanied by fever in the acute stage, which is usually low-grade but could be high.

Diagnostic Tests
Bone Scan
A radionuclide (technetium-labeled) three-phase bone scan is the mainstay of early diagnosis. It shows increased marker uptake in the first and second stages of the scan, indicating hyperemia and blood pooling, in the first few weeks. Activity on the bone scan decreases with maturity of the HO.

Imaging
Plain films are of limited value in early diagnosis since they are often normal for the first few weeks till calcification occurs. A fluffy or pop-corn appearance may be seen in the periarticular region. In the hip it is often around the antero-medial aspect between the anterior superior iliac spine and the lesser trochanter.

Ultrasound can detect changes earlier than plain films in the form of echogenic shadows (reflecting bone formation) within a soft tissue mass.

Magnetic resonance imaging (MRI) can also be used to visualize the HO. Computed tomography (CT) is not useful for early diagnosis, but MRI or CT can supplement information regarding extent and anatomical relationship with nerves and blood vessels that is required for operative planning.

Laboratory Studies
Alkaline phosphatase is commonly elevated after 2 to 3 weeks and can be a useful indicator of HO, but is relatively nonspecific. It may remain elevated till the bone is mature and has been used as a supplementary tool to determine maturity and timing for resection, although its utility in this regard may be limited. The erythrocyte sedimentation rate (ESR) is often elevated, sometimes to very high levels, in the first few days or weeks. C-reactive protein (CRP) can also be elevated.

Creatinine kinase may be increased due to damage to surrounding muscle. Prostaglandin E2 (PGE2) levels in 24-hour urine samples can be elevated and has been suggested as a useful marker though is not commonly done.

Differential Diagnosis
Local limb swelling, sometimes associated with fever, can also occur with limb fractures, venous thrombosis, and cellulitis. The occasional occurrence of high fever and significantly elevated ESR can raise possibility of systemic infection.

Management

Range of Motion
The role of ROM in patients with HO is controversial. Gentle ROM is recommended at all stages, and may help prevent occurrence and progression of HO and HO-related ankylosis and functional impairment. Forceful ROM, however, should be avoided; it has been suggested as possibly contributing to HO formation perhaps through local trauma and micro-hemorrhage.

Pharmacological Prophylaxis
Routine bisphosphonate use for HO prophylaxis after SCI was suggested in the past. However, it is currently not typically recommended given the possibility of HO to develop after bisphosphonate prophylaxis is stopped, and weighing potential side-effects versus the relatively low frequency of HO with serious functional limitations.

Nonsteroidal anti-inflammatory drugs (NSAIDs) have been studied for prevention of HO after SCI, and for treatment in the early stage when inflammatory markers such as CRP and ESR are elevated. While indomethacin was shown to be effective in reducing HO, it is not routinely used in practice given its side-effect profile. The use of cyclooxygenase 2 (COX-2) inhibitors like celecoxib has been suggested as a potential prophylactic option with fewer side-effects than indomethacin, and merits further research.

Pharmacological Treatment
The first generation bisphosphonate, etidronate, is often used for treatment of HO, with a recommendation to start treatment early after diagnosis. Lack of

randomized controlled trials limits ability to make definitive recommendations. The suggested starting dose is typically 20 mg/kg/day. Practice regarding continued dosage and duration varies, with some continuing at the same dose for six months to decrease recurrence, and others reducing the dose to 10 mg/kg/day after a period of time. Etidronate seems to act primarily by blocking mineralization of the bone matrix versus inhibiting its production, so there is potential that HO progression may resume after the drug is stopped. It does not affect HO that has already formed. Side-effects, primarily gastrointestinal, can affect tolerance but may be limited by giving the medication in divided doses.

Newer generation bisphosphonates are more potent and have lesser side effects. A small study suggested pamidronate may be effective; however further research on newer agents is needed.

Radiation Therapy
Radiation therapy has been shown to be effective, although the studies in SCI are small and low quality. Given the potential for side-effects, radiation is typically not used as a primary treatment, but is used postoperatively after resection, with a goal to reduce recurrence.

Surgical Resection
HO that is causing significant functional limitation or other complications may require consideration for surgical resection. Anterior wedge resection of HO at the hip is the usual procedure. The surgery can be difficult, and associated with significant blood loss. It is generally recommended to delay surgery till the HO is mature, based on bone scan and lab testing prior to resection, because of the very high rate of recurrence with resection of immature HO. There are some reports, however, of good results with earlier resection prior to full maturity. Attention to post-operative positioning is important. Gentle passive ROM can be initiated after 3 to 4 days, but more aggressive therapy should be delayed. Post-operative radiation and/or drug treatment with NSAIDs or bisphosphonates is sometimes used, but needs further study for definitive recommendations.

KNOWLEDGE GAPS AND EMERGING CONCEPTS

There are significant knowledge gaps regarding the pathophysiology, prevention, and treatment of HO. Some recommendations are based on HO developing after hip arthroplasty; SCI-specific research is needed. Trials with newer bisphosphonates are ongoing, with a need for further study. Warfarin has been suggested as a potential prophylactic agent based on positive results from an observational study and postulated role on inhibition of bony matrix formation; however, this needs further evaluation before being considered in practice. New potential treatment avenues, for example, involving inhibition of BMP receptors, may be identified with research to further understand the pathogenesis of HO.

SUGGESTED READING

Aubut JA, Mehta S, Cullen N, Teasell RW; ERABI Group; Scire Research Team. A comparison of heterotopic ossification treatment within the traumatic brain and spinal cord injured population: an evidence based systematic review. *NeuroRehabilitation.* 2011;28(2):151-160.

Banovac K, Sherman AL, Estores IM, Banovac F. Prevention and treatment of heterotopic ossification after spinal cord injury. *J Spinal Cord Med.* 2004;27(4):376-382.

Cipriano CA, Pill SG, Keenan MA. Heterotopic ossification following traumatic brain injury and spinal cord injury. *J Am Acad Orthop Surg.* 2009;17(11):689-697.

Citak M, Suero EM, Backhaus M, et al. Risk factors for heterotopic ossification in patients with spinal cord injury: a case-control study of 264 patients. *Spine.* 2012;37(23):1953-1957.

Sakellariou VI, Grigoriou E, Mavrogenis AF, Soucacos PN, Papagelopoulos PJ. Heterotopic ossification following traumatic brain injury and spinal cord injury: insight into the etiology and pathophysiology. *J Musculoskelet Neuronal Interact.* 2012;12(4):230-240. Review.

Sullivan MP, Torres SJ, Mehta S, Ahn J. Heterotopic ossification after central nervous system trauma: a current review. *Bone Joint Res.* 2013;2(3):51-57.

Teasell RW, Mehta S, Aubut JL, et al. A systematic review of the therapeutic interventions for heterotopic ossification after spinal cord injury. *Spinal Cord.* 2010;48(7):512-521.

CHAPTER 39

Metabolic and Endocrine Issues: Overview

GENERAL PRINCIPLES

Several metabolic and endocrine abnormalities may occur in people with spinal cord injury (SCI). Consensus on several of these SCI-related metabolic and endocrine consequences is well established and uniformly accepted, although some aspects of their underlying mechanism and management are unclear. Examples of such conditions include changes in body composition with loss of lean body mass, modifications in energy expenditure, alterations in calcium metabolism, and osteoporosis with significant loss of bone.

For several other metabolic and endocrine conditions, there is varying degree of agreement, and additional evidence is needed to establish the causation, association and significance of those conditions in SCI.

CLINICAL CONSIDERATIONS

Potential metabolic and endocrine consequences, and related considerations are summarized in Table 39.1. Several of the conditions are discussed in further detail in other sections, which are referenced in Table 39.1. Effects of SCI on drug metabolism are summarized in Table 39.2.

Table 39.1

Metabolic and Endocrine Issues in SCI

Condition	Considerations
Body composition changes	- Loss of lean tissue mass - Increased relative adiposity - See Chapter 39A for details
Reduced energy expenditure	- Reduced basal metabolic rate (due to reduced muscle mass and, especially in injury above T6, reduced sympathetic activity) - Reduced energy expenditure of activity - See Chapter 39A for details
Carbohydrate metabolism	- Impaired glucose tolerance and possible increase in diabetes mellitus and metabolic syndrome (although consensus on contribution of SCI vs other demographic or co-existing factors is currently lacking) - See Chapter 33D regarding contribution to cardiovascular risk and Chapter 39A for discussion about metabolic syndrome in SCI
Lipid metabolism	- Prevalence of low levels of HDL seems higher than the general population - Potential cardiovascular risk factor (See Chapter 33D)
Bone loss and calcium metabolism	- Hypercalcemia in acute stage (See Chapter 39B, Table 39B.1 for details) - High rate of skeletal resorption and bone loss below the injury, leading to severe osteoporosis and fracture risk. See Chapter 39B for details
Anabolic hormone deficiency	- Growth hormone responses to provocative stimulation have been shown to be blunted. Pathogenesis and significance is not well established. Could be potential additional contributing factor to losses of lean tissue mass - Higher prevalence of testosterone deficiency has been reported in men with chronic SCI. See Chapter 35
Hypoalbuminemia, anemia	- Relatively common in SCI, but if significant, it should not be simply considered a normal consequence of SCI, and should prompt consideration of secondary complications (e.g., infection, inflammation, malnutrition)

(continued)

Table 39.1

Metabolic and Endocrine Issues in SCI (*continued*)

Condition	Considerations
Hyponatremia	- Sometimes seen in individuals with chronic tetraplegia. Pathogenesis is not clear. Altered regulation of the anti-diuretic hormone (ADH) level may be involved. High fluid intake could be a contributing factor but does not explain by itself without abnormality of free water excretion. May need fluid restriction if severe
Effect of SCI on pre-existing conditions	- Management of pre-existing diabetes may be complicated by immobility, weight gain, glucocorticoid/methyl-prednisone administration, acute stress, or infections resulting from SCI, in addition to the effect of reduction in muscle mass and related insulin resistance
Effect of SCI on drug metabolism	- See Table 39.2

Abbreviations: HDL, high-density cholesterol; SCI, spinal cord injury.

Table 39.2

Potential Effects of SCI on Drug Metabolism

SCI-Related Change	Impact on Pharmacokinetics
Delayed gastric emptying	- Rapid absorption of acidic drugs - Delayed absorption of basic drugs
Reduced gastrointestinal motility	- Increased absorption of drugs that undergo enterohepatic circulation - Decreased bioavailability of drugs that are destroyed by gut bacteria
Reduced blood flow to skin and muscle	- Less reliable transcutaneous, subcutaneous, and intramuscular drug absorption below injury level
Increased percentage of body fat	- Effect on fat- and water-soluble drug distribution
Reduced plasma protein level	- Increased free fraction of protein-bound drugs
Impaired kidney function	- Reduced renal elimination of drugs

Abbreviation: SCI, spinal cord injury.

SUGGESTED READING

Bauman WA, Korsten MA, Radulovic M, Schilero GJ, Wecht JM, Spungen AM. 31st g. Heiner sell lectureship: secondary medical consequences of spinal cord injury. *Top Spinal Cord Inj Rehabil.* 2012;18(4):354-378.

Bauman WA, Spungen AM, Adkins RH, Kemp BJ. Metabolic and endocrine changes in persons aging with spinal cord injury. *Assist Technol.* 2001;11:88-96.

Mestre H, Alkon T, Salazar S, Ibarra A. Spinal cord injury sequelae alter drug pharmacokinetics: an overview. *Spinal Cord.* 2011;49(9):955-960.

Energy Consumption and Body Composition After SCI

GENERAL PRINCIPLES

Energy Expenditure in SCI

Total daily energy expenditure (TDEE) includes three main components: basal metabolic rate (BMR), energy expenditure of activity, and thermic effect of food. After the postacute phase, TDEE is reduced in spinal cord injury (SCI) (Table 39A.1). The reduction in energy expenditure is related to the level and completeness of injury, with rates being lower for those with tetraplegia than for those with paraplegia.

BMR is the minimum amount of energy required for the anabolic and catabolic processes in the body at rest. It is generally expressed as kcal/24 hours and typically accounts for 60% to 75% of TDEE. Fat-free mass (muscle, bone, and organs) primarily contributes to BMR. Difference in skeletal muscle mass is major reason for individual differences in BMR. BMR is reduced after SCI due to reduction in both muscle mass and sympathetic activity.

Energy expenditure of activity or exercise is also reduced in SCI. Large body segments require more energy to move than smaller segments, for example, legs versus arms. Muscle paralysis, especially of the large lower extremity muscles, and reduced cardiovascular inotropic and chronotropic responses to activity related to lower sympathetic activity, result in reduced energy expenditure of activity after SCI.

Body Composition in SCI

Body composition includes fat mass (FM) and fat free mass (FFM). FFM includes water, proteins, and minerals. Determination of body composition using hydro-densitometry is based on this two-component model of FM and FFM and the known differences in density of these two components.

SCI affects body composition in multiple ways (Table 39A.2). Lean muscle mass is reduced after SCI. Reduced lean muscle mass results in reduced

Table 39A.1

Energy Metabolism and Effect of SCI

Total daily energy expenditure is reduced in SCI due to reduction in both BMR and in energy expenditure of exercise or activity

Reduced BMR occurs in SCI secondary to
- Reduced muscle mass
- Reduced sympathetic activity (in SCI above T6)

Reduced energy expenditure of activity occurs due to
- Muscle paralysis, especially of lower extremity large muscles
- Reduced cardiovascular inotropic and chronotropic reactions to activity related to blunted sympathetic response

Abbreviations: BMR, basal metabolic rate; SCI, spinal cord injury.

Table 39A.2

Effect of SCI on Body Composition and Body Mass Index

Body Composition

SCI can affect body composition in several ways.
- Reduced lean muscle mass resulting in reduced total body water
- Decreased bone mineral content
- Relative increase in % BF
- Because of the above changes, the two-component model may give inaccurate assessment of body composition underestimating % BF

BMI and Obesity

- BMI or body weight may not accurately reflect adiposity in SCI using the designated thresholds for able-bodied individuals, given the increased percent body fat after SCI
- Lower BMI cut-off for overweight has been suggested to be used in people with SCI (e.g., 22 kg/m² instead of 25 kg/m² to consider overweight)
- Ideal body weight may need to be adjusted downward by 5% to 10% for those with paraplegia and 10% to 15% for those with tetraplegia
- Lower caloric intake than recommended by standard guidelines based on body weight may be more appropriate in SCI (based on neurological level and completeness of injury)

Abbreviations: BF, body fat; BMI, body mass index; SCI, spinal cord injury.

total body water. In addition there is decreased bone mineral content (from SCI-related osteoporosis), as well as a relative increase in percent body fat (BF). Because of these changes, the two-component model may give inaccurate assessment of body composition underestimating percent BF.

Body Mass Index and Obesity

Body mass index (BMI) assesses weight in relation to height squared (kg/m²). BMI is considered to be reflective of adiposity. In the general population, BMI greater than 25 kg/m² is considered overweight, and BMI greater than 30 kg/m² is considered obese.

In SCI, BMI or body weight may not accurately reflect adiposity using the designated thresholds for able-bodied individuals, given the increased percent of BF. It has been suggested that a lower BMI cut-off for overweight be used in people with SCI (e.g., 22 kg/m^2 instead of 25 kg/m^2 to consider overweight). Lower caloric intake than recommended by standard guidelines based on body weight may be more appropriate in SCI, depending on neurological level and completeness of injury.

In addition to cardiovascular risk, excess weight and obesity can have multiple detrimental effects on people with SCI including reduced functional capability, greater susceptibility to overuse injuries, and worsening of respiratory compromise.

Metabolic Syndrome

Although not conclusively established, the risk of metabolic syndrome may be increased after SCI. The metabolic syndrome is associated with a proinflammatory and prothrombotic state that is thought to promote cardiovascular disease. Abdominal/visceral adipose tissue has been shown to secrete inflammatory cytokines that cause direct and indirect vascular endothelial injury as well as prothrombotic agents that inhibit fibrinolysis, so the increased adiposity after SCI may create increased cardiovascular risk.

CLINICAL CONSIDERATIONS

Assessment

It has been suggested that ideal body weight may need to be adjusted downward by 5% to 10% for those with paraplegia and 10% to 15% for those with tetraplegia. As mentioned above, BMI may underestimate adiposity in people with SCI so lowered cut-off levels for overweight are suggested. Other anthropometric measurements such as arm-circumference or skin-fold thickness are also considered to be inaccurate in people with SCI.

Effects of SCI may confound diagnosis of metabolic syndrome and its individual components (Table 39A.3). Components of the metabolic syndrome, as defined by the National Cholesterol Education Project Adult Treatment Panel III (NCEP ATP III) include:

- Central obesity (waist circumference >102 cm in males, >88 cm in females)
- Atherogenic dyslipidemia (Triglyceride >150 mg/dL, and/or high-density lipoprotein (HDL)-c <40 mg/dL in men, <50 mg/dL in women)
- Hypertension (Blood pressure >130/85 mmHg)
- Insulin resistance and hyperglycemia (fasting glucose >110 mg/dL)

In SCI, abdominal muscle paralysis may increase waist circumference measurement so that may not be an accurate assessment of central obesity. Neurogenic hypotension or autonomic dysreflexia may confound blood pressure readings.

Table 39A.3
Metabolic Syndrome in SCI

Diagnosis

Effects of SCI may confound diagnosis of metabolic syndrome:
- Abdominal muscle paralysis may increase waist circumference measurement so that may not be an accurate assessment of central obesity
- Neurogenic hypotension or autonomic dysreflexia may confound blood pressure readings

Management

SCI may impact management of metabolic syndrome:
- Typical parameters for caloric intake based on weight or BMI may not be accurate in SCI. Caloric requirements may be lower and need to be calculated accordingly
- Physical activity and exercise options are limited in SCI. Muscle paralysis and reduced sympathetic response may limit effectiveness of exercise. While exercise should be prescribed, optimal exercise regimens are not fully established for people with SCI
- Choice of pharmacological management may need to be adapted in SCI. E.g., a thiazide diuretic for hypertension may not be an appropriate option in those who perform intermittent catheterizations for bladder management.

Abbreviations: BMI, body mass index; SCI, spinal cord injury.

Laboratory tests for specific aspects of nutritional assessment include lipid profile, prealbumin and albumin levels for assessment of protein status, and Vitamin D levels to identify deficiency and need for replacement.

Management

The presence of SCI impacts dietary and exercise recommendations for general health, and influences the management of metabolic syndrome (Table 39A.3).

Important aspects of management of metabolic syndrome include:

- Dietary modifications: (a) Reduced caloric intake for sustainable weight loss and weight management, and (b) Minimizing saturated and trans fats, foods or beverages with high glycemic index, and added sugar or salt
- Increased physical activity
- Pharmacological management as needed (in conjunction with lifestyle management) for hypertension, lipid modification, and glucose control

Diet and Nutrition

Typical parameters for caloric intake based on weight or BMI may not be accurate in SCI. While differences in age, gender, body habitus, and activity need to be taken into account to determine ideal caloric intake, on average daily caloric requirement may need to be based on ideal body weight that is 5% to 10% below standard for individuals with paraplegia and between 10% to 15% less than standard for those with tetraplegia. Average estimated energy requirements are reported to be ~23 kcal/kg/day in people with tetraplegia and ~28 kcal/kg/day in those with paraplegia.

In addition to appropriate caloric intake, nutritional counseling should stress increased fruit and vegetable intake and decreased intake of saturated fat and refined carbohydrates. While protein requirements are considerably higher during the acute hyper-catabolic stage in the initial weeks after SCI when a negative nitrogen balance is typical, protein requirements after the post-acute phase are similar to the general population at ~0.8 g/kg. The presence of pressure ulcers increases protein requirements, especially with Stage III and IV wounds.

Activity and Exercise
Physical activity and exercise options are limited in SCI. Muscle paralysis and reduced sympathetic response may limit effectiveness of exercise. While exercise should be prescribed, optimal exercise regimens are not fully established for people with SCI. Exercise after SCI is further discussed in Chapter 43.

Pharmacological Management
The presence of SCI may influence choice of pharmacological management of hypertension or other components of the metabolic syndrome. For example, thiazide diuretics, typically prescribed as first line agents for hypertension, may not be appropriate for individuals who perform intermittent catheterizations for bladder management.

KNOWLEDGE GAPS AND EMERGING CONCEPTS

Additional studies are needed to establish the risk and consequences of metabolic syndrome in people with SCI.

Research to develop and evaluate optimal ways to measure body composition and obesity in SCI is ongoing.

SUGGESTED READING

Bauman WA, Spungen AM. Metabolic changes in persons after spinal cord injury. *Phys Med Rehab Clin North Am.* 2000;11:102-140.

Gater DR. Obesity after spinal cord injury. *Phys Med Rehabil Clin North Am.* 2007;18(2):333-351.

Groah SL, Nash MS, Ljungberg IH, et al. Nutrient intake and body habitus after spinal cord injury: an analysis by sex and level of injury. *J Spinal Cord Med.* 2009;32(1):25-33.

Khalil RE, Gorgey AS, Janisko M, Dolbow DR, Moore JR, Gater DR. The role of nutrition in health status after spinal cord injury. *Aging Dis.* 2013;4(1):14-22.

Laughton GE, Buchholz AC, Martin Ginis KA. Lowering body mass index cutoffs better identifies obese persons with spinal cord injury. *Spinal Cord.* 2009;47(10):757-762.

Price M. Energy expenditure and metabolism during exercise in persons with spinal cord injury. *Sports Med.* 2010;40:681-696.

Spungen AM, Adkins RH, Stewart CA, et al. Factors influencing body composition in persons with spinal cord injury: a cross-sectional study. *J Appl Physio.* 2003;95:2398-2407.

Calcium Metabolism and Osteoporosis After SCI

GENERAL PRINCIPLES

Etiology

Spinal cord injury (SCI) results in a loss of the normal coupling of bone formation and bone resorption, primarily due to a significant increase in bone resorption. Bone loss starts within days to weeks after injury, and continues at an accelerated pace for the first 6 to 12 months, at a peak rate of up to 4% loss of bone mineral density (BMD) per month. After that time, bone loss continues at a slower rate for several years before stabilizing.

The excess bone resorption occurs only below the level of injury. Trabecular bone seems to be especially susceptible (e.g., in proximal and distal femoral and tibial epiphysis, and diaphysis), although both cortical and trabecular bone loss occurs.

Calcium released by bone is excreted by kidneys, with hypercalciuria developing within the first week and continuing for 6 to 18 months. Hypercalcemia can also occur, peaking between 1 and 6 months (Table 39B.1).

Epidemiology

As a result of the bone loss, pathological fractures are common. The sites of greatest bone loss, and of fracture risk, are the distal femur and proximal tibia, with a reported bone loss of 50% to 60% at those sites by 5 to 7 years in people with complete SCI. The upper limb is affected only in people with tetraplegia, but not in paraplegia. The spinal column is relatively spared.

Those with a motor complete injury are at much higher risk for bone loss and fracture. Other risk factors for fractures include paraplegia versus tetraplegia (probably related to differences in levels of activity), whites, females, and greater time since injury.

Pathophysiology

The precise pathophysiology of SCI-related osteoporosis is not fully understood. Mechanical, hormonal, and neurological factors all likely play a part.

Table 39B.1

Hypercalcemia After SCI	
Risk factors	- Adolescents and young males - Complete tetraplegia - Prolonged immobilization
Time course	- Peaks between 1–3 months postinjury
Presentation	- Nausea, vomiting, abdominal pain (if some preserved sensation) - Polyuria, polydipsia - Confusion, behavioral changes, psychosis - Presentation may be vague; high index of suspicion warranted for those at risk
Tests	- Serum calcium (often >12 mg/dL) (In presence of hypoalbuminemia, total calcium may underestimate ionic calcium level) - Renal function tests, since renal insufficiency can occur
Management	- Hydration with intravenous fluids (with indwelling catheter in place) - Loop diuretics—furosemide (not thiazides, which cause hypercalcemia) - Bisphosphonate—Pamidronate, single intravenous dose

Abbreviation: SCI, spinal cord injury.

The absence of mechanical stress on bone, as a result of paralysis, has been considered an important factor in bone loss, as is immobility. Hormonal influences are also important; there is some evidence of a role of parathyroid hormone, as well as possible contribution of decreased testosterone levels. Bone is richly innervated by autonomic fibers, and blunted sympathetic response after SCI may also play a part, perhaps through bone perfusion changes.

Complications and Associated Conditions

Pathological fractures are the primary complication of osteoporosis. Fractures can be associated with additional problems such as skin breakdown, increased spasticity, autonomic dysreflexia, mal-union, and additional potential impairments in mobility and positioning.

CLINICAL CONSIDERATIONS

The main clinical consequences of dysfunction of calcium and bone metabolism after SCI are:

- Immobilization hypercalcemia, and
- Secondary osteoporosis with fracture risk

Clinical considerations related to immobilization hypercalcemia after SCI are summarized in Table 39B.1.

The remainder of this chapter focuses on clinical aspects of osteoporosis and fractures.

Assessment

History and Physical Examination
Osteoporosis without fractures is asymptomatic, and is not apparent on clinical assessment till fractures occur. Additional secondary causes of osteoporosis (e.g., smoking, malnutrition, inflammatory bowel disease, medications, hyperthyroidism) may be identified during assessment. History of previous fracture may be present. Old fractures may be identified incidentally without known history of a fracture episode.

Fractures may occur with trivial injury, often during transfers, range of motion, or minor slip or fall. In some cases, there may be no identified history of overt injury. Insensate patients may feel no pain and present with nonspecific symptoms of feeling unwell or increased spasticity, and the diagnosis may be overlooked initially. Individuals with SCI above T6 neurological level may present with autonomic dysreflexia due to the noxious stimulus resulting from fracture, even in the absence of any pain sensation. Examination may show painless swelling or deformity.

Diagnostic Tests
Bone Mineral Density
The primary diagnostic test to diagnose osteoporosis is measurement of BMD through dual-energy X-ray absorptiometry (DXA). Test results are in the form of two scores: T score (BMD compared with a young adult of the same gender with peak bone mass; a score above −1 is considered normal, between −1 and −2.5 is classified as osteopenia, and below −2.5 is defined as osteoporosis. The T score is used to estimate fracture risk); and Z score (BMD compared with other people of same age group, size and gender).

However, the standard osteoporotic diagnostic criteria and BMD measurement have not been adequately evaluated in people with SCI, and may not be appropriate since standard DXA does not evaluate the distal femur and proximal tibia, the sites of greatest risk in SCI. Consensus about the precise clinical role of routine DXA in people with SCI is not established at this time, given the above limitations and lack of currently established good treatment options.

Imaging
Plain films show advanced osteoporosis, but are of limited value in early diagnosis since they may be normal till 30% BMD is lost. They are sometimes useful in chronic SCI, for example, to evaluate risk prior to initiating a new weight-bearing program. Plain x-rays are also indicated for diagnosing and evaluating pathological fractures, although hairline fractures may be missed.

Quantitative computed tomography (qCT) may be a more valid tool to evaluate osteoporosis, but currently has very limited availability beyond the research setting.

Laboratory Studies
Vitamin D levels should be checked. Laboratory tests may identify other secondary or contributing causes. Biomarkers of bone turnover include hydroxyproline, C-telopeptide, and N-telopeptide, among others; however, their role in clinical management is unclear at this time.

Differential Diagnosis
The possibility of lower limb pathological fracture should always be kept in mind in patient presentation with swelling of one leg. Other causes of unilateral leg swelling in someone with SCI include heterotopic ossification, venous thrombosis, and cellulitis.

Management

Identification and Treatment of Secondary Contributing Factors
Vitamin D deficiency should be identified and treated. Prevalence of Vitamin D deficiency is increased in people with SCI. Reduced sunlight exposure, lifestyle changes, and medications have been suggested as potential contributing factors, as well as an impaired ability to convert Vitamin D to its active form. At this time there are no evidence-based SCI-specific guidelines for Vitamin D and calcium supplementation in people with SCI beyond those available for the general population.

Role of Medications/Bisphosphonates in Treating SCI-Related Osteoporosis
Bisphosphonates have a strong affinity for bone and inhibit osteoclastic resorption. Some studies suggest positive effects of bisphosphonate treatment for osteoporosis in SCI, including recent reports with newer agents such as zoledronic acid. However, the results are mixed and several other studies have shown no benefit, including a trial of pamidronate treatment for SCI-related osteoporosis. In general, studies in this area are limited by small sample sizes, issues with study design, or lack of full consideration of confounding factors. Larger randomized trials are needed to establish the role of bisphosphonate to prevent and/or reduce SCI-related osteoporosis. No definitive guidelines or consensus currently exist, and presently there is considerable variation in opinion and practice in this regard.

Role of Exercise and Activity
Prolonged immobility should be avoided. Passive weight bearing has been shown to be largely ineffective for SCI-related osteoporosis. Some small studies have suggested benefit with functional electrical stimulation (FES)-assisted cycling or other forms of exercise, but again, the results have been mixed and

sustainability of improvement has not been demonstrated. This is an area of further study both to establish benefit and to define optimal exercise protocols.

Reducing Risk of Falls and Injuries

Given the high lifetime risk of fractures, precautionary measures to reduce fall risk should be stressed, including safety in transfers, which is one of the high-risk activities for injury. Caution should be applied when considering initiation of new weight-bearing activities for someone with chronic SCI and severe osteoporosis.

Management of Osteoporotic Fractures

In general, a nonsurgical approach is followed for nonambulatory patients, except in those with severe displacement or other complications. Fractures around the knee are typically treated with a knee immobilizer or a well-padded splint. Circular casts should be avoided because of risk of underlying skin breakdown; if used, they should be well padded and bi-valved to allow for regular skin inspection (Table 39B.2). Elevation of the extremity may be needed to minimize edema; for the lower extremity this may mean using an elevated leg-rest for the wheelchair, which may temporarily reduce maneuverability and wheelchair access and may need to be considered in the treatment and discharge plan.

Increased spasticity may need temporary medication adjustment. The effect of the fracture and related deformity and/or immobilization on function, transfers, and wheelchair seating should be considered and addressed as appropriate.

Severely displaced fractures with rotational deformities may be considered for surgical treatment, but there are often problems with fixation and healing due to the poor quality of the bone. In the rare extreme case, amputation may be considered.

Table 39B.2

Key Considerations in Management of Osteoporotic Fractures in SCI

- Avoid circular casts; if used they should be well padded and bi-valved
- Surgery is typically not indicated, in the absence of severe deformity, and is problematic due to bone quality
- Temporary increase in spasticity and/or autonomic dysreflexia should be anticipated and addressed as appropriate
- The effect of fracture-related deformity and/or immobilization on wheelchair access, function, transfers, and wheelchair seating should be considered and addressed

Abbreviation: SCI, spinal cord injury.

KNOWLEDGE GAPS AND EMERGING CONCEPTS

There are several avenues of ongoing research regarding bone metabolism and osteoporosis in SCI, with promising initial results. However, many gaps remain for evidence-based practice in this area, both in early diagnosis and in management. The role and optimal type and frequency of exercise intervention including FES-exercise, as well as the potential role of newer bisphosphonates in SCI-related osteoporosis needs further study with well-designed trials of sufficient power to generate conclusive results. Among areas of ongoing research are: combined mechanical and pharmacological approaches to prevent or reduce bone loss, study of the role of sclerostin in osteoporosis after SCI, and pharmacological approaches to target and inhibit receptor activator of nuclear-kβ ligand (RANKL), that has a prominent role in osteoclastic activity.

SUGGESTED READING

Bauman WA, Schnitzer TJ, Chen D. Management of osteoporosis after spinal cord injury: what can be done? Point/counterpoint. *PM R.* 2010;2(6):566-572.

Biering-Sørensen F, Hansen B, Lee BS. Non-pharmacological treatment and prevention of bone loss after spinal cord injury: a systematic review. *Spinal Cord.* 2009;47(7):508-518.

Charmetant C, Phaner V, Condemine A, Calmels P. Diagnosis and treatment of osteoporosis in spinal cord injury patients: a literature review. *Ann Phys Rehabil Med.* 2010;53(10): 655-668.

Dionyssiotis Y. Spinal cord injury-related bone impairment and fractures: an update on epidemiology and physiopathological mechanisms. *J Musculoskelet Neuronal Interact.* 2011;11(3):257-265.

Dolbow DR, Gorgey AS, Daniels JA, Adler RA, Moore JR, Gater DR. The effects of spinal cord injury and exercise on bone mass: a literature review. *NeuroRehabilitation.* 2011;29(3):261-269.

Giangregorio L, McCartney N. Bone loss and muscle atrophy in spinal cord injury: epidemiology, fracture prediction, and rehabilitation strategies. *J Spinal Cord Med.* 2006;29(5): 489-500.

Maïmoun L, Fattal C, Sultan C. Bone remodeling and calcium homeostasis in patients with spinal cord injury: a review. *Metabolism.* 2011;60(12):1655-1663.

Morse LR, Giangregorio L, Battaglino RA, et al. VA-based survey of osteoporosis management in spinal cord injury. *PM R.* March 2009;1(3):240-244.

Qin W, Bauman WA, Cardozo CP. Evolving concepts in neurogenic osteoporosis. *Curr Osteoporos Rep.* 2010;8(4):212-218.

CHAPTER 40

Aging With a Spinal Cord Injury

GENERAL PRINCIPLES

Life expectancy of persons with spinal cord injury (SCI) has progressively increased. Mean age of the SCI population as well as mean age at injury have increased, in association with overall aging of the general population. Consequently, issues related to aging with SCI are increasingly encountered by individuals with SCI, their caregivers, and health care providers.

Suggested Accelerated Aging Trajectory After SCI

Ongoing research has suggested occurrence of early aging in individuals with SCI, often with atypical features. The body's reserve capacity of its organ systems begins to decline at a rate of approximately 1% per year in able-bodied people after their mid-20s. Because of the normal excess reserve in most body systems, this decline does not present a significant problem to meet daily life needs for the average person even up to age 70 years. It has been suggested that for certain body systems and functions, SCI may accelerate this age-related decline.

Various factors could contribute to this suggested alteration in aging trajectory. For example, lack of mobility, muscle activity and weight-bearing after SCI lead to changes in body composition with decreased proportion of muscle mass and increased adipose tissue, reduced bone mineral density, and potential increase in cardiovascular risk factors. Similarly upper extremity overuse over time can lead to accelerated musculoskeletal problems.

It is important to differentiate factors that are associated with aging from those related to duration of injury, although there is often an overlap. Respiratory complications, for example, are related more to aging than to duration of injury.

CLINICAL CONSIDERATIONS

Particular attention is warranted in anticipating and managing new problems, minimizing secondary complications, and maintaining health, function, and quality of life as people age with SCI.

A complicating factor is that clinical manifestations related to interaction of SCI and aging in various body systems may present with atypical or nonspecific features resulting in diagnostic confusion, and delayed identification and treatment.

Interaction Between Aging and SCI

Aging and SCI both affect all body systems. There is considerable interaction and overlap between effects of SCI and age-related factors that affect both diagnosis and management, as discussed below for each system and summarized in Table 40.1.

Respiratory

Because of higher risk of pneumonia with older age, pneumococcal and yearly influenza vaccinations are especially important, as is smoking cessation.

Late onset ventilatory failure may occur in people with tetraplegia who were previously ventilator-free. Contributing factors may include age-related decrease in chest wall and lung compliance, decreased alveoli, and decreased vital capacity that may decompensate borderline ventilators, progressive spinal deformity with thoracic kyphoscoliosis, excess weight gain and obesity, or neurological deterioration due to progressive posttraumatic syringomyelia.

Cardiovascular

Heart disease is now a major cause of mortality and morbidity in people with SCI, and with the aging of this population, ischemic heart disease (IHD)-related issues have become increasingly important in the care of these individuals. It has been suggested that the prevalence of IHD is increased after SCI compared to the general population, although universal consensus in that regard is currently lacking.

Individuals with SCI above T5 may not perceive chest pain with angina. They may present atypically with episodic dyspnea, nausea, unexplained autonomic dysreflexia, syncope, or changes in spasticity. There may also be confusion in the interpretation of physical signs, with difficulty in differentiating congestive heart failure from dependent edema or from lung crackles caused by atelectasis, both of which are common in SCI.

Similarly, a delay in diagnosis of peripheral arterial disease (PAD) may occur in patients with SCI because of the lack of the cardinal symptom of intermittent claudication. Symptoms of more advanced limb ischemia, such as rest pain or numbness, may also be absent, and patients may first present with advanced disease.

Table 40.1
Potential Interactions Between Effects of SCI and Effects of Aging

Organ System	Effects of SCI	Effects of Aging
Respiratory	- Impaired cough→ retention of secretions, atelectasis, mucus plugs, pneumonia - Impaired ventilation (with high tetraplegia) - Sleep disordered breathing	- Decreased chest wall and lung compliance - Decreased alveoli - Decreased vital capacity - Can decompensate borderline ventilators

Cardiovascular	- Early, but could be ongoing:
	  • Orthostatic hypotension
	  • Venous thromboembolism
	- Ongoing issues:
	  • Autonomic dysreflexia
	  • ↓ Cardiovascular fitness
	  • Cardiovascular effects of medications in SCI
	- Influence of SCI on coronary artery disease and peripheral vascular disease
	  • ↑ Risk factors e.g., ↓ HDL, ↑ %body fat and insulin resistance, ↓ physical activity
	  • Diagnostic limitations (confusing or absent signs, exercise stress test not feasible)
		- ↑ Prevalence of cardiovascular disease including ischemic heart disease (IHD) peripheral arterial disease (PAD)

Metabolic	- Pharmacokinetic effects of SCI/ effect of SCI on drug metabolism and bioavailability (absorption, distribution, metabolism, excretion) - Effect on carbohydrate and lipid metabolism (see above)	- Polypharmacy potential - Impact of aging on drug pharmacokinetics (e.g., age related decline in hepatic metabolism and renal elimination) and pharmacodynamics
Genitourinary	- Loss of voluntary control - Detrusor sphincter dyssynergia - ↑ Urinary tract pressure - Bladder stones - Urinary tract infection (UTI) - ↑ Bladder cancer (indwelling chronic catheter, smokers) - Erectile dysfunction	- ↓ Bladder capacity - ↑ Uninhibited detrusor contractions - ↓ Kidney function - ↑ Nocturia, change in diurnal urine output - ↑ UTI - Prostate enlargement - Erectile dysfunction due to co-morbidities

(continued)

Table 40.1

Potential Interactions Between Effects of SCI and Effects of Aging (*continued*)

Organ System	Effects of SCI	Effects of Aging
Gastrointestinal	- Loss of voluntary bowel control - Anorectal dyssynergia - ↓ Rectal expulsive force - Anorectal problems (hemorrhoids, fissures, proctitis, prolapse) - Gallstones - False +ve stool testing may complicate colorectal cancer screening	- ↓ GI motility - ↓ Acid secretion - Need for colon cancer screening
Skin/ Integument	- ↑ Risk for pressure ulcers (immobility, lack of sensation, spasticity) - Marjolin's ulcer (squamous cell carcinoma) risk in chronic ulcers	- Skin atrophy - ↓ Elasticity, vascularity and collagen content - ↓ Tolerance to shear
Neurological	- Paralysis, sensory loss - Entrapment neuropathies (median nerve at wrist, ulnar at elbow) - Posttraumatic syringomyelia - May have cognitive impairment from coexisting brain injury	- ↓ Muscle mass/strength - ↓ Coordination/agility - Impaired balance/gait - Prolonged reaction time
Musculoskeletal	- Overuse syndromes including shoulder/rotator cuff problems - Chronic pain (nociceptive and/or neuropathic) - Heterotopic ossification - Secondary osteoporosis and pathologic fractures	- Degenerative arthritis - Age-related osteoporosis
Psychosocial	- Increased potential for stress, depression, isolation - Quality of life is related more with participation rather than degree of impairment	- Aging caregivers/spouse - Loss of social support - Impact on social participation

Abbreviation: HDL, high-density lipoprotein.

Metabolic/Endocrine

Changes in body composition and energy metabolism with aging may compound changes secondary to SCI.

Hypothyroidism should be kept in the differential diagnosis of new onset of fatigue in the aging person with SCI.

Drug metabolism, including clearance, is affected by both SCI and aging and there is particular risk of drug interactions and drug-related side-effects.

Genitourinary

Benign prostatic hyperplasia is very common in older males and may confound assessment and management of SCI-related genitourinary dysfunction.

Patients with long-standing indwelling catheters are at higher risk for bladder cancer and may require periodic screening.

Arthritic changes with loss of hand dexterity and decreased mobility may affect previous ability to perform intermittent catheterization.

Gastrointestinal

Decreased gastrointestinal motility with aging may worsen constipation.

Further loss of dexterity and mobility with aging may interfere with ability to perform proper digital stimulation, requiring modification of the previously established bowel program.

Bleeding from local anorectal problems or trauma that may occur in SCI may interfere with stool testing for colon cancer screening, which is recommended at age over 50 years as in able-bodied individuals. Colonoscopy for cancer screening requires special bowel preparation to enable adequate visualization, which may be especially cumbersome for people with SCI.

Because of difficulty in performing adequate dental hygiene on a regular basis, people with tetraplegia may be at higher risk of developing dental disease as they age.

Skin

Loss of tissue elasticity and increased tendency for skin dryness with aging may add to risk of skin breakdown, so proper attention to those aspects is warranted.

Neurologic

Posttraumatic syringomyelia should be considered in the differential diagnosis of new onset of neurological and functional decline instead of automatically ascribing it to age-related decline.

Age-related decrease in balance and coordination can further compound gait problems in ambulatory individuals with SCI.

Loss of visual acuity with aging (cataracts, macular degeneration) may significantly reduce function in those who were previously relying on vision to partly compensate for SCI-related sensory impairment.

Sleep patterns change with aging and may need attention.

Ability for new learning is affected by aging to a variable degree and should be kept in mind while planning educational and training programs for these individuals. Poor retention, overstimulation, or frustration may occur if the material is not focused and too much information is included at one time.

Musculoskeletal

Degenerative arthritis may significantly worsen ability to perform activities of daily living and mobility, and decrease functional independence.

Overuse syndromes in the upper extremity are common and may worsen with aging.

Age-related changes in bone metabolism may compound SCI-related osteoporosis.

Use of nonsteroidal anti-inflammatory drugs (NSAIDs) for pain or SCI-related overuse injury should be particularly judicious in older adults given the higher risk of gastrointestinal bleeding.

Function

Functional decline with aging is accelerated in people with SCI. It has been reported that, on average, additional assistance for function is required at age 49 years for individuals with tetraplegia and age 55 years in those with paraplegia compared to 70 years or older for the general population. Modifications in the way activities are performed and/or use of adaptive equipment or other technology can facilitate preservation or maintenance of functional independence.

Psychosocial

Aging or death of spouse or companion in conjunction with the individual's own decline in functional ability can lead to loss of independent living and potential for social isolation and reduced participation. Particular efforts to address these issues are needed, as are measures to ensure caregiver support.

Advanced care planning and opportunity to discuss thoughts and fears about death and dying as appropriate should be facilitated.

It is important to realize, however, that reported quality of life does not necessarily decline with aging in SCI. Some studies have suggested that overall depression rates decline with aging after peaking between 25 and 45 years of age in people with SCI, and that rates decline in those living with SCI for more than 20 years. Risk of depression in the older population is associated with presence of other illnesses and with significant decline in function, further underscoring the need to adequately address those issues.

KNOWLEDGE GAPS AND EMERGING CONCEPTS

Increasing survival and progressively increasing lifespan are relatively recent phenomena. Aging with SCI is an evolving but important multidimensional area for research.

Research is needed to better understand and differentiate the effect of aging versus duration of injury.

Greater understanding of the aging trajectory after SCI is needed, with identification of specific factors that have the greatest impact on psychological and physical functioning, participation, and quality of life.

There is a need for systems of care for people aging with SCI, and for providers and health care teams who are knowledgeable about age-related changes in SCI so that appropriate assessment, follow-up, and management can be provided.

SUGGESTED READING

Capoor J, Stein AB. Aging with spinal cord injury. *Phys Med Rehabil Clin N Am*. 2005;16(1): 129-161.

Charlifue S, Jha A, Lammertse D. Aging with spinal cord injury. *Phys Med Rehabil Clin N Am*. 2010;21(2):383-402.

Groah SL, Stiens SA, Gittler MS, Kirshblum SC, McKinley WO. Spinal cord injury medicine. 5. Preserving wellness and independence of the aging patient with spinal cord injury: a primary care approach for the rehabilitation medicine specialist. *Arch Phys Med Rehabil*. 2002;83(3 suppl 1):S82-S89, S90-S98.

VI. Psychosocial Issues and Life Participation After SCI

CHAPTER 41

Psychological Considerations Following SCI

GENERAL PRINCIPLES

To provide effective care, an awareness of psychological considerations in spinal cord injury (SCI) is important for all clinicians involved in care of people with SCI, regardless of discipline. While psychologists bring unique and necessary expertize to the SCI treatment team, attention to psychological health is shared by all members of the team.

Response to Spinal Cord Injury

The response to SCI varies significantly between individuals, and each person goes through a unique adjustment process that unfolds over time. Previous belief, based on stage theories of response to loss, is not supported by available research in SCI. In fact, after SCI people often don't go through sequential stages of denial, anger, bargaining, depression, and acceptance, but can go directly to any one or more of those or other emotional states, and may sometimes remain in any of those states for a prolonged period of time.

Nonspecific distress and shock of recent SCI is common in the acute stage, but is often not sustained for a prolonged period. In some cases there is no evident psychological dysfunction. Research shows a significant discrepancy between the more negative perceptions of health care workers with an over-estimation and expectation of sustained negative emotions and distress after SCI, and the reported experience and outlook of people with SCI. Studies have suggested several factors that influence the response to SCI (Table 41.1).

Depression Following SCI

While not the rule, depression is reported in a significant proportion of people with SCI, with the incidence estimated at 20%–30% although that varies between studies. The risk of major depressive symptoms in individuals with SCI is greater than in able-bodied control subjects.

Table 41.1

Potentially Modifiable Risk Factors for Depression After SCI

Risk Factor	Description	Potential Therapeutic Intervention
Low environmental rewards	Lack of pleasurable and positive experiences	Identifying and increasing participation in pleasurable activities; managing barriers to participation; overcoming avoidant tendencies
External (vs. internal) locus of control	Perceiving one's life and personal situation to be largely at the mercy of outside forces or chance; being less confident in own ability to manage and influence one's condition or to keep it from interfering from things one wants to do	Coping effectiveness training, skills training in self-management and problem-solving
Chronic pain	Often associated with "catastrophizing" and/or feelings of helplessness	Teaching skills to identify negative thoughts and feelings related to pain and help modify maladaptive behaviors.
Alcohol and substance abuse	Shown to be a risk for depression	Alcohol and substance abuse counseling and treatment

Abbreviation: SCI, spinal cord injury.

Risk Factors for Depression After SCI

Risk factors for depression after SCI can be grouped as nonmodifiable and modifiable. Nonmodifiable risk factors include a prior history of depression, family history of depression or suicide, preinjury family fragmentation with poor support structure, being less than 5 years postinjury, and co-existing traumatic brain injury (TBI). A consistent association has not been found between the extent of injury and risk of depression.

Potentially modifiable risk factors, based on research in SCI, include reduced participation in rewarding activities, an external (instead of internal) locus of control (i.e., perceiving one's situation to be largely at the mercy of outside forces or chance and being less confident in one's own ability to manage and influence one's condition), chronic pain, especially if associated with feelings of helplessness and/or "catastrophizing," and alcohol and substance abuse. Knowledge about potentially modifiable risk factors is especially important for informing development of effective therapeutic strategies that may reduce or prevent depression and foster positive adaptation and coping strategies (Table 41.1).

Suicide Ideation and Risk
The risk of suicide in people with SCI is estimated to be three to five times that of the general population. The risk is greatest between 2 to 5 years of injury. It is reported to be higher in people with complete paraplegia in some studies. One explanation put forward for this seemingly counter-intuitive association of suicide with lower level of injury is that because less support is provided to people with paraplegia, the perceived burden of coping may be greater than with tetraplegia.

Refusal or Request for Removal of Life-Sustaining Treatment
Refusal or request for removal of life-sustaining treatment (e.g., a ventilator in a person with high tetraplegia who is unable to breathe on his own) is, fortunately, an infrequent occurrence, but one that is associated with significant ethical tensions. The patient's decision-making capacity should be assessed. Underlying depression should be assessed and treated, if present. This challenging situation is discussed further in Chapters 8 and 48.

Posttraumatic Stress Disorder

The traumatic event leading to SCI may be associated with development of posttraumatic stress disorder (PTSD). It is reported at a higher rate in active duty service members and Veterans who are injured in a war theater, but is also seen in some cases of civilian injuries.

Diagnostic criteria for PTSD include a history of exposure to a traumatic event that meets specific stipulations, and symptoms from each of the following four symptom clusters: intrusion (e.g., recurrent, involuntary, and intrusive memories, traumatic nightmares, and/or flashbacks); effortful avoidance of trauma-related thoughts or external reminders; negative alterations in cognitions and mood that begin or worsen after the traumatic event (e.g., feeling numb and detached from others, dissociative amnesia of the traumatic event unrelated to head injury); and alterations in arousal and reactivity (e.g., hyper-vigilance, exaggerated startle response, problems in concentration, sleep disturbance, irritable or aggressive behavior). To make the diagnosis, symptoms should persist for more than one month, cause significant distress or functional impairment, and should not be attributable to a medication, substance use, or medical illness.

Other Maladaptive Behaviors After SCI

Alcohol and Substance Abuse
The incidence of alcohol and substance abuse is higher after SCI than in the general population. In addition to the direct deleterious medical effects of alcohol or drug abuse, associated impaired judgment or cognition may lead

to secondary problems such as pressure ulcers from neglecting to do pressure relief, or urinary problems from bladder distension. It can lead to impulsivity and unsafe behaviors, and is associated with increased risk of depression and significant negative impact on physical as well as psychosocial functioning, relationships, and economic well-being.

Dysfunctional Behavior
Behavioral issues may involve anger and hostility towards others, including the treatment team. Excess dependency on others may develop, interfering with maximizing functional abilities and achievable outcomes. Noncompliance with recommended care and reduced motivation to participate in self-care and rehabilitation may be related to limited understanding of the consequences or an effort to exert control, but these may also be associated with depression or substance abuse. Issues related to behavioral and compliance problems are also discussed in Chapter 48.

Dual Diagnosis: Traumatic Brain Injury and SCI

While estimates vary (ranging from 15% to 60%) depending on the criteria used, a significant proportion of people with SCI sustain a concomitant TBI at the time of trauma. Concomitant TBI is especially common with high-velocity impact, and may be evident by history of loss of consciousness, impaired Glasgow Coma Scale (which assesses eye opening, verbal response, and best motor response), and/or imaging findings. The presence and duration of posttraumatic amnesia (PTA) is related to functional outcomes after TBI and can be assessed with tests such as the Galveston Orientation and Amnesia Test (GOAT).

Those with more severe TBI may develop posttraumatic complications such as hydrocephalus and/or seizures. Cerebrally mediated autonomic dysfunction (also known as autonomic storming or dysautonomia) may occur during the early recovery phase of those with severe TBI or brainstem injury, and present with paroxysmal tachycardia, tachypnea, hypertension, fever, rigidity, and sweating. While paroxysmal increase in blood pressure and sweating that occur with dysautonomia overlap with signs of SCI-related autonomic dysreflexia, the other accompanying distinctive clinical features help differentiate the two conditions.

Often, TBI, especially mild TBI, presents with more subtle findings such as difficulty in new learning. Neuropsychological testing, incorporating a battery of tests administered by a qualified mental health practitioner, is indicated in patients with cognitive problems or impaired learning, or in anyone with suspected or diagnosed TBI. Motor impairment due to SCI may not allow completion of tests that involve writing or drawing, so testing needs to be adapted accordingly.

The presence of TBI can significantly interfere with the new learning and follow-through required during rehabilitation, and lead to poor frustration tolerance. Tasks may have to be simplified or broken into small components for practice, with avoidance of multi-tasking. Impaired attention and/or memory can affect compliance, with a need for reminders, repetition, and/or written back-up. Overstimulation should be avoided, and patients often function best in quiet nondistracting environments. TBI can also contribute to fatigue and depression. Sleep disturbance is also common, and can worsen symptoms. Trazodone, 25–50 mg at night, may be helpful for insomnia in this setting. Benzodiazepines can worsen cognitive function and should be avoided in these patients.

Psychogenic Paralysis

Psychogenic or hysterical paralysis is a form of conversion disorder that may have a presentation that is superficially similar to SCI. The patient presents with an apparent neurological deficit that does not correlate with other clinical or radiological findings. It is a diagnosis of exclusion, and also needs to meet criteria for a conversion disorder. A stressful event often precedes the onset of symptoms suggesting that psychological factors are involved. The patient does not consciously or intentionally feign the symptoms in a conversion disorder, unlike the case in factitious disorder (in which patients assume a voluntary sick role) or malingering (intentional fabrication for external gain) which can also present similarly.

Distribution of neurological deficit may be inconsistent with an anatomical distribution. Rectal tone, muscle stretch reflexes, and superficial reflexes are typically preserved. Specific physical examination maneuvers may assist in the diagnosis. These include the Spinal Injuries Center (SIC) test, in which the examiner lifts the knees of the patient to a passively flexed position with the feet flat on the bed. The test is positive if the patient maintains the knees in the flexed position after support is withdrawn. In cases where patients present with unilateral leg paralysis, the Hoover's sign or test can be helpful. While the examiner supports both limbs from under the heels with the patient in a supine position, the patient is asked to attempt to raise each leg. The sign is positive when pressure is felt under the heel of the paralyzed leg when the nonparalyzed leg is raised, and no pressure is felt under the non-paralyzed leg (which should normally be felt) when the patient is trying to raise the paralyzed leg.

Neurological testing should be carefully repeated with review of baseline imaging. More definitive tests, such as magnetic resonance imaging (MRI) or motor evoked potential testing should be considered if the patient fails to start improving in 2 to 3 days to avoid missing an organic cause of paralysis.

A mental health assessment might confirm the presence of contributing psychological symptoms in case of a conversion disorder, which may need to be addressed separately. Direct confrontation of the patient about the source of symptoms may not be productive with a conversion disorder, where the patient is not consciously faking the deficit. The patient should be gently encouraged to resume normal function, minimizing focus on the disability. If symptoms do not spontaneously remit, a short rehabilitation stay with strategic, behaviorally-based intervention may be helpful.

CLINICAL CONSIDERATIONS

Assessment

Routine screening for depression should be performed in people with SCI. Symptoms suggestive of major depressive disorder (MDD) include depressed mood or a loss of interest or pleasure in daily activities that lasts for more than two weeks and represents a change from the person's baseline, impaired functioning, significant weight change or change in appetite, change in sleep (insomnia or hypersomnia), psychomotor retardation, fatigue or loss of energy, feelings of worthlessness or excessive or inappropriate guilt, diminished ability to think or concentrate, and thoughts of death or suicidal ideation or plan.

Risk factors for depression should be identified. Secondary factors that could contribute to or worsen depression should be determined, for example, the effect of medications, pain, or disturbed sleep. Suicide risk is assessed with inquiry about suicidal ideation, plan or intent, and any previous attempts.

While bereavement or grief reaction after SCI may appear similar to depression, that does not usually involve prolonged feelings of guilt, self-reproach, worthlessness, or thoughts of death as seen in depressive disorders.

Depression Screening Measures
It is important to keep in mind that these measures do not replace a clinical interview for a diagnosing MDD. Nonspecific effects of SCI (e.g., fatigue, reduced energy) and the hospital environment (e.g., disturbed sleep) can lead to spurious inflation of scores on depression measures (Table 41.2).

Several depression screening measures are available but are lengthy and inefficient as screening tools. Among the most common depression scales currently used in people with SCI is the Patient Health Questionnaire (PHQ)-9. It consists of nine items and is shorter than most depression measures. It has been validated in multiple nonpsychiatric medical conditions, including SCI. Its overall accuracy as an indicator of MDD in SCI has been reported to be better than other depression screening.

Table 41.2

Distinguishing Somatic Symptoms of Depression From Medical Illness

Symptom	Characteristic
Sleep disturbance	Early morning awakening is characteristic of primary depression
Fatigue	Fatigue due to primary depression is often worse in the morning
Weight loss	Weight loss with a normal appetite suggests a medical condition

The PHQ-2, comprises the first two items of the PHQ-9, and can be administered as a prescreen (Table 41.3). It inquires about the degree to which an individual has experienced depressed mood and loss of interest over the past two weeks. Those symptoms are based on the two essential criteria for the diagnosis of MDD. It has been suggested that physicians could include the PHQ-2 as part of their review of systems. Any positive response to the two questions would be an indication for more in-depth assessment for depression by the rehabilitation psychologist or other mental health professional.

Management

The Clinical Team's Role in Promoting Adjustment to SCI

Supportive and positive engagement by the rehabilitation team, by fostering success and control during rehabilitation, can be a significant factor in promoting adjustment to injury and confidence in individuals with SCI. It is often best to provide medical and prognostic information matter-of-factly, yet at the same time leave room for hope. Unfounded assumptions that overrate depression and underestimate positive outlook are common in clinical staff including the rehabilitation team, and should be watched for and minimized. Expressions of hope should be respected and direct confrontations of denial concerning probable implications of the injury should be avoided. Feelings of hope have been shown to assist with a future orientation and help patients move forward through the recovery process. Over time, the hope becomes more realistic, though the time frame differs among individuals. Helping patients and family identify effective coping strategies that have aided them in the past is useful.

Rehabilitation psychologists are indispensable members of the treatment team for identifying and treating psychological impairments and facilitating improved psychological outcomes and progress. They can also be a valuable

Table 41.3

Prescreening for Depression With Patient Health Questionnaire-2 (PHQ-2)[a]

Over the past 2 weeks, how often have you been bothered by any of the following problems?

- Little interest or pleasure in doing things
  0 = Not at All
  1 = Several Days
  2 = More Than Half the Days
  3 = Nearly Every Day
- Feeling down, depressed, or hopeless
  0 = Not at All
  1 = Several Days
  2 = More Than Half the Days
  3 = Nearly Every Day

[a]PHQ-2 score of ≥3 is often the recommended cut-off score requiring further evaluation (e.g., with PHQ-9) but, depending on the clinical context, any positive response may be an indication for mental health evaluation.

resource for assisting other team members to work effectively with individuals with SCI and their families.

Significant psychological dysfunction should be promptly identified and appropriately addressed.

Management of Depression
Despite extensive research on the importance of addressing depression in SCI, under-treatment of depression persists. Clinical depression should be promptly and aggressively treated.

Sixty to seventy percent of patients respond to any of the commonly used antidepressant drugs if given in an adequate dose for 6 to 8 weeks. Mild to moderate depression has been shown to respond to cognitive behavior therapy (CBT) or interpersonal therapy alone but takes longer than medications. Antidepressant medication in combination with either CBT or interpersonal therapy seems to be the most effective approach.

Pharmacological Treatment
General principles of pharmacological treatment of depression are summarized in Table 41.4. Antidepressant medications include selective serotonin uptake inhibitors (SSRIs), serotonin and norepinephrine reuptake inhibitors (SNRIs), tricyclic antidepressants (TCAs), monoamine oxidase inhibitors (MAOIs), and other antidepressants such as bupropion and trazodone.

Table 41.4

General Principles in Pharmacological Treatment of Depression

Antidepressants improve depressive symptoms. 60%–70% of patients respond to any of the commonly used antidepressant drugs if given in an adequate dose for 6–8 weeks

There are no significant differences in effectiveness among most antidepressants. Medication choice is based on known previous response, side effect profile, convenience, cost, patient preference, and drug interaction risk

The primary advantages of SSRI over TCA and MAOI are safety and tolerability

Usually started at low dose and increased every 5–7 days to target dose

Response usually takes 2–3 weeks

Antidepressants should not be stopped abruptly except in an emergency

Patients taking antidepressants should be monitored for side effects, suicide risk, and effectiveness

Problem side effects may require temporary decrease in dose or/and adjunctive treatment

If unacceptable side effects occur, the drug should be tapered over a week and a new drug initiated, considering potential drug interaction in the choice

Response should be evaluated after 6 weeks at target dose. If response is inadequate, a further step-wise increase in dose may be considered as tolerated

Trial at adequate dose for 6–8 weeks is needed before considering the treatment ineffective. Compliance issues should also be considered in nonresponders

If there is inadequate response after maximal dose, taper and switch to a different drug

Once remission is achieved, treatment should be continued for at least 6–12 months to prevent relapse

Abbreviations: MAOI, monoamine oxidase inhibitors; SSRIs, selective serotonin uptake inhibitors; SNRI, serotonin and norepinephrine reuptake inhibitors; TCA, tricyclic antidepressants.

Choice of agent is based on known previous response, side effect profile, convenience, cost, patient preference, and drug interaction risk. The primary advantages of SSRI over TCA and MAOI are safety and tolerability. MAOIs are now rarely used for depression. TCAs have anticholinergic side effects, and pose a higher risk of cardiovascular events in patients with heart disease. Moreover, they are highly lethal in overdoses compared to SSRIs so should be avoided in those who are at risk for suicide. Trazodone is primarily used as a sleep aid due to sedation and short duration. Of the SSRIs, fluoxetine and paroxetine are most prone to cause drug interactions because of inhibition of metabolism of other medications through the P450 system. Unlike most SSRIs which are activating and so taken during the day, paroxetine is sedating, and usually taken at night. Table 41.5 lists SSRIs and SNRIs commonly used to treat depression.

Cognitive Behavioral Therapy and Other Psychotherapeutic Interventions
CBT includes interventions to help individuals identify negative or distorted thoughts and feelings, and refocus on more realistic and productive thinking.

Table 41.5

SSRI and SNRI Antidepressant Agents	
Medication	Daily Dose Range
SSRI	
Citalopram (Celexa)	20–60 mg
Escitalopram (Lexapro)	10–20 mg
Fluoxetine (Prozac)	20–80 mg
Paroxetine (Paxil)	20–50 mg
Paroxetine CR (Paxil CR)	25–62.5 mg
Sertraline (Zoloft)	50–200 mg
SNRI	
Desvenlafaxine (Pristiq)	50 mg
Duloxetine (Cymbalta)	30–120 mg
Mirtazapine (Remeron)	15–45 mg
Venlafaxine, extended release (Effexor ER)	37.5–225 mg

Abbreviations: SSRI, selective serotonin uptake inhibitors; SNRI, serotonin and norepinephrine reuptake inhibitors.

It includes skills training to modify maladaptive behaviors, and practice positive coping and problem-solving strategies. CBT has been demonstrated to be effective in treating depression and for addressing factors that contribute to distress such as chronic pain. It can also help in relapse prevention.

KNOWLEDGE GAPS AND EMERGING CONCEPTS

While there has been considerable research in psychological factors impacting SCI, much of it is based on small or cross-sectional studies. Well-designed longitudinal research in needed. In particular, research is needed to identify specific aspects of interventions that would be most effective in promoting positive adjustment to SCI and in preventing and treating psychological dysfunction and emotional distress. Additional research would be helpful to further refine development of depression measures in people with SCI, and to address interpretation, after accounting for nondepressive somatic symptoms, to further improve validity of these measures.

SUGGESTED READING

Bombardier CH, Fann JR, Tate DG, et al. An exploration of modifiable risk factors for depression after spinal cord injury: which factors should we target? *Arch Phys Med Rehabil.* 2012;93(5):775-781.

Chevalier Z, Kennedy P, Sherlock O. Spinal cord injury, coping and psychological adjustment: a literature review. *Spinal Cord.* 2009;47(11):778-782.

Consortium for Spinal Cord Medicine. *Depression Following Spinal Cord Injury. Clinical Practice Guidelines for Health Care Professionals.* Washington, DC: Paralyzed Veterans of America; 1998.

Kirschner KL, Smith GR, Antiel RM, Lorish P, Frost F, Kanaan RA. "Why can't I move, Doc?" Ethical dilemmas in treating conversion disorders. *PM R.* 2012;4(4):296-303.

Macciocchi S. Co-occurring traumatic brain injury and acute spinal cord injury rehabilitation outcomes. *Archives Phys Med Rehabil.* 2012;93(10):1788-1794.

Mehta S, Orenczuk S, Hansen KT, et al. An evidence-based review of the effectiveness of cognitive behavioral therapy for psychosocial issues post-spinal cord injury. *Rehabil Psychol.* 2011;56(1):15-25.

Peter C, Müller R, Cieza A, Geyh S. Psychological resources in spinal cord injury: a systematic literature review. *Spinal Cord.* 2012;50(3):188-201.

Post MW, van Leeuwen CM. Psychosocial issues in spinal cord injury: a review. *Spinal Cord.* 2012;50(5):382-389.

Sommer JL, Witkiewicz PM. The therapeutic challenges of dual diagnosis: TBI/SCI. *Brain Inj.* 2004;18(12):1297-1308.

van Leeuwen CM, Kraaijeveld S, Lindeman E, Post MW. Associations between psychological factors and quality of life ratings in persons with spinal cord injury: a systematic review. *Spinal Cord.* 2012;50(3):174-187.

Wegener ST, Adams LL, Rohe D. Promoting optimal functioning in spinal cord injury: the role of rehabilitation psychology. *Handb Clin Neurol.* 2012;109:297-314.

CHAPTER 42

Socioeconomic Consequences and Quality of Life

GENERAL PRINCIPLES

Beyond its many medical consequences, a major life event like spinal cord injury (SCI) has a significant impact on the individual and family, with important social, psychological, and economic implications. This chapter focuses on societal and economic implications of SCI, and the related concepts of participation and quality of life (QOL).

Economic Considerations

Costs of SCI Care
SCI is associated with extraordinarily high costs, both to the individual and to society. The largest identified categories of care-related costs over the long term are inpatient care, followed by attendant care. Costs have greatly increased over the years, attributable to both improved life expectancy and increased costs of care over time.

Acute care charges in inflation-adjusted dollars have increased significantly over time despite decreased length of stay. Rehabilitation charges per day have also increased but not as much as acute care charges per day. Rehospitalizations add significantly to costs. The leading causes of rehospitalization after SCI are urinary tract infections (UTIs), followed by pressure ulcers, and respiratory conditions, with pressure ulcers being the most expensive cause of rehospitalization.

Average yearly health care and living expenses that are directly attributable to SCI vary significantly based on the SCI level and completeness, as defined by the American Spinal Injury Association (ASIA) Impairment Scale (AIS), and also with the time since injury, with first year expenses being much greater than expenses in subsequent years. Published estimates for persons served in the federally designated SCI Model Care systems (which may not necessarily be representative of the SCI population as a whole), report average first year expenses in 2012 dollars for persons with high tetraplegia

(C1–C4) AIS A, B, or C to be $1,044,197, low tetraplegia (C5–C8) AIS A, B, or C to be $754,524, paraplegia AIS A, B, or C to be $508,904, and incomplete motor functional at any level, AIS D, to be $340,787. Corresponding average yearly expenses for each subsequent year are reported to be $181,328 for those with high tetraplegia, $111,237 for those with low tetraplegia, $67,415 for those with paraplegia, and $41,393 for those with incomplete motor functional SCI at any level.

The above estimates do not include indirect costs such as loss of wages, fringe benefits, and productivity which are calculated to be an average of $70,575 per year in February 2013 dollars, but vary considerably based on education, severity of injury, and preinjury employment history.

Estimated costs and expenses are helpful guides for life care planning. Estimates of life-time costs obviously vary with age at injury and life expectancy, with lower life-time cost estimates for older age at injury compared to younger.

Impact of SCI on Societal Roles and Relationships

SCI affects not just the individual, but the entire family, with disruption of "normal" preinjury life. Family reaction may include anxiety, denial, anger, resentment, frustration, fatigue, and/or guilt. In addition there is often a financial burden after a disability both from reduced earnings and from additional expenses for needed resources. Divorce rates after SCI are higher than in the general population. Parenting tasks may have to be relearned or modified, although some studies have shown no substantial differences in parental satisfaction and outcomes of children of parents with and without SCI. Spouses or significant others may have to deal with role-reversal, and with role-confusion related to being both a partner and a caregiver. Caregivers may have little time to attend to their own needs with potential negative impact on their own health, decreased socialization, and lack of leisure time.

Despite the potential challenges, many people with SCI participate in meaningful social roles and establish fulfilling relationships. Facilitating developmentally and culturally appropriate social roles after a significant injury or illness is an important goal of rehabilitation.

Impact of SCI on employment is discussed in Chapter 44.

Participation and Community Reintegration After SCI

Participation refers to involvement in life activities and life situations. Participation allows individuals to fulfill various societal roles. Participation in life activities and social integration correlates significantly with subjective QOL, and is an important aspect of rehabilitation.

Measures of Participation
The most widely used measure of participation after SCI is the Craig Handicap Assessment and Reporting Technique (CHART), which has demonstrated

validity and reliability in people with SCI and available normative data. The CHART provides subscores in six domains including physical independence, mobility, occupation, social integration, economic self-sufficiency, and, in its updated version, cognitive independence. One limitation of CHART is that it does not consider personal values and preferences. Another instrument is the Life Satisfaction Questionnaire (LiSat) which measures satisfaction with participation in various life domains.

Environmental Measures
Given the importance of environmental factors on participation, measures of environmental influences on participation have been developed. An example of such a measure, which has been tested in people with SCI with acceptable demonstrated reliability, is the Craig Hospital Inventory of Environmental Factors (CHIEF).

Quality of Life After SCI

Improved QOL is a broad overall goal of SCI care and rehabilitation, but it is a difficult concept to measure and define with precision or consistency. In addition, utility of several popular measures of QOL is limited in people with SCI, for example, because of inappropriate questions for individuals with motor impairments such as those related to walking.

Many components contribute to QOL, of which health-related quality of life (HRQOL) is only one. Example of an instrument that measures HRQOL is the Short Form (SF)-36, which is also available in modified versions. A different aspect of QOL is the sense of subjective well-being and life satisfaction. An instrument that has been used to describe overall subjective well-being is the Diener Satisfaction with Life Scale (SWLS) for which normative data are available from the SCI Model Systems and other sources.

Table 42.1 lists examples of commonly used measures for different aspects of participation and QOL for which normative data is available for people with SCI.

Factors Affecting QOL
QOL and life satisfaction among people with SCI has been shown to relate positively to social participation, social support, and to perceived control over one's life. On the other hand, consistent or strong associations have not been found between QOL and biomedical factors such as completeness of injury or extent of impairment.

CLINICAL CONSIDERATIONS

Discharge Planning and Community Integration

Preparation for discharge following SCI includes assessment of available options based on evaluation of the extent of impairment and functional

Table 42.1

Examples of Measures of Participation and Quality of Life After SCI[a]

Domain	Measure	Description
Participation	Craig Handicap Assessment and Reporting Technique (CHART)	Provides subscores in six domains including physical independence, mobility, occupation, social integration, cognitive independence, and economic self-sufficiency
Environmental factors	Craig Hospital Inventory of Environmental Factors (CHIEF)	Assesses frequency and magnitude of perceived social, attitudinal, policy, and physical/architectural barriers to participation
Health-related quality of life (HRQOL)	Short Form (SF)-36	Provides scores for eight health-related parameters: physical function, social function, physical role, emotional role, mental health, energy, pain, and general health perceptions
Overall satisfaction with life (subjective)	Diener Satisfaction with Life Scale (SWLS)	Five-item scale that measures life satisfaction from the global perspective of the individual

Abbreviation: SCI, spinal cord injury.
[a]Several other measures exist for each of these domains. This table includes examples of the more commonly used ones for which normative data is available.

limitations, comorbidities, care needs, goals and preferences, and available support and resources. The vast majority of individuals with SCI are able to return back to their community following an SCI. Discharge planning includes ensuring appropriate patient and family education, planning for emergencies and contingencies, coordinating needed follow-up and support, provision of appropriate durable medical equipment, and home assessment and home modifications as needed.

Home Modifications

Modifications to the home to accommodate wheelchair access and other limitations are an important aspect of discharge planning. In some cases, permanent modifications may not be feasible by the time of discharge and interim measures may be needed. Modifications may be needed to entrances, doors, hallways, bathroom, bedroom, kitchen, stair access, or other spaces. Some require few resources (e.g., removing unnecessary clutter, eliminating throw rugs, and rearranging furniture) while others may involve considerable expense. Examples of some important requirements for wheelchair access include: ramps that provide at least 12″ of length for every 1″ in rise (i.e., are not too steep), doorways that are a minimum of 32" to 36" in width depending on the type of wheelchair (32" for manual, 34" for power, and 36" if a turn is involved), and light switches at a height less than or equal to 36".

Emergency Planning
Police and fire departments should be notified that an individual with disability resides in the home. Back-up power source is needed for ventilator-dependent individuals. Emergency telephone numbers should be readily accessible. A kit with medications, catheters, and other supplies is helpful to keep in case of emergencies that require quick evacuation. The American Red Cross website "Evacuation Planning for Persons with Disabilities and Caregivers" is a good resource for guidance about emergency preparedness.

Facilitating Community Integration
Additional important aspects of community integration and participation, covered elsewhere in this book, include driving and transportation access (Chapter 45), education and employment (Chapter 44), and recreational activities and adaptive sports (Chapter 43). Maintaining community integration for people aging with SCI is another important consideration (Chapter 40).

Facilitating Awareness and Access to Benefits and Resources

Assisting individuals and families with awareness and access to potential resources, and advocating for them as appropriate, is of crucial importance to address the socioeconomic and participation challenges that are encountered following SCI. At the same time, patients should not be viewed as passive recipients of support and dependent on others, but fostered to be actively and independently engaged in shaping their lives.

Various publically funded and/or community resources may be accessible to people with SCI depending on their circumstances. Table 42.2 lists some sources of benefits designed to provide assistance to people with disabilities that may be available to individuals with SCI, if they meet specific eligibility criteria. These include benefits administered through Social Security Administration (Social Security Disability Insurance [SSDI], and Supplemental Security Income [SSI]), Medicaid, Medicare, Veteran benefits, Worker's compensation, and Rehabilitation Services Administration (RSA) administered programs.

Life Care Planning

A life care plan is a comprehensive interdisciplinary document that specifies future medical and rehabilitation needs of the person with SCI, and is a useful tool for planning and long-term management. The International Academy of Life Care Planners has defined a life care plan as a dynamic document based on published standards of practice, comprehensive assessment, data analysis, and research, which provides an organized, concise plan for current and future needs, with associated costs, for individuals who have experienced catastrophic injury or have chronic health care needs.

Table 42.2

Benefit Programs and Sources Based on Eligibility

Program	Description/Benefits	Eligibility
Social Security Disability Insurance (SSDI)	Wage replacement income that pays benefits to the individual with disability and some family members. Administered by the Social Security Administration (SSA)	Meets criteria for disability (inability to engage in substantial gainful activities because of a medically determinable impairment that has lasted or is expected to last ≥12 months) Legal resident of the United States Sufficient work credits by paying taxes to qualify based on age at disability onset
Supplemental Security Income (SSI)	Monthly payments to individuals with very little income or resources, provided as supportive income. Is also administered by SSA	Meets above criteria for disability Not based on prior work or work credits (unlike SSDI) At or below the specified criteria for income and resources
Medicaid (Medical Assistance Program)	Administered by states to provide medical care for public assistance recipients with medical needs. Covers a broad range of services, but coverage differs from state to state	Specified financial and nonfinancial criteria that vary by state
Medicare	Health insurance program administered by the federal government	Individuals who are 65 and older, or those <65 yrs who meet criteria for a disability (and have received SSDI for ≥24 months)
Veteran benefits	Benefits may include disability compensation, pension, education/training, home loans, health care, burial, and benefits for dependents and survivors. Additional benefits for Veterans with service-connected disability can include home adaptation grants, vocational rehabilitation and employment, and education assistance. Administered by the US Department of Veterans Affairs	US Veteran Specific benefits vary based on Service connection and/or income-based eligibility

(continued)

Program	Description/Benefits	Eligibility
Worker's compensation	State-regulated insurance program that provides wage replacement and medical benefits. Plans differ among jurisdictions	Individuals injured in the course of employment, regardless of who was at fault
Rehabilitation Services Admin-istration (RSA) administered programs	Various grant programs and projects to assist individuals with disabilities, including a variety of independent living services through Centers for Independent Living and vocational reha-bilitation (VR) programs implemented by state VR agencies	Criteria vary based on the specific program, and target those with significant disabilities. Also, see Chapter 44 for employment-related resources

Components of a comprehensive life care plan often include: projected evaluations, projected therapeutic modalities, diagnostic testing, wheel-chair needs, accessories and maintenance, other mobility-related equipment needs, orthotics, aids for independent functioning, home equipment and accessories, medication and supplies, home care and facility care (including attendant care, residential care, and/or transitional care), future projected medical care, potential complications, transportation, architectural renova-tions, health maintenance and recreational needs, and vocational/educa-tional plan.

Personal Assistance Services

Personal assistance services may be obtained through several different means: provided by family or friends, publicly-funded agencies, or privately funded. Personal assistants can help with activities of daily living (ADL) such as bath-ing, dressing, grooming, transfers, and bowel and bladder care, as well as with instrumental ADL such as meal preparation, laundry, transportation, and shopping. This assistance can be crucial not only for physical health and func-tion, but also to enable participation in life activities for individuals with SCI. However, funding can be an obstacle, and finding and retaining personal assis-tance services can be a challenge. Teaching individuals with SCI about various aspects of hiring and retaining personal assistants is an important facet of care.

Caregiver Support

Caregiver stress and burden should be addressed as an ongoing part of reha-bilitation and SCI care. Marital and family counseling, caregiver support including peer support groups, respite care, and access to supportive services and resources can be very helpful.

KNOWLEDGE GAPS AND EMERGING CONCEPTS

Longitudinal research is needed to examine targeted interventions and innovative measures to enhance participation and QOL of people with SCI. An example of such innovations is the increasing availability and incorporation of telemedicine technology, including various forms of home telehealth, that provide promising avenues of facilitating transition and support for community integration after discharge from rehabilitation.

SUGGESTED READING

Beauregard L, Guindon A, Noreau L, Lefebvre H, Boucher N. Community needs of people living with spinal cord injury and their family. *Top Spinal Cord Inj Rehabil*. 2012;18(2):122-125.

Boakye M, Leigh BC, Skelly AC. Quality of life in persons with spinal cord injury: comparisons with other populations. *J Neurosurg Spine*. 2012;17(1 suppl):29-37.

Cao Y, Chen Y, DeVivo M. Lifetime direct cost after spinal cord injury. *Top Spinal Cord Inj Rehabil*. 2011;16:10-16.

Charlifue S, Post MW, Biering-Sørensen F, et al. International Spinal Cord Injury Quality of Life Basic Data Set. *Spinal Cord*. 2012;50:672-675.

Cooper RA, Cooper R. Quality-of-life technology for people with spinal cord injuries. *Phys Med Rehabil Clin N Am*. 2010;21(1):1-13.

DeVivo M, Chen Y, Mennemeyer ST, Deutsch A. Costs of care following spinal cord injury. *Top Spinal Cord Inj Rehabil*. 2011,16(4):1-9.

French D, Campbell RR, Sabharwal S, Nelson AL, Palacios PA, Gavin-Dreschnack D. Healthcare costs for patients with chronic spinal cord injury in the Veterans Health Administration. *J Spinal Cord Med*. 2007;30(5):477-481.

Gurcay E, Bal A, Eksioglu E, Cakci A. Quality of life in patients with spinal cord injury. *Int J Rehabil Res*. 2010;33(4):356-358.

Hill MR, Noonan VK, Sakakibara BM, Miller WC; SCIRE Research Team. Quality of life instruments and definitions in individuals with spinal cord injury: a systematic review. *Spinal Cord*. 2010;48(6):438-450.

National Spinal Cord Injury Statistical Center. Spinal cord injury: facts and figures at a glance, Feb 2013. *J Spinal Cord Med*. 2013;36(4):394-395.

Priebe MM, Chiodo AE, Scelza WM, Kirshblum SC, Wuermser LA, Ho CH. Spinal cord injury medicine. 6. Economic and societal issues in spinal cord injury. *Arch Phys Med Rehabil*. 2007;88(3 suppl 1):S84-S88.

Scelza WM, Kirshblum SC, Wuermser LA, Ho CH, Priebe MM, Chiodo AE. Spinal cord injury medicine. 4. Community reintegration after spinal cord injury. *Arch Phys Med Rehabil*. 2007;88(3 suppl 1):S71-S75.

Stiens SA, Fawber HL, Yuhas SA. The person with a spinal cord injury: an evolving prototype for life care planning. *Phys Med Rehabil Clin N Am*. 2013;24(3):419-444.

Ullrich PM, Spungen AM, Atkinson D, et al. Activity and participation after spinal cord injury: state-of-the-art report. *J Rehabil Res Dev*. 2012;49(1):155-174.

Weitzenkamp DA, Whiteneck GG, Lammertse DP. Predictors of personal care assistance for people with spinal cord injury. *Arch Phys Med Rehabil*. 2002;83(10):1399-1405.

CHAPTER 43

Exercise and Sports After SCI

GENERAL PRINCIPLES

Benefits of Exercise and Sports Participation After Spinal Cord Injury

Regular physical activity, exercise, and sports participation has many benefits. This is true of people with spinal cord injury (SCI) as well as the general population. The United States Department of Health and Human Services has published *"Physical Activity Guidelines for Americans"* that includes a section on physical activity guidelines for individuals with disabilities (Table 43.1). It concludes that "Overall, the evidence shows that regular physical activity provides important health benefits for people with disabilities. The benefits include improved cardiovascular and muscle fitness, improved mental health, and better ability to do tasks of daily life. Sufficient evidence now exists to recommend that adults with disabilities should get regular physical activity."

Research on benefits of exercise and sports participation after SCI is primarily based on small studies of variable quality and design and the evidence in many areas is still inconclusive, though promising. However, taken together, the literature consistently reports benefits of exercise and sports participation after SCI in enhancing physical fitness in measures of physical capacity (e.g., maximal oxygen consumption), body composition (increased lean mass), and functional performance (improved mobility and select activities of daily living), and in enhancing psychological well-being, community integration, and participation. There is also encouraging literature on the role of exercise in preventing chronic disease and ameliorating cardiovascular and metabolic disease risk factors (e.g., lipid profile, glucose metabolism) in people with SCI, although the optimal intensities, duration, and specific types of physical activities to reduce disease risk are not established.

Barriers to Physical Activity and Exercise After SCI

Significant physical, psychological, and access barriers to regular physical exercise after SCI exist.

Table 43.1

Physical Activity Guidelines for Adults With Disabilities (U.S. Department of Health and Human Services)[a]

Adults with disabilities should strive to get at least 150 mins a week of moderate-intensity, or 75 mins a week of vigorous-intensity, aerobic activity, or an equivalent combination of moderate- and vigorous-intensity aerobic activity. Aerobic activity should be performed in episodes of at least 10 mins, and preferably, it should be spread throughout the week.

Adults with disabilities, who are able to, should also do muscle-strengthening activities of moderate or high intensity that involve all major muscle groups on 2 or more days a week. These activities provide additional health benefits.

When adults with disabilities are not able to meet these guidelines, they should engage in regular physical activity according to their abilities and should avoid inactivity.

Adults with disabilities should consult their health care provider about the amounts and types of physical activity that are appropriate for their abilities.

[a]NCHPAD: 2008 Physical Activity Guidelines for Adults with Disabilities—National Center on Health, Physical Activity, and Disability (www.ncpad.org, Accessed 7/30/13).

Physical Factors
Exercise capacity in SCI is limited by two primary physiological factors: muscle paralysis, and the blunted sympathetic response to exercise. In addition autonomic dysreflexia, orthostatic hypotension, impaired thermoregulation, insensate and fragile skin, and musculoskeletal overuse and injury can be significant SCI-related factors that can impact activity and exercise and need to be addressed (Table 43.2).

Psychological Factors
Lack of motivation, lack of adherence, reduced energy, depression, concern about physical limitations, fear of embarrassment, lack of self-confidence, and worry about exercise being too difficult, can all be potential barriers to regular exercise.

Access Factors
Reduced access to exercise after SCI is a significant factor in multiple ways. Exercise facilities with wheelchair-accessible equipment and adequate transfer space may not be readily available. There may be difficulty operating exercise equipment independently. Environmental barriers to outdoor physical activity can include steep or uneven terrain, poorly maintained or absent sidewalks, lack of curb cuts, and inclement weather. Lack of readily available transportation to exercise facilities can be another barrier. Financial barriers may preclude access to specialized equipment or gym access. In addition, access can be hampered by lack of awareness of exercise and adapted sports programs, lack of SCI-specific knowledge amongst fitness professionals, and failure of clinicians to address options for regular physical activity.

Sports and Exercise Options for People With SCI

Adapted Exercise and Sports Equipment
Advances in equipment innovation have led to development of increasing variety of equipment, which can facilitate participation in physical activity

Table 43.2

Potential Complications With Exercise and Sports Participation in SCI

Problem	Prevention/Management
Overuse injury	- Incorporate flexibility exercise into the overall fitness program, including glenohumeral and pectoral stretching - Resistance training including strengthening of posterior shoulder and scapular muscles - Proper wheelchair positioning - Proper technique and equipment - Rest and injury-specific principles of care after musculoskeletal injury, gradual return, and progression of exercise program
Abrasions, burns, and blisters	- Protective gear, gloves, taping - Treat and protect open cracks and blisters - Avoid contact of insensate skin with potentially hot metal equipment
Falls and contact injuries	- Equipment safety - Appropriate padding and protective gear - Low threshold to check for fractures
Skin breakdown	- Proper seating and cushion, regular pressure relief - Regular skin inspection - Avoid training or participation with open wounds
Hyper- or hypothermia from impaired thermoregulation	- Avoid training in hot and humid weather (or in very cold conditions) - Maintain hydration - Wear clothing appropriate to the weather - Cooling spray or cooling vests in hot weather - Seek assistance, remove from outside environment, cooling for hyperthermia, cover for hypothermia
Orthostatic hypotension	- Avoid exercise in hot weather or immediately after meals - Wear elastic stockings and/or abdominal corset while exercising - Proper hydration - Recline at onset of symptoms
Autonomic dysreflexia	- Empty bladder/bowel fully before exercise - Never try to induce dysreflexia ("boosting"); the practice is specifically banned by sporting organizations including the International Paralympic Committee - Initiate measures to relieve immediately if occurs and seek treatment emergently

Abbreviation: SCI, spinal cord injury.

and exercise for people with different levels of motor function. Commercially available equipment is now increasingly available for individuals and facilities that can be accessed and adjusted for use by individuals with tetraplegia or paraplegia. This includes different forms of upper body aerobic exercise equipment, strength training equipment, and full body seated exercise equipment.

Functional electrical stimulation (FES) can be combined with residual voluntary movement for exercise, and has been incorporated into various exercise equipment including FES-assisted cycling, rowing, arm ergometry, and systems for standing and walking.

Specialized equipment is needed for several adapted sports. The typical daily-use wheelchair is not appropriate for sporting events. Sport-specific wheelchairs are available for racing, tennis, basketball, rugby, and hand-cycling.

Sports and Physical Activity Participation Options
There is a plethora of options for recreational and/or competitive activities and adapted sports for people with SCI and other disabilities. These include archery, athletics, aviation, baseball, basketball, billiards, boating, bowling, curling, cycling, dancing, fencing, fishing, golf, hockey, horseback riding, kayaking, powerlifting, racing, rock climbing, rugby, sailing, scuba diving, shooting, skiing, sled hockey, snowmobiling, table tennis, tennis, and track and field events. Some are more organized than others, and most are supported and facilitated by various organizations. The National Veterans Wheelchair Games are among the largest wheelchair sporting events in the world. Several other competitive sporting venues are available at the local, regional, national, and international levels.

CLINICAL CONSIDERATIONS

Assessment

Preparticipation Screening
Screening is recommended to provide appropriate exercise prescription and to identify conditions that may require further evaluation and management, special precautions (Table 43.2), or modified participation in exercise and sports. Baseline strength and endurance should be assessed. Depending on the clinical context additional testing such as determination of bone mineral density to screen for fracture risk, pulmonary function testing, and/or exercise stress testing (e.g., with arm-crank ergometry, wheelchair ergometry, or field testing) may be warranted.

Classification of Athletes With SCI for Competitive Sports
Rehabilitation professionals with the required knowledge and expertise may be involved in panels for evaluation and classification of athletes with SCI and other disabilities for many competitive sports. Classification systems

that incorporate consideration of functional abilities have been put in place for many competitive sports, and are continuing to evolve. Classification is sport-specific because impairments affect the ability to perform in different sports to a different extent. Observation of movement and function during performance is often a part of the classification system. Athletes with similar level of disability are grouped together in one classification to ensure fair competition. The Paralympic sports website (www.paralymic.org) provides information about adapted sporting events and includes details about sports-specific classification systems.

Management

Counseling Individuals With SCI for Exercise and Sports Participation

Clinicians play a key role in counseling people with SCI about the benefits of exercise and sports participation, and for enabling participation by initiating appropriate referrals and providing information and facilitating access to resources.

Based on available evidence, SCI clinicians should promote sports and exercise as means to improve physical fitness. It may be helpful to explain the importance of participating in strength and endurance activities for performing activities of daily living, maintaining independence, and mitigating some physical effects of SCI. Potential psychosocial outcomes of activity, such as reduced pain and stress, or enhanced mood and self-esteem, and improved quality of life may also be motivating factors.

Exercise Prescription

Optimal intensity, duration, frequency, and mode of exercise for reducing disease risk in people with SCI are not established, but may be extrapolated from available guidelines for able-bodied individuals. The Federal guidelines included in Table 43.1 provide a framework for prescription, as do those developed by the American College of Sports Medicine. Prescription with specified and quantifiable goals can facilitate motivation and improve adherence to exercise programs.

Endurance training can be provided by several modes including arm-crank ergometry, wheelchair ergometry, swimming, and hybrid FES systems. Strength training can be incorporated in task-specific functional activities and can be supplemented as appropriate by an adapted program using weights and/or elastic bands. Circuit training can provide both strength and endurance benefits. While training of weak muscles may follow the same principles as training muscles with normal strength, the training protocol may need to be modified. Resistive strength training should be individualized and progressive, and should include posterior shoulder and scapular stabilizing muscles. Flexibility exercises, including regular stretching of shoulder and pectoral muscles should be incorporated to minimize risk of overuse injury. Adequate warm-up and cool-down should be an integral part of the exercise prescription.

Preventing and Managing Medical Complications Related to Physical Activity
Although there may be some risks associated with physical activity participation, the benefits generally substantially outweigh the risks. Individualized
counseling about risk prevention and prompt identification and management
of SCI-specific medical complications that could be precipitated or exacerbated
by physical and athletic activity, is important (Table 43.2).

KNOWLEDGE GAPS AND EMERGING CONCEPTS

Additional research is needed to more conclusively demonstrate the various
benefits of exercise and sports participation in people with SCI. Demonstrating the value of these programs is especially important for advocating and
securing the needed resources in an environment with increasing constraints
to ensure value-based health care interventions. Research is also needed to
establish optimal mode, duration, frequency, and intensity of exercise for cardiovascular and metabolic risk reduction in people with SCI.

SUGGESTED READING

Cowan RE, Nash MS. Cardiovascular disease, SCI, and exercise: unique risks and focused
    countermeasures. *Disabil Rehabil.* 2010;32:2228-2236.
Cowan RE, Nash MS, Anderson KD. Exercise participation barrier prevalence and associ-
    ation with exercise participation status in individuals with spinal cord injury. *Spinal
    Cord.* 2013;51(1):27-32.
Jacobs PL. Effects of resistance and endurance training in persons with paraplegia. *Med Sci
    Sports Exerc.* 2009;41:992-997.
Martin Ginis KA, Jörgensen S, Stapleton J. Exercise and sport for persons with spinal cord
    injury. *PM R.* 2012;4(11):894-900.
National Center on Health, Physical Activity, and Disability – NCHPAD. 2008 Physical Activity
    Guidelines for Adults with Disabilities. http://www.ncpad.org. Accessed July 30, 2013.

CHAPTER 44

Employment After SCI

GENERAL PRINCIPLES

Employment Status After Spinal Cord Injury

People with spinal cord injury (SCI) have much lower employment rates than the general population. Reported employment rates in individuals with SCI vary widely in the literature, likely due to differences in study population, study design, and how employment is defined, but on an average paid employment after SCI is estimated to be around 35%. A much smaller percent return to their preinjury job.

Positive Correlates of Employment
In addition to the obvious economic benefits, employment after SCI has been correlated with several positive outcomes related to health status, function, self-esteem, life satisfaction, and quality of life.

Predictors of Employment After SCI
Factors associated with employment after SCI include education, age at injury, preinjury occupation, severity of injury, and race/ethnicity. Educational attainment is one of the strongest predictors of employment after SCI; people with a 4-year or graduate degree after injury are most likely to return to work. Being younger at time of injury is associated with better employment outcomes. Those in white-collar jobs are more likely to return to work. Whites have higher rates of employment after SCI than minorities, mirroring racial disparity patterns in the general population. While people with paraplegia are more likely to return to work than those with tetraplegia, some studies suggest that, once employed, those with tetraplegia may be equally likely to sustain employment as those with paraplegia. Among those who are employed, percent of time worked after injury is significantly higher in ambulatory individuals.

Barriers to Employment After SCI
Several SCI-related conditions impose potential challenges to employment, for example, impaired mobility, impaired arm and hand function, bowel and

bladder dysfunction with possible incontinence, risk for pressure ulcers, and neuropathic pain syndromes. Psychological factors including fear or anxiety about return to work can play a significant role, as can concern or fear of losing economic or public health benefits. Low expectations regarding employment capabilities on part of the individual with SCI, family, society, employers, and/ or the treating team can create significant attitudinal barriers. Lack of readily available accessible transportation is reported to be a significant perceived barrier to employment.

The Americans With Disabilities Act

The Americans with Disabilities Act (ADA), a federal law passed in 1990, prohibits discrimination against people with disabilities in employment, public transportation, public services, public accommodations, and telecommunications. Title I of the ADA prohibits discrimination in employment and requires employers to provide reasonable accommodations for employees with disabilities.

Reasonable Accommodation
Under the ADA, employers with more than 15 employees are required to make reasonable accommodations for qualified candidates with disabilities unless such accommodation would impose undue hardship. The ADA requires reasonable accommodation in three aspects of employment: (1) to ensure equal opportunity in the application process, (2) to enable a qualified individual with a disability to perform the essential functions of a job, and (3) to enable an employee with a disability to enjoy equal benefits and privileges of employment. Examples of reasonable accommodations include making existing facilities accessible, job restructuring, part-time or modified work schedules, and acquiring or modifying equipment.

Table 44.1 provides examples of reasonable accommodation that commonly apply to workers with SCI.

Table 44.1

Examples of Reasonable Accommodations in the Workplace for People With SCI

Work Issue	Possible Solutions
Standard desk may not allow wheelchair access under it	- Work surface modification (e.g., raising the desk or changing its shape)
Inability to use a standard keyboard/ mouse	- Trackball for mouse function - Adapted keyboard - Voice recognition software
Access into the facility	- Access to reserved disabled parking - Accessible route/ramp into facility - Automatic door openers - Easy-access door handles

(continued)

Work Issue	Possible Solutions
Access within the facility	- Widening of narrow doorways to at least 32" or adding offset hinges for additional 1-2" clearance
	- Maintain at least 36" clear path of travel
	- Use lower shelves for frequently accessed material for wheelchair access
Bathroom access	- Grab bars
	- Raised toilet seat
	- Lowered mirrors and paper towel dispensers, automated hand dryers
	- Knee clearance for sinks
Morning routine/bowel and bladder care	- Flexible schedule
	- Part-time work
	- Telecommuting
	- Breaks as needed

Abbreviation: SCI, spinal cord injury.

Legislation to Encourage Return to Work After Disability Without Loss of Health Benefits

The Ticket to Work and Work Incentives Improvement Act (TWWIIA), signed in 1999, reduces barriers that require people with disability to choose between health care coverage and work. It expands Medicaid and Medicare coverage for eligible individuals who work, and provides them greater choice and control.

CLINICAL CONSIDERATIONS

The goal of vocational rehabilitation is to enable individuals with disabilities to engage in gainful employment. SCI clinicians play an important role in the process by positively engaging the individual with SCI about work, initiating appropriate referrals, facilitating awareness of and access to resources, providing support and encouragement, allaying anxiety and fears about employment, and working in conjunction with the vocational specialist and the individual with SCI at different points during the process as needed, to problem-solve and address clinical issues that could impact work performance.

A hospital-based vocational counselor or vocational rehabilitation specialist may be available through consultation or as part of the rehabilitation team. Referrals may also be made to government programs for which the individual is eligible, such as State vocational rehabilitation agencies, and to community agencies and resources.

Approaches to Vocational Rehabilitation After SCI

A variety of approaches has been used for vocational rehabilitation that include traditional methods and alternative approaches, such as supported employment (SE).

Traditional Approaches to Vocational Rehabilitation

Following a referral to vocational rehabilitation, the traditional approach includes an initial screening followed by more detailed evaluation, vocational testing to assess level of general intelligence, aptitude, achievement, interest, and work skills, followed by development of a vocational goal, providing relevant training and other pre-employment or reentry programs, with subsequent job placement and follow-up. Follow-up is typically time-limited, after which it is discontinued, for example, at 60 to 90 days following placement, or if a determination is made that employment is not feasible.

Traditional approaches may also include placement in intermediate programs such as sheltered workshops that provide some work experience and limited income or day programs that provide supervised day activities, but don't lead to competitive employment.

Supported Employment (Table 44.2)

Evidence-based practice of SE is an alternative approach to vocational rehabilitation that has been implemented with some reports of significantly greater success than with traditional methods. While the greatest experience with this approach has been implemented in populations with mental illness, there are increasing reports about positive experience with implementation of the SE model in people with other disabilities, including SCI.

The principles underlying evidence-based SE, also known as the individualized placement and support model, include: competitive employment as the goal, zero exclusion, rapid job search, integrated approach working closely with the treatment team, personal preferences are honored, ongoing individualized support, and benefits counseling. These principles are further described in Table 44.2.

Table 44.2

Principles of Evidence-Based Supported Employment

Principal	Description	Rationale[a]
Competitive employment	The focus is on competitive employment as an attainable goal, rather than intermediate activities such as day treatment or volunteer work.	Targeted efforts toward competitive employment may be more effective than indirect strategies; intermediate activities may not contribute to and may interfere with competitive employment.
Zero exclusion/individual choice	No one is excluded who wants to participate. The only requirement is a desire to work in a competitive job.	Belief that success is possible regardless of severity or type of disability. People with severe disabilities can obtain and succeed in competitive jobs.

(continued)

Principal	Description	Rationale[a]
Rapid job search	Emphasis is on immediate assistance with job finding rather than lengthy prevocational assessment, training or counseling.	Training can be provided concurrently with SE. Training provided after job placement can be personalized to the job situation to improve work performance.
Integrated treatment	Integration of SE program with the SCI team. SE staff participate in treatment team meetings and interact with team members outside of these meetings.	This integrated approach is associated with better communication, increased awareness and focus of clinicians on employment, and incorporation of clinical information into vocational plans.
Attention to individual preferences	Services are based on the individual's preferences and choices, rather than providers' judgments.	Increased chance of finding jobs uniquely tailored to the individual's strengths and preferences, including unconventional, not-easy-to-categorize positions.
Ongoing individualized support	Follow-along supports continue for a time that fits the individual rather than terminating at a set point after a job is started.	Continued on-the-job support and support for problem-solving facilitates success. Additionally, it is important not to give up too early on those who do not benefit initially.
Benefits counseling	Ongoing planning and guidance regarding Social Security, Medicaid, and other benefits and government entitlements.	A major barrier to employment can be fear of losing benefits. Clarifies misconceptions and helps individuals make well-informed choices.

Abbreviations: SCI, spinal cord injury; SE, supported employment.
[a] Much of the rationale for these principles is validated in populations other than SCI.

In this model, the vocational rehabilitation specialist, working in an integrated manner with the treatment team provides several forms of support for career planning, job search and job development, on the job support, and job retention (Table 44.3).

Table 44.3

Supported Employment Activities of the Vocational Rehabilitation Specialist

Career Planning

- Recommend and provide support for career exploration activities
- Gather information on the individual's personal abilities and support needs
- Assist with determining transportation options for employment

Job Search and Job Development

- Identify and arrange for meetings with potential employers
- Meet with employers to discuss abilities and qualifications for work
- Meet with employers to discuss on the job and ongoing support services
- Refer the individual to interviews with prospective employers
- Discuss the pros and cons of particular work opportunities with the job seeker
- Provide assistance with the pre-employment process (i.e., completing job applications, disclosure, testing, interviewing, etc.)

On the Job Support

- Facilitate additional on-the-job skills training
- Offer ideas for assistive technology and other types of accommodations
- Provide feedback to the employee on his or her performance
- Model positive interactions with customers, coworkers, and supervisors
- Promote communication and rapport between the employee with the disability and workplace staff
- Facilitate the use of existing workplace supports

Job Retention Services

- Assist the person with arranging medical appointments outside of work hours
- Problem-solve with the person what to do if their transportation to work is late or how to make alternative arrangements
- Teach the person how to ask for time off from work
- Provide referral to a benefits specialist to ensure use of available work incentives
- Assist the individual with resolving workplace problems related to job performance, getting along with coworkers, or supervisors
- Assist the individual with identifying and/or requesting new accommodations from the employer

Adapted from Targett, P., & Wehman, P. 2003. Successful work supports for persons with spinal cord injury. *SCI Psychosocial Process*, 16(1), 5–11.

KNOWLEDGE GAPS AND EMERGING CONCEPTS

Additional research is needed to validate the encouraging experience from initial reports of implementation of evidence-based practice of SE in the SCI setting. Focused research is also needed to evaluate specific program components and to determine best practices that lead to increased employment and positive work-related outcomes for people with SCI.

SUGGESTED READING

Bruyère SM, ed. *Employing and Accommodating Individuals with Spinal Cord Injuries.* [Brochure]. Ithaca, NY: Cornell University; 2000. (Original work written 2000 by N. Somerville & D. J. Wilson)

Krause JS, Reed KS. Barriers and facilitators to employment after spinal cord injury: underlying dimensions and their relationship to labor force participation. *Spinal Cord.* 2011;49(2):285-291.

Krause JS, Saunders LL, Acuna J. Gainful employment and risk of mortality after spinal cord injury: effects beyond that of demographic, injury and socioeconomic factors. *Spinal Cord.* 2012;50(10):784-788. Doi: 10.1038/sc.2012.49.

Ottomanelli L, Lind L. Review of critical factors related to employment after spinal cord injury: implications for research and vocational services. *J Spinal Cord Med.* 2009;32(5):503-531.

Ottomanelli L, Goetz LL, Suris A, et al. Effectiveness of supported employment for veterans with spinal cord injuries: results from a randomized multisite study. *Arch Phys Med Rehabil.* 2012;93(5):740-747.

Targett P, Wehman P. Successful work supports for persons with spinal cord injury. *SCI Psychosoc Proc.* 2003;16(1):5-11.

CHAPTER 45

Driving and Transportation Access After SCI

GENERAL PRINCIPLES

Accessible transportation is a crucial element of independence after spinal cord injury (SCI). Transportation is one of the major barriers to community participation and access cited by people with SCI.

Transportation Options and Barriers

Depending on the level and completeness of injury, presence of other impairments, available resources and capabilities, options for transportation after SCI may include: driving a regular or adapted vehicle, being a passenger in an adapted or regular personal vehicle, taking accessible public transportation, or specialized transportation and shared ride services.

Cost and available funding sources may be important factors impacting transportation options. While vehicular adaptions for someone with paraplegia may sometimes be accomplished for under $1,500, purchase of a highly specialized, adapted van for someone with C5 tetraplegia can cost upward of $80,000. Cost of special transportation services may only be covered by funding sources for certain purposes of the trip (e.g., for medical or therapy appointments, or for education), but may not be otherwise covered. Availability of accessible public transportation, including hours of service and the service area, varies widely depending on the location and community.

Special modes of transportation are associated with their own challenges. For example, air travel is associated with issues related to transfer to another chair for boarding the aircraft, access to the toilet during travel, and transportation of personal wheelchairs.

Driving Options Based on Level of Injury

Driving ability and options depend on the level and completeness of SCI (Chapter 26, Tables 26.3 to 26.5). Patients with C1 to C4 complete tetraplegia are unable to drive themselves and require attendant-driven accessible transportation (e.g., a van with a wheelchair lift and tie-downs). For patients with complete SCI, the highest level of injury at which independent driving is possible is C5, and these individuals require a highly specialized modified van. Patients with C6 complete injury can drive a modified van with lift, tie-downs, and hand controls. Many patients with C7 tetraplegia will also need to drive a modified van, though, for some a modified car may be an option. Those with complete SCI at C8 and below can drive a modified car with hand controls. For patients with incomplete injury, driving options depend on the extent and distribution of weakness.

CLINICAL CONSIDERATIONS

Driving Evaluation and Training

Driving assessment and training are important components of SCI rehabilitation, and are typically carried out by a trained and certified driver rehabilitation specialist, working in conjunction with others in the SCI team as needed.

The process includes predriving interview and clinical assessment, seating assessment, static behind the wheel assessment and training, driving simulation, dynamic on-the-road assessment and training, prescription for vehicular modification, consideration of transportation alternatives, and follow-up services.

Predriving Assessment
Evaluation of muscle strength, sensation, sitting balance, transfers, spasticity, range of motion, and coordination are important aspects of physical assessment for driving after SCI. Visual, perceptual, and cognitive evaluation is included, and is especially pertinent in those with concomitant traumatic brain injury, elderly individuals, and those with multiple sclerosis.

Behind-the-Wheel Assessment and Training
Static behind-the-wheel assessment and training includes evaluation and consideration of options for entry and exit from the vehicle, steering, braking and acceleration, and secondary controls including lights, wipers, and horn. Driving simulators have become increasingly available with advances in technology. These provide risk-free opportunities for interactive evaluation and training in response to various simulated scenarios. Once the individual is assessed to be appropriate and ready, progression is made to driving on the open road.

Vehicle/Equipment Selection and Prescription
Considerations in vehicular and equipment selection and prescription include vehicle entry and egress, seat safety, wheelchair securement or storage, driving

position including visibility and leg clearance, steering options, acceleration and brakes, and secondary controls (Table 45.1).

Preparation for Driving
As needed, documentation and assistance is provided to fulfill state-specific medical clearance and licensing requirement and for disabled parking application. Patients should be counseled about driving safety to

Table 45.1
Vehicle and Equipment Options for Driving After SCI

Options	Considerations
Vehicle type	
Van	- Attendant-driven van for C1–C4 complete SCI; drivers with C5, C6, and many C7 LOI need modified van - May need to lower van floor to accommodate and provide seated visibility to driver or passenger in power wheelchair
Car	- C8 and lower LOI (and some C7) can drive an adapted car - For those who have a choice of either option, lifestyle, family transportation needs, and preferences may influence selection
Steering	
Spinner knob	- Requires close to normal grip capacity - Provided to facilitate steering with one hand, with other hand used for hand controls
Tri-pin steering device	- Commonly used steering device for people with tetraplegia who have wrist extension (or orthotic wrist support) but no grip strength
V-grip or palm-grip	- Require some finger/grip strength
Acceleration and brakes	
Push-pull hand controls	- Mounted on the steering column in cars - Can be floor mounted in vans
Vacuum-assisted hand control	- Requires good hand strength and is more costly, but may be an option when less installation space is available
Highly specialized systems	- Electronic acceleration and braking or power-assisted controls may be required for higher LOI (C5), but can be costly and high maintenance

(continued)

Options	Considerations
Secondary controls	
For headlights, horn, heating and cooling, signals	- Can be touch pad systems, auditory signals, or voice-activated for higher LOI
Balance and postural control	
Chest straps, lateral stabilizers, lumbar support	- May be needed for those with impaired trunk control and seated balance
Wheelchair access and storage	
Lift, ramp, loading device	- Platform lift or ramp required for power wheelchairs - Manual wheelchair users who can transfer to driver seat may be able to fold or disassemble chair for storage, or require a loading device or lift
Wheelchair security	
Manual or automatic lock-downs or tie-downs	- Required for passenger or driver in wheelchair, or for securing wheelchair being transported in the main cabin

Abbreviations: SCI, spinal cord injury; LOI, level of injury.

address SCI-related issues such as skin care and pressure relief while driving, and to be careful about contact with hot surfaces on insensate skin. Teaching and problem-solving about situations such as spasms that may be triggered by sharp turns or bumps, or onset of autonomic dysreflexia while driving, is needed. Proactive planning for emergencies or breakdown that could occur while driving, becomes especially important after SCI.

Transportation Alternatives

At any point during the evaluation process, it may be determined that independent driving is not a feasible or appropriate option. Planning for alternative transportation options is needed. Those who are able to drive independently should also be aware of the options and resources available for alternative transportation. Community access via public transportation is often initiated and practiced during initial rehabilitation to allay anxiety and help problem-solve prior to discharge.

KNOWLEDGE GAPS AND EMERGING CONCEPTS

The use of driving simulators and advances in virtual reality technology has enhanced ability for risk-free driving evaluation and training. Additional research is needed in this area to demonstrate validity and correlation with on-road performance and driving.

SUGGESTED READING

Akinwuntan AE, Devos H, Stepleman L, et al. Predictors of driving in individuals with relapsing-remitting multiple sclerosis. *Mult Scler.* 2013;19(3):344-350.

Carlozzi NE, Gade V, Rizzo AS, Tulsky DS. Using virtual reality driving simulators in persons with spinal cord injury: three screen display versus head mounted display. *Disabil Rehabil Assist Technol.* 2013;8(2):176-180.

Kiyono Y, Hashizume C, Matsui N, Ohtsuka K, Takaoka K. Car-driving abilities of people with tetraplegia. *Arch Phys Med Rehabil.* 2001;82(10):1389-1392.

Marcotte TD, Rosenthal TJ, Roberts E, et al. The contribution of cognition and spasticity to driving performance in multiple sclerosis. *Arch Phys Med Rehabil.* 2008;89(9):1753-1758.

VII. Systems-Based Practice

CHAPTER 46

Systems of Care for SCI

GENERAL PRINCIPLES

Spinal Cord Injury System of Care Needs and Gaps

Spinal cord injury (SCI) requires optimal care from onset to prevent second-ary complications that can negatively affect long-term outcomes. Individuals with spinal SCI experience increased health needs and risks for secondary conditions that begin at the time of injury and continue for the remainder of their lives. While they may be otherwise healthy, they have been characterized as having a thinner margin of health that requires additional vigilance and timely access to health services.

People with SCI are reported to have better outcomes with a specialized and systematic approach to care. Coordinated and integrated systems of care have been shown to reduce SCI complications, length of stay in hospital, and costs, and improve outcomes.

Gaps in Care and Services

While some coordinated systems of care exist, the care for majority of indi-viduals with SCI is quite fragmented, with poor care coordination and several potential gaps in service. Access to adequate primary care and related health services can be especially problematic, with default to repeated emergency room visits for ongoing health care needs in many instances. Several factors have been reported as contributing to disparities in access to primary care (Table 46.1).

Established SCI Systems of Care in the United States

Spinal Cord Injury Model Systems Program

The Spinal Cord Injury Model Systems (SCIMS) program began in 1970, with funding from the National Institute on Disability and Rehabilitation Research (NIDRR) in the U.S. Department of Education, to demonstrate a comprehensive care system for SCI and also to conduct research to improve the health and quality of life of persons with SCI. It has evolved over the past three decades into a program in which SCI centers in the United States compete for awards based on their system of care ("medical, vocational, and other rehabilitation services") having rehabilitation integrated with acute care, and demonstrating

Table 46.1

Barriers to Adequate Primary Care for People With SCI

Domain	Factors
Knowledge barriers	Primary care physicians often lack SCI-specific knowledge
	SCI specialists may provide aspects of primary care in some cases, but often have limited primary care training
	Clinicians with lack of knowledge and expertise about the needed durable medical equipment and assistive technology may provide inadequate or inappropriate prescription
Physical access barriers	Lack of height-adjustable exam tables
	Small exam rooms with limited accommodation for wheelchairs
	Inadequate accessible parking and ramp access
	Imaging tables may not allow easy transfer
Attitudinal barriers	Reluctance and apprehension to position and move patients for physical exam may result in inadequate examination
	May avoid seeing patients in wheelchairs, who may be seen as requiring more time
	Inappropriate attribution of all problems to SCI, even if unrelated
System of care barriers	Fragmented systems with incentives for cost-cutting and cost-shifting, instead of an investment in long-term outcomes
	Transportation for appointments may be a barrier
	Health plans may view people with SCI as high-cost, high-risk, and may be reluctant to enroll them in the absence of incentives

Abbreviation: SCI, spinal cord injury.

improved outcomes, participation in a national database that monitors medical and secondary complications as well as neurological and functional recovery, participation in independent and collaborative research, and provision of continuing education related to SCI.

SCIMS data is entered in the National SCI Statistical Center, and is estimated to capture approximately 13% of all new SCIs occurring in the United States. At time of this writing, there were 14 funded SCI Model System grantees.

While providing comprehensive and integrated rehabilitation programs, many SCI Model Systems provide relatively limited scope of ongoing health care services after the postrehabilitation period, so that subsequent primary and specialty care is often still fragmented.

Department of Veterans Affairs (VA) SCI System of Care

VA has the largest single network of SCI care in the nation. It provided a full range of care to nearly 26,000 veterans with spinal cord injuries and disorders in 2008 and SCI specialty care to about 13,000 of these veterans. A study conducted by a major consulting firm in 2000 comparing VA's SCI services to those funded by several private and public health insurers showed that VA's coverage was more comprehensive.

VA's system of care provides a coordinated lifelong continuum of services for eligible veterans with SCI of all ages, including emergency care, medical and surgical stabilization, rehabilitation, primary care, preventive care, specialty sustaining care, surgical care, outpatient care, home care, and long-term care. VA's SCI specialty care focuses on the prevention or early detection of complications of SCI, with multidisciplinary teams providing annual comprehensive evaluations.

VA services are delivered through a "hub and spoke" system of care, extending from 24 regional SCI centers, offering primary and specialty care by multidisciplinary teams, to the approximately 134 SCI primary care teams or support clinics at local VA medical centers. Each primary care team has a physician, nurse, and social worker, and those with support clinics may have additional team members. Newly injured Veterans and Active Duty Service Members are referred to a VA SCI center for rehabilitation after being stabilized at a trauma center. Each year, approximately 450 newly injured Veterans and Active Duty Service Members receive rehabilitation at VA SCI centers.

CLINICAL CONSIDERATIONS

SCI Rehabilitation Teams

Teamwork is the cornerstone of SCI care. Teams can be characterized as multidisciplinary or interdisciplinary. In multidisciplinary teams, different disciplines work independently or sequentially, from their own disciplinary-specific perspectives. One team member is affected very little by the efforts of the other team members. Interdisciplinary team members, on the other hand, work jointly on goals, though from each of their respective disciplinary perspectives, to try to achieve the best outcomes for the patient, who is at the center of the team. The interdisciplinary team model, if properly implemented, is typically considered more effective in the rehabilitation setting.

The potential challenges of health care teams include resolution of different perspectives or conflicts, potential for perceived erosion of autonomy, and issues related to communication and coordination of the multiple aspects of care (see Chapter 48). SCI rehabilitation teams typically include physicians, nurses, physical, occupational, speech, and recreational therapists, psychologists, and social workers/case managers, and may include or consult with specialists in nutrition, vocational counseling and rehabilitation, orthotics, drivers training, and/or rehabilitation engineering.

Health Care Maintenance and Disease Prevention After SCI

There is general consensus that comprehensive preventive health evaluations for individuals with SCI are important, although uniform agreement about optimal frequency and specific elements is lacking. Because all body systems are potentially affected by SCI, ongoing long-term health care management needs to be comprehensive.

- Measures such as smoking cessation and pneumonia and annual influenza vaccinations are important for reducing respiratory problems (Chapter 32). Respiratory infections should be promptly identified and treated. It is important to recognize and address worsening ventilatory function that may occur with aging or after other complications.
- Primary and secondary prevention of cardiovascular disease includes smoking cessation, diet and weight control, lipid management, screening for and treatment of hypertension and glucose intolerance or diabetes, and individualized exercise program (Chapter 33D). Autonomic dysreflexia is a life-threatening emergency, and persons with SCI above T6 neurological level can be at lifelong risk (Chapter 33C).
- Ongoing monitoring of bladder management is needed to ensure low pressure and complete voiding, minimize urinary tract complications, preserve upper urinary tracts, and be compatible with the individual's lifestyle (Chapter 34A). There should be predictable and effective bowel elimination without bowel incontinence (Chapter 36A).
- Continued education of the patient and reinforcement to ensure regular pressure relief practices and skin inspection, and appropriate prescription, maintenance, and monitoring of support surfaces are important for prevention of pressure ulcers (Chapter 37).
- Neurologic function should be periodically reassessed on an ongoing basis, and any worsening (e.g., due to syringomyelia or carpal tunnel syndrome) identified, investigated and addressed appropriately (Chapter 38B). Spasticity should be monitored and treated as needed (Chapter 38A).
- Measures for upper extremity preservation after SCI should be followed lifelong. These include optimization of equipment and wheelchair to minimize upper extremity stresses, activity modification to minimize repetitive or excessive upper extremity forces during daily activities and transfers, and individualized exercise program incorporating appropriate flexibility and strengthening components (Chapter 27). It is important to recognize and to address contributing factors to pain, which is often multifactorial (Chapter 38C). Fall prevention is important to prevent injuries.

▩ Monitoring, identification, and timely treatment of depression or mal-adaptive behavior may be needed (Chapter 41).

▩ It is important to address environmental barriers, promote self-efficacy, and optimize participation and community integration in response to changes in the living situation and social support, functional decline, and/or aging (Chapter 42). Ongoing rehabilitation interventions are often indicated to address changes in neurologic status, new goals, changes in living situation, or functional decline associated with medical complications and comorbidities, and aging (Chapter 40).

Noncompliance with follow-up for scheduled periodic preventive health evaluations may result from concerns about out-of-pocket cost of the visit and medical tests, availability of transportation, time, distance and inconvenience factors, or belief that follow-up was not necessary or of value. Aspects of routine evaluation that have been reported to be of greatest perceived value by people with SCI include getting their medications and supplies refilled and ability to make equipment changes.

KNOWLEDGE GAPS AND EMERGING CONCEPTS

Innovations and increasing implementation of technologies for virtual access, including secure messaging with health care providers, and telemedicine, including teleconsultation and home telehealth, provide potential solutions to enhance access. Clinical information systems and electronic medical records have potential to improve coordination and communication between transitions to different care settings or providers. Implementation and effectiveness research will be helpful to demonstrate value and increase adoption of these innovations.

Aspects of health care reform have particular relevance to individuals with a chronic disability such as SCI, and, depending on specifics of implementation going forward, may incorporate improved access (such as provisions for prohibiting exclusion of insurance coverage of those considered high-risk), and financial incentives and provisions for improved care coordination and avoidance of preventable complications.

SUGGESTED READING

Chen Y, Deutsch A, DeVivo MJ, et al. Current research outcomes from the spinal cord injury model systems. *Arch Phys Med Rehabil.* 2011;92(3):329-331.

Choi H, Binder DS, Oropilla ML, et al. Evaluation of selected laboratory components of a comprehensive periodic health evaluation for veterans with spinal cord injury and disorders. *Arch Phys Med Rehabil.* 2006;87(5):603-610.

Collins EG, Langbein WE, Smith B, Hendricks R, Hammond M, Weaver F. Patients' perspective on the comprehensive preventive health evaluation in veterans with spinal cord injury. *Spinal Cord.* 2005;43(6):366-374.

Curtin CM, Suarez PA, Di Ponio LA, Frayne SM. Who are the women and men in Veterans Health Administration's current spinal cord injury population? *J Rehabil Res Dev.* 2012;49(3):351-360.

DeJong G. Primary care for persons with disabilities. An overview of the problem. *Am J Phys Med Rehabil.* 1997;76(3 suppl):S2-S8.

DeJong G, Hoffman J, Meade MA, et al. Postrehabilitative health care for individuals with SCI: extending health care into the community. *Top Spinal Cord Inj Rehabil.* 2011;17(2): 46-58.

Kirshblum SC. Clinical activities of the model spinal cord injury system. *J Spinal Cord Med.* 2002;25(4):339-344.

New PW, Townson A, Scivoletto G, et al. International comparison of the organisation of rehabilitation services and systems of care for patients with spinal cord injury. *Spinal Cord.* 2013;51(1):33-39.

Sabharwal S, Fiedler IG. Increasing disability awareness of future spinal cord injury physicians. *J Spinal Cord Med.* 2003;26(1):89-92.

Sinclair LB, Lingard LA, Mohabeer RN. What's so great about rehabilitation teams? An ethnographic study of interprofessional collaboration in a rehabilitation unit. *Arch Phys Med Rehabil.* 2009;90(7):1196-1201.

VA fact sheet. www1.va.gov/opa/publications/factsheets/fs_spinal_cord_injury.pdf. Accessed August 5, 2013.

CHAPTER 47

Patient Safety in SCI Care

GENERAL PRINCIPLES

Increased Focus on Patient Safety

Since the publication of the Institute of Medicine (IOM) report "To Err Is Human: Building a Safer Health System" in 1999, which highlighted the scope and enormity of medical errors and patient safety concerns in health care, there has been a significantly increased focus on patient safety. The Joint Commission established National Patient Safety Goals (NPSGs) in 2002 that accredited health care organizations must comply with, and these are updated annually. The 2013 NPSG are summarized in Table 47.1.

Prevention of harm to patients is the primary rationale for patient safety initiatives. Errors also diminish patient trust and satisfaction. Additionally, attention to patient safety has major financial implications. Patient errors are costly, significantly increase lengths of stay, and pose liability for malpractice claims. There is also an increasing movement from payers to impose financial penalties and limit reimbursement for health care costs that relate to avoidable errors and complications.

Major Patient Safety Concerns and Medical Errors

Errors in health care can relate to:

- Diagnosis (error or delay in diagnosis, failure to perform indicated tests, failure to act on results of monitoring or testing)
- Treatment (error in the performance of a procedure, error in administering the treatment, error in the dose or method of using a drug, avoidable delay in treatment, inappropriate care that is not indicated)
- Prevention (failure to provide prophylactic treatment, inadequate monitoring or follow-up)
- Other factors (failure of communication, equipment failure, other system failure)

Serious patient safety concerns identified in the IOM report include issues such as adverse drug events and improper transfusions, surgical injuries and wrong-site surgery, suicides, restraint-related injuries or death, falls, burns, pressure ulcers, and mistaken patient identities.

Table 47.1
2013 National Patient Safety Goals (The Joint Commission)[a]

Accuracy of patient identification
- Use at least two patient identifiers when providing care, treatment, and services.
- Eliminate transfusion errors related to patient misidentification.

Effective communication among caregivers
- Report critical results of tests and diagnostic procedures on a timely basis.

Medication safety
- Label all medications and solutions in perioperative and other procedural settings.
- Reduce harm associated with the use of anticoagulant therapy.
- Maintain and communicate accurate patient medication information.

Reduce risk of health care-associated infections
- Comply with the current CDC or WHO hand hygiene guidelines.
- Evidence-based practices to prevent health care-associated infections due to multidrug-resistant organisms in acute care hospitals.
- Evidence-based practices to prevent central line-associated bloodstream infections.
- Evidence-based practices for preventing surgical site infections.
- Evidence-based practices to prevent indwelling CAUTI.

Reduce falls
- Reduce the risk of falls (applicable to home care and long-term care).

Prevent health care-associated pressure ulcers
- Assess and periodically reassess risk for developing a pressure ulcer and take action to address any identified risks (applicable to long-term care).

Suicide risk assessment
- Identify patients at risk for suicide (applicable to patients being treated for emotional or behavioral disorders in hospital).

Risk assessment
- Identify risks associated with home oxygen therapy, e.g., home fires (applies to home care).

Universal protocol for preventing wrong site, wrong procedure, wrong person surgery
- Conduct a preprocedure verification process.
- Mark the procedure site.
- A time-out is performed before the procedure.

Abbreviations: CAUTI, catheter-associated urinary tract infections; CDC, Centers for Disease Control and Prevention; WHO, World Health Organization.

[a]The National Patient Safety Goals for each program, with additional information is available on The Joint Commission website at www.jointcommission.org

Unique Vulnerabilities in Spinal Cord Injury Care Regarding Patient Safety

Spinal cord injury (SCI) can increase vulnerability to patient safety concerns and risk of medical errors for several reasons (Table 47.2).

Atypical or nonspecific presenting symptoms, potential for limited physical examination due to difficulty in positioning, and lack of knowledge about unique SCI-related conditions all contribute to increased risk of diagnostic errors. Medication-related adverse events are among the most common patient safety concerns, and the need for multiple medications as well as several mechanisms that alter pharmacokinetics (Table 47.3) make individuals with SCI especially susceptible. Special vulnerabilities apply to risk of major complications such as pressure ulcers, falls and injuries, suicide risk, and infections in various settings. Failure to adequately apply indicated preventive measures can lead to a variety of SCI-specific complications such as spinal instability, venous thrombo-embolism, and bladder, bowel, or skin problems. Increased episodes of transition between different care settings, especially in the context of fragmented health care systems (Chapter 46), increase vulnerability to inadequate patient hand-offs. Special risks are also imposed by potential

Table 47.2
Special Vulnerabilities Regarding Patient Safety in SCI Care

Patient Safety Concern	SCI-Related Considerations
Diagnostic errors	- Absence of typical presentations is common in SCI, increasing potential for diagnostic errors (e.g., lack of limb pain with osteoporotic fracture, or absent chest pain with myocardial infarction) - Nonspecific symptoms can be misattributed (e.g., fatigue can be the presenting or only symptom of several medical problems after SCI, such as urinary infection, but may be misattributed to nonspecific causes or poor sleep) - Difficulty in positioning or transferring people with SCI on exam table increases risk of inadequate physical exam - Lack of knowledge about conditions unique to SCI (e.g., autonomic dysreflexia) can result in misdiagnosis and inappropriate treatment
Medication-related adverse events	- Polypharmacy is common after SCI, increasing risk of drug interactions and medication reconciliation errors - Altered pharmacokinetics after SCI (see Table 47.3) increase unpredictability and potential for medication-related adverse effects

(continued)

Table 47.2

Special Vulnerabilities Regarding Patient Safety in SCI Care (*continued*)

Patient Safety Concern	SCI-Related Considerations
Falls and fall-related injuries	- Unlike other high-risk groups, falls among wheelchair-users may be higher in more active patients, and occur most often during transfers - Patients ambulating with assistive devices (e.g., incomplete SCI) are at increased risk of falls - Underlying SCI-related osteoporosis increases risk of fracture even with minor injuries or falls
Pressure ulcers	- High-risk for PUs due to SCI-related motor and sensory impairment - Traditional risk assessment tools have limited utility in stratifying risk in a universally high-risk group for PU such as SCI - Inadequate pressure relief or turning schedule, suboptimal support surface/seating prescription, or inadequate monitoring of bony prominences, can all increase risk of PU after SCI - Hospital-acquired PU may occur outside the SCI unit (e.g., lying on a hard surface while waiting for a test)
Hospital-acquired infections	- Asymptomatic bacteriuria that is common in SCI should not be confused with CAUTI - Prolonged or repeated antibiotic use (sometimes inappropriate, e.g., to treat asymptomatic bacteriuria) increases risk of infections with multi-resistant organisms or *Clostridium difficile* - Isolation procedures and contact precautions may need to be reconciled with rehabilitation and participation goals - Elevating head end of the bed, which is recommended for reducing VAP, may conflict with risk of skin shear or breakdown
Burns and injuries	- Lack of sensory feedback increases risk of injuries (e.g., from contact with a hot surface)
Inadequate preventive measures	- In the acute or postoperative period, inadequate immobilization or spinal precautions can result in neurological deterioration - Delayed or inadequate thrombo-prophylaxis in the first few weeks after SCI increases risk of potentially fatal venous thrombo-embolism - Failure to monitor and prevent high urinary bladder pressure and postvoid residual volume can lead to silent renal complications - Inadequate preventive maintenance of wheelchair and seating system can lead to pressure ulcers (e.g., from bottomed out or punctured seat cushion)

(*continued*)

Patient Safety Concern	SCI-Related Considerations
Suicide risk	- Suicide risk is 3–5 times higher in people with SCI, and is highest in years 2–5 postinjury - Somatic symptoms of depression, such as low energy, anorexia, and/or sleep disturbance may be misattributed to SCI-related medical problems without inquiry about mood changes
Inadequate patient handoffs	- Transitions of care between different care settings are more common in SCI, increasing potential for errors in handoffs - Fragmented systems of care increase risk of errors in transition with inadequate communication and coordination
Equipment malfunction	- People with SCI use a variety of equipment, including life sustaining equipment such as ventilators. Failure to prevent and promptly address equipment failure, or lack of back-up plans, can have disastrous consequences - Baclofen pump malfunction can lead to serious, even life-threatening, withdrawal reaction
Environmental safety risks	- Emergency evacuation for natural or other disasters requires special considerations in SCI due to impaired mobility and medical needs - Sustained power outage at home poses serious safety risk for users of power equipment such as ventilators, power wheelchair, or electric bed - Extreme environmental temperature can cause hypo or hyperthermia due to impaired thermoregulation, especially in those with high, complete SCI

Abbreviations: CAUTI, catheter associated urinary tract infection; SCI, spinal cord injury; PU, pressure ulcer; VAP, ventilator-associated pneumonia.

equipment malfunction and environmental factors, including power outages or extreme temperatures.

CLINICAL CONSIDERATIONS

Addressing Patient Safety in SCI Practice

There are several evidence-based strategies that have been evaluated with demonstrated effectiveness. Many can be adopted at this time, at the level of individual practitioners, and at organizational and system of care levels, to promote patient safety and minimize risks due to medical errors.

Examples include: Hand hygiene (practiced at key points in time to disrupt the transmission of microorganisms to patients including: before patient contact; after contact with blood, body fluids, or contaminated surfaces, even if gloves are worn; before invasive procedures; and after removing gloves); barrier precautions; preprocedure checklists; adherence to the do-not-use list for hazardous abbreviations; medication reconciliation and standardized hand-off

Table 47.3

Potential Effects of SCI on Pharmacokinetics

SCI-Related Change	Impact on Pharmacokinetics
Delayed gastric emptying	- Rapid absorption of acidic drugs - Delayed absorption of basic drugs
Reduced gastrointestinal motility	- Increased absorption of drugs that undergo enterohepatic circulation - Decreased bioavailability of drugs that are destroyed by gut bacteria
Reduced blood flow to skin and muscle	- Less reliable transcutaneous, subcutaneous, and intramuscular drug absorption below injury level
Increased percentage of body fat	- Effect on fat- and water-soluble drug distribution
Reduced plasma protein level	- Increased free fraction of protein-bound drugs
Impaired kidney function	- Reduced renal elimination of drugs

Abbreviation: SCI, spinal cord injury.

communications; use of clinical pharmacists to reduce adverse drug events; computerized provider order entry; and use of simulation exercises in patient safety training. Patients should be taught and encouraged to become active participants in efforts to reduce errors and improve safety, and ask pertinent questions about their care.

Attention to the special vulnerabilities, listed in Table 47.2, for patient safety among individuals with SCI, with consideration of specific practices and interventions that minimize risk related to each of those areas is an integral and vital part of SCI practice.

Fostering a Patient Safety Culture

A positive patient safety climate has been reported to be associated with improved patient safety. The system should facilitate a culture of learning, promote reporting, and focus on system vulnerabilities rather than on blame. Reporting should include not only actual adverse events but also near-miss reporting of events that didn't harm a patient but provide an opportunity to understand vulnerabilities in the system.

As specified in the IOM report, the majority of medical errors do not result from individual recklessness or the willful actions of particular individuals. More commonly, errors are caused by faulty systems, processes, and conditions that lead people to make mistakes or fail to prevent them. Thus, mistakes can best be prevented by designing the health system at all levels to make it safer to make it harder for people to do something wrong and easier for them to do it right. Of course, people still must be vigilant and held responsible for their actions. But when an error occurs, blaming an individual does little to make the system safer and prevent someone else from committing the same error.

KNOWLEDGE GAPS AND EMERGING CONCEPTS

Specific research to apply patient safety practices in SCI care is rudimentary, although there is emerging research in focused areas, for example, hospital-acquired infections in SCI populations. Given the unique patient safety vulnerabilities of people with SCI, additional SCI-specific research in patient safety is crucial.

Implementation research to identify most effective ways to incorporate evidence-based practices in various areas of patient safety is also much needed. Research should focus on strengthening the evidence around effectiveness of strategies to improve patient safety and promote a patient safety culture.

SUGGESTED READING

DeVivo MJ, Black KJ, Richards JS, Stover SL. Suicide following spinal cord injury. *Paraplegia.* 1991;29(9):620-627.

Evans CT, LaVela SL, Weaver FM, et al. Epidemiology of hospital-acquired infections in veterans with spinal cord injury and disorder. *Infect Control Hosp Epidemiol.* 2008;29(3):234-242.

Hammond FM, Horn SD, Smout RJ, et al. Acute rehospitalizations during inpatient rehabilitation for spinal cord injury. *Arch Phys Med Rehabil.* 2013;94(4 suppl):S98-S105.

Kohn LT, Corrigan JM, Donaldson MS, eds. *To Err is Human: Building a Safer Health System.* Washington, DC: National Academy Press, Institute of Medicine;1999.

Kwan JL, Lo L, Sampson M, Shojania KG. Medication reconciliation during transitions of care as a patient safety strategy: a systematic review. *Ann Intern Med.* 2013;158(5 pt 2):397-403.

Mestre H, Alkon T, Salazar S, Ibarra A. Spinal cord injury sequelae alter drug pharmacokinetics: an overview. *Spinal Cord.* 2011;49(9):955-960.

McDonald KM, Matesic B, Contopoulos-Ioannidis DG, et al. Patient safety strategies targeted at diagnostic errors: a systematic review. *Ann Intern Med.* 2013;158(5 pt 2):381-389.

Nelson A, Fitzgerald SG, Palacios P, et al. Wheelchair-related falls in veterans with spinal cord injury residing in the community: a prospective cohort study. *Arch Phys Med Rehabil.* 2010;91(8):1153-1312.

Shekelle PG, Pronovost PJ, Wachter RM, et al. The top patient safety strategies that can be encouraged for adoption now. *Ann Intern Med.* 2013;158(5 pt 2):365-368.

Siefferman JW, Lin E, Fine JS. Patient safety at handoff in rehabilitation medicine. *Phys Med Rehabil Clin N Am.* 2012;23(2):241-257.

Sullivan N, Schoelles KM. Preventing in-facility pressure ulcers as a patient safety strategy: a systematic review. *Ann Intern Med.* 2013;158(5 pt 2):410-416.

Weaver SJ, Lubomksi LH, Wilson RF, Pfoh ER, Martinez KA, Dy SM. Promoting a culture of safety as a patient safety strategy: a systematic review. *Ann Intern Med.* 2013;158 (5 pt 2):369-374.

CHAPTER 48

Ethical Issues in SCI Practice

GENERAL PRINCIPLES

Ethical concerns and tensions arise in spinal cord injury (SCI) care in a variety of situations. In some instances there are clear right or wrong answers. However, in many instances, the issues are not as straightforward and there are conflicts between values on either side of an ethical dilemma. For example, respecting a patient's refusal of treatment may conflict with acting in the patient's best interest. Balancing these principles and resolving ethical tensions to try and arrive at the best course of action is an inherent part of clinical practice.

Ethical Principles and Terms

Certain fundamental ethical principles are especially relevant to health care and clinical practice. These include: respect for persons (respecting autonomy, maintaining confidentiality, and avoiding deception and nondisclosure), acting in the best interest of patients, and allocating resources justly. Even though they are not considered absolute, and are sometimes in conflict with each other, these principles serve as important guidelines in clinical practice.

Autonomy
Clinicians must respect a patient's right to make decisions regarding his medical care. Competent, informed patients have the right to choose among treatment options and refuse any unwanted medical interventions. By providing informed consent and following patients' wishes, clinicians demonstrate their respect for the patient's autonomy.

Beneficence
Clinicians must act in the best interests of their patients. Clinicians must put the interests of their patients ahead of their own interests. Market forces, societal pressures, and administrative exigencies must not compromise this principle.

Nonmaleficence
This principle relates to "do no harm" to patients. It requires that clinicians not intentionally create a needless harm or injury to the patient, either through acts of commission or omission. Clinicians must refrain from providing ineffective treatments or acting with malice toward patients.

Confidentiality
Clinicians must maintain the confidentiality of medical information. Confidentiality respects patient autonomy and encourages patients to be candid. However, confidentiality can be overridden in certain situations to protect third parties when there is the potential for serious, foreseeable harm to third parties. For example, legally mandated reporting includes child or elder abuse, and domestic violence.

Justice
The principle of distributive justice deals with issues of treating patients equally. Distributive justice aims at ensuring that everyone has access to necessary care based on the ethical principles of equity and solidarity. In the face of limited health care resources, clinicians should practice cost-effective medicine. Clinicians should make recommendations and decisions based on ethically pertinent considerations.

Professional Codes as a Source of Guidance

Professional codes are among the sources that serve to provide guidance about ethical conduct and professionalism. For example, one of the most widely accepted of these for physicians and adopted by multiple medical organizations is the Physician Charter jointly authored by the American Board of Internal Medicine Foundation, American College of Physicians Foundation and the European Federation of Internal Medicine in 2002. It presents ten professional responsibilities or physician commitments, based on three fundamental principles (Table 48.1).

Common Conflicts Between Ethical Principles

Some of the most common and difficult ethical issues in practice arise when the patient's autonomous decision conflicts with the physician's beneficent duty to look out for the patient's best interests. In general, as long as the patient meets the criteria for decision-making capacity, the patient's decisions should be respected even while trying to convince the patient otherwise.

Another potential ethical dilemma is the balancing of beneficence and nonmaleficence. This balance is one between the benefits and risks of treatment and comes into play in medical decisions. By providing informed consent, physicians give patients the information necessary to understand the scope and nature of the potential risks and benefits in order to make a decision.

VII. Systems-Based Practice

Physician Charter on Professionalism

Fundamental Principles

Primacy of patient welfare

A Set of Commitments

Commitment to professional competence.

Commitment to honesty with patients.

Commitment to patient confidentiality.

Commitment to maintaining appropriate relations with patients.

Commitment to improving quality of care.

Commitment to improving access to care.

Commitment to a just distribution of finite resources.

Commitment to scientific knowledge.

Commitment to maintaining trust by managing conflicts of interest.

Commitment to professional responsibilities.

The potential benefits of proposed interventions must outweigh the risks in order for the action to be ethical.

Informed Consent and Decision-Making Capacity

Informed consent is the process by which a fully informed patient can participate in choices about his or her health care. It is generally accepted that complete informed consent includes the following elements: the nature of the decision/procedure, reasonable alternatives to the proposed intervention, the relevant risks, benefits, and uncertainties related to each alternative, assessment of patient understanding, and the acceptance of the intervention by the patient. In order for the patient's consent to be valid, the patient must be considered to have decision-making capacity and consent must be voluntary.

While often used interchangeably, technically there is a distinction between the terms "competency" and "decision-making capacity." Competency is a legal term; the ultimate decision to determine an individual to be incompetent is made by a court of law. Decision-making capacity is a clinical determination. Evaluation of decision-making capacity generally includes assessment of the patient's ability to: understand his or her situation, understand the consequences and risks associated with the decision at hand, and communicate a decision based on that understanding. When this is unclear, a psychiatric consultation can be helpful. However, just because a patient refuses a treatment does not in itself mean the patient is incompetent or lacks decision-making capacity.

CLINICAL CONSIDERATIONS

Table 48.2 lists examples of some situations in SCI practice, where ethical tensions and challenges are especially relevant. Each of those situations are further discussed below.

Breaking Bad News—About Prognosis After SCI

There is no one right way to discuss prognosis with a newly injured patient, but certain principles apply. In communicating prognosis it is important to remember that, while truth-telling and honesty with patients is always important, there is a difference between being truthful and being blunt. The conversation should not be rushed; the setting should be private, ideally with the physician seated at the level of the patient. It is often helpful to start with finding out what the patient understands and what the patient has been already told. It is also important to consider how much the patient wants to hear, consider the individual situation, and tailor the message accordingly. It is often helpful to give the information in small chunks and to stop between each chunk to evaluate the patient's reaction and understanding. Being attentive and responsive to the patient's reaction (or asking what the individual is feeling if it is not apparent), validating emotions, and responding with empathy appropriately are important aspects of communication in this situation.

Table 48.2

Scenarios in SCI Practice Where Ethical Tensions Commonly Arise

- **Breaking bad news—about prognosis after SCI**
  (Balancing truth-telling with compassion and preservation of hope)

- **Requests to withdraw life-sustaining treatment**
  (Patients with high cervical injury who ask to be taken off the ventilator)

- **Nonadherence to indicated treatments**
  (Individuals who don't follow pressure relief measures despite worsening pressure ulcers)

- **Interdisciplinary team conflicts**
  (Disagreements between the treatment team, addressing unprofessionalism, or perceived incompetence from others in the team)

- **Confidentiality**
  (Special confidentiality issues may arise in setting of team care, or in communication with families)

- **Disclosing errors**
  (Increased vulnerability in SCI for errors, e.g., related to knowledge deficits, lack of consideration of atypical presentations, or system issues)

- **Difficult, abusive, or hateful patient behavior**
  (Need to balance patient safety and vulnerability with concern for staff and other patients)

- **Maintaining professional boundaries**
  (Especially relevant in the face of a vulnerable patient population)

(continued)

Table 48.2

Scenarios in SCI Practice Where Ethical Tensions Commonly Arise (*continued*)

- **Requests for inappropriate treatments**
  (Stretch needed resources and take away from indicated treatments)

- **Equitable access to care and resource allocation**
  (Knowledge, physical, attitudinal, and system-based barriers)

- **Patients who seek unproven "cures" for SCI**
  (Importance of separating hope from hype)

It is often best to provide medical and prognostic information matter-of-factly, yet at the same time leave room for hope. Expressions of hope should be respected and direct confrontations of denial concerning probable implications of the injury should be avoided. Feelings of hope have been shown to assist with a future orientation and help patients move forward through the recovery process. Over time, the hope becomes more realistic, though the time frame differs among individuals.

Requests to Withdraw Life-Sustaining Treatment

Requests for withdrawal of life-sustaining treatment (e.g., a ventilator in someone with high, complete tetraplegia), while an infrequent occurrence, is one of the most ethically challenging situations in SCI practice.

An honest and sincere response, acknowledging the patient's suffering, is appropriate if such requests are expressed, and an ongoing dialogue about the recovery process and the likelihood of returning to a meaningful life after SCI should be maintained. A number of factors must be balanced when considering an overt refusal or a request for withdrawal of treatment including the patient's right to self-determination and the health care provider's duty to benefit the patient and prevent harm. Underlying depression should be assessed and treated. The patient's decision-making capacity should be assessed.

For competent patients who express an explicit unwavering request to withdraw life-sustaining treatment such as a ventilator, negotiating a time-limited trial (TLT) has been suggested as an option. This is a mutual agreement between the physician/treatment team and the patient to revisit goals of treatment and the potential for treatment cessation after a predefined period. It allows opportunity for patient reflection, adaptation to life with SCI, palliation of symptoms and suffering, time to build trust, goal setting, evaluation of trends and progress, recruitment of supportive resources, and rehabilitation and functional improvement. Trying to understand and addressing the patient's unmet needs is important; keeping in mind that the needs may be social rather than primarily medical. Helping the patient regain control over as many aspects of their life as feasible, to promote self-determination, is often helpful in fostering positive adaptation.

The institution's ethics committee should be consulted when appropriate, and legal counsel consult may be needed if conflict continues or if there is any uncertainty regarding the patient's request. Caregiver interests may occasionally not align with those of the patient. Potential caregiver burdens and conflicts of interest should be considered, especially when proxies are making decisions.

Nonadherence to Indicated Treatments

Competent patients have a right to refuse medical intervention. Dilemmas may arise when a patient refuses or does not adhere to indicated medical interventions, but does not withdraw from the role of being a patient. An example is the patient with SCI who is admitted for healing an ischial pressure ulcer but refuses to avoid sitting on the wound or perform regular pressure relief. Simply labeling such patients "noncompliant" is usually not productive. Compliance may be improved by using shared decision making, incorporating aspects of motivational interviewing, rather than negative labeling, lecturing, or confrontation.

Interdisciplinary Team Conflicts

Conflicts can arise in the SCI interdisciplinary team because of disagreements about various aspects of patient care or from perceived threats to autonomy. There may be hierarchical issues and inequality in authority, which could lead to reluctance to voice legitimate concerns and lead to potentially negative patient outcomes. Disagreements are common and expected, given the different backgrounds, expertise, and perspectives of various team members. While these may be resolved in a number of ways, a necessary component of professionalism is mutually respectful behavior, including duly considering the input of other professionals. Respect is demonstrated through language, gestures, as well as actions. There should be appropriate mechanisms in place for airing differences in perspectives and opinions.

Confidentiality

In the interdisciplinary team setting there may be special issues with confidentiality. In contrast to settings where a single provider is involved, working in clinical teams creates increased potential for confidentiality breaches requiring vigilance and due attention to auditory and visual privacy. Computerized patient records pose new and unique challenges to confidentiality. Answering questions from the family can also create confidentiality issues. It is usually best to explicitly confirm with the competent patient about how much and with whom information should be shared.

Disclosing Errors

Errors are inevitable in medical practice. As discussed in Chapter 47 there are several vulnerabilities in SCI care that can especially increase risk of potential for errors and adverse events. Most errors are not the result of negligence, but may be related to knowledge deficits, lack of consideration of atypical presentations, errors in judgment or perception, lapses in attention, or related to system issues. In general, when an error occurs one should explicitly acknowledge that an error occurred and offer an apology to the patient. An explanation of the error and its consequences should be provided. This should be followed by an explanation of what can and will be done to mitigate the resulting harm to the patient and to prevent the error from recurring. Giving only a partial explanation may be viewed as being evasive. While there may be a loss of trust as a result of disclosure of the error, it is likely to be considerably less than if a patient feels that something is being hidden from them. While there may be a fear of litigation, it has been shown that patients are less likely to consider a malpractice suit when the physician has been honest with them about mistakes.

Difficult, Abusive, or Hateful Patient Behavior

Considering the therapeutic needs of the hateful or difficult patient on the one hand (who may in fact be especially vulnerable because of alienating caregivers with hateful behaviors), and at the same time balancing it with concern for staff and other patients (e.g., if there is any threat or actual physical violence) can create ethically challenging situations. Creating a behavioral plan, with engagement of the patient as much as feasible, that includes clearly outlined and ethically appropriate enforceable consequences for continued inappropriate behaviors, without endangering patient safety, can be helpful. Rehabilitation staff should learn about how to defuse volatile situations. Communication and consistency of response within the team is especially important in these situations.

Maintaining Professional Boundaries

Vigilance in maintaining professional boundaries may be especially pertinent in the SCI rehabilitation setting, where there are often long-term therapeutic partnerships with patients, and a patient population that may be especially vulnerable. Ethical issues arise if professional, therapeutic relationships with patients blur with personal relationships.

Requests for Inappropriate Treatments

There is no obligation to offer treatments that are not expected to benefit patients. In situations where the patient or family requests an intervention that the health care team considers futile or even potentially harmful, open communication and explanation of the rationale for not offering those treatments is necessary. Dilemmas may arise, for example, when patients with high complete injuries want to focus exclusively on walking rather than focusing on wheelchair skills and activities of daily living.

A related issue is that of promoting emerging treatments and technologies to patients. While emerging technologies hold considerable promise and there are exciting new developments, it is important that patients are aware of the limitations and extent of demonstrated efficacy so they can make fully informed decisions about participation, including consideration of the time commitment and costs involved. It is also important to keep in mind reports suggesting that creating sustained unrealistic expectations, which are not met, may adversely affect longer-term adjustment after SCI.

Equitable Access to Care and Resource Allocation

Disparities in care and decreased access to primary care services, as discussed in Chapter 46, runs counter to the ethical principle of distributive justice, which aims to ensure that everyone has access to necessary care. Addressing and advocating for access by minimizing the knowledge, physical access, attitudinal, and system of care barriers that are listed in Chapter 46, Table 46.1, may be required of clinicians in SCI practice.

Health care professionals are generally not good at predicting what life with disability is like and have been consistently shown to be more negative in their predictions than the actual reported experience of people living with SCI. In some cases, erroneous beliefs amongst health care professionals, and biases about disability may contribute to certain treatments not being offered. As an extreme example, this could even apply to life-sustaining treatments. In the case of high tetraplegia, and there is evidence to suggest that acute medical and emergency personnel may significantly underestimate the potential quality of life for these patients. Therefore, any decision to withdraw life support soon after SCI needs to be scrutinized carefully.

Patients Who Seek Unproven "Cures" for SCI

Given the lack of proven or effective strategies for reversing SCI, there is concern that patients may be willing to try nonvalidated experimental treatments for SCI that have not been adequately tested for safety and efficacy. Desperate patients may also be prone to victimization by individuals or organizations offering questionable treatments for material gain or for-profit, or to stem cell tourism.

Clinicians should be prepared to offer advice or to direct patients to the appropriate source for guidance if they are considering experimental treatments. A document titled "Experimental Treatments for Spinal Cord Injury: What you should know" published by the International Campaign for Cures of Spinal Cord Injury Paralysis provides guidance on questions that should be asked by those considering such treatments. In addition to issues around informed consent that pertain to all clinical research, particular concern about therapeutic misconception may occur in patients desperate for any treatment. It refers to the belief or hope on part of the study subject, that direct benefit will occur when it is neither expected nor the intent of research. It is important to make sure that patients fully understand the risks involved and the extent of any potential benefits, and to steer them away from non-validated, unregulated interventions that don't meet the criteria for a well-designed clinical trial.

KNOWLEDGE GAPS AND EMERGING CONCEPTS

There has been an increasing recognition of the need for addressing professionalism, interpersonal communication, and awareness of ethical issues that commonly arise in health care, with new and emerging efforts for teaching and evaluating related skills at the medical school, postgraduate, and continued professional development level. These efforts are especially pertinent to SCI practice where juxtaposition of medical and ethical issues is common in various situations throughout the care continuum. Additional study is warranted to identify and implement effective measures that enhance skills and attitudes to promote professionalism and ethical practice in the potentially challenging SCI-specific situations discussed in this chapter.

SUGGESTED READING

ABIM Foundation; ACP-ASIM Foundation; European Federation of Internal Medicine. Medical professionalism in the new millenium: a physician charter. *Ann Intern Med.* 2002;136:243-246.

Baile WF, Buckman R, Lenzi R, Glober G, Beale EA, Kudelka AP. SPIKES-A six-step protocol for delivering bad news: application to the patient with cancer. *Oncologist.* 2000;5(4):302- 311.

Blight A, Curt A, Ditunno JF, et al. Position statement on the sale of unproven cellular therapies for spinal cord injury: the international campaign for cures of spinal cord injury paralysis. *Spinal Cord.* 2009;47(9):713-714.

Cashman S, Reidy P, Cody K, Lemay C. Developing and measuring progress toward collaborative, integrated, interdisciplinary health care teams. *J Interprof Care.* 2004;18(2):183-196.

DeVivo MJ, Black KJ, Richards JS, Stover SL. Suicide following spinal cord injury. *Paraplegia.* 1991;29(9):620-627.

Haas LJ, Leiser JP, Magill MK, Sanyer ON. Management of the difficult patient. *Am Fam Physician.* 2005;72(10):2063-2068.

Harvey L, Wyndaele JJ. Are we jumping too early with locomotor training programs? *Spinal Cord.* 2011;49(9):947.

Kirschner KL. Ethical-legal issues in physiatrics. *PM R.* 2009;1(1):81.

Kirshblum S, Fichtenbaum J. Breaking the news in spinal cord injury. *J Spinal Cord Med.* 2008;31(1):7-12.

Kirschner KL, Kerkhoff TR, Butt L, et al. 'I don't want to live this way, doc. Please take me off the ventilator and let me die.' *PM R.* 2011;3(10):968-975.

Sabharwal S. Teaching professional communication in SCI practice: multidimensional perspectives. *Am J Phys Med Rehabil.* March 2013;92(3):a13-a14.

Sabharwal S, Fiedler IG. Increasing disability awareness of future spinal cord injury physicians. *J Spinal Cord Med.* Spring 2003;26(1):45-47.

Savage TA, Parson J, Zollman F, Kirschner KL. Rehabilitation team disagreement: guidelines for resolution. *PM R.* 2009;1(12):1091-1097.

Tuszynski MH, Steeves JD, Fawcett JW, et al. Guidelines for the conduct of clinical trials for spinal cord injury as developed by the ICCP Panel: clinical trial inclusion/exclusion criteria and ethics. *Spinal Cord.* 2007;45(3):222-231.

Wu A, Cavanaugh TA, McPhee SJ, Lo B, Micco GP. To tell the truth: ethical and practical issues in disclosing medical mistakes to patients. *J Gen Intern Med.* 1997;12:770-775.

Index

Printed in the United States
By Bookmasters